How to Keep Yourself and Your Loved Ones Out of Harm's Way

Our Toxic WORLD

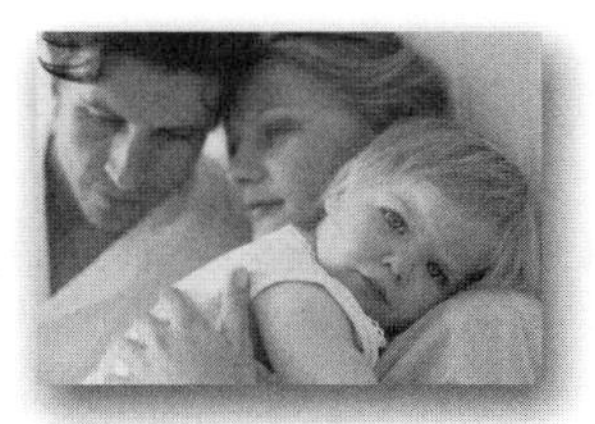

A Wake Up Call

CHEMICALS DAMAGE YOUR BODY, BRAIN, BEHAVIOR AND SEX

by

Doris J. Rapp, MD

New York Times Best Selling Author
Board Certified in Environmental Medicine,
Pediatrics and Allergy

Our Toxic World
A Wake Up Call
by Doris J. Rapp, MD
Website: www.drrapp.com
Phone 800-787-8780

Prepublication Printing: October, 2003

Published in U.S.A. by
Environmental Medical Research Foundation
PO Box 60, Buffalo, NY 14223
1-800-787-8780
fax: (716) 875-5399
website: www.drrapp.com

ISBN: 1-880509-08-3

DISCLAIMER(S)

This book is intended to provide you with enough insight and background knowledge so you will recognize your own possible need to seek a knowledgeable physician's advice and help. All your medical decisions should be thoroughly discussed with your own personal doctor. This book relates how others have been helped and it cannot be interpreted as personal medical advice for you or your family.

If you have any questions regarding any statements or claims in this book, please check them out personally, but know that the author has repeatedly striven to be certain that all information and references were as reliable, accurate and current as possible. Not all references are from peer-reviewed journals and many web sites are included so it is easy for readers to check numerous articles related to any topics of particular interest.

Printed in the United States of America

This book is dedicated to:

- The many patients and parents who so generously allowed the videos of their personal responses during allergy testing with chemicals to be shared with others. Words can never convey what is clearly evident in a few minutes of video. They shared their private health challenges in a genuine effort to help others recognize what can and unfortunately does happen. I am truly forever grateful to every one of them.

- Theron Randolph, M.D. in the 1940's recognized chemical sensitivities and no one listened in spite of all his publications, books and successes with patients when others had failed. He led the way but unfortunately was so far ahead of his times that he not only unappreciated, but he was persecuted and ridiculed, much like Semmelweis. Bless him for all he taught to so many about this illness that has become the modern day plague rapidly devastating all forms of life on our planet. His movie of one astounding patient was so compelling and convincing that I too made movies and eventually videos to document the incredible.

- My beloved Teddy, who will be forever loved and missed.

ACKNOWLEDGEMENTS

This book required more assistance and time than anyone could possibly imagine. I am particularly grateful and appreciative of the following:

- Katherine Sansone, who was cheery, helpful, and positive. Gabriel Kramarenko did the final critical part.
- Lillian Scala, Ph.D., for her virgoean edit of some references.
- Smiling Carolyn Landers for her endless typing and retyping, and never ending assistance in finding references.
- Kalpana Patel, M.D., Joan Nielson, M.D. and Martha Stark, M.D. for reading the manuscript and making suggestions.
- Hershal Fryd is a computer "doctor" and without his unique and extensive expertise, this book could never have been completed.
- Special reference sleuths who helped when we were desperate. Cindy Rose, Julius Anderson, M.D., Missy Trzeciak-Kerr and Randy Landers.
- Scott Spiegel who provided current needed information almost on a daily basis.
- Robyn Tom who assisted the editor, Katherine Sansone.
- David Clubb, Photographer 602.678.7090.
- Laara DeLain, Paula Weirather and Jackie Alexander for the initial typing and secretarial help.
- Irin Smith, Barbara Ketover and Connie Wilson who provided suggestions for possible titles.
- Christopher Hegarty was always there providing his special in depth wisdom and spiritual advice.
- Sara O'Meara, Linda Sands and others who knew about this book and prayed for a proper and timely completion.

With thanks and gratitude I acknowledge the immense spiritual comfort and help I received to smooth out the many challenges that, at times, seemed to effectively and totally block the creation of this book. This book really is not mine, but "ours." On difficult days I often needed and clung to the following:

Good Morning, This is God.
I will be handling all your problems today.
I will not need your help. So have a good day.

PREFACE

This book was written to increase your awareness about the potentially tragic, harmful effects of the numerous chemicals to which we are all exposed on a daily basis. Scientific proof is presented to illustrate the frightening changes that chemicals consistently appear to cause in many forms of our wildlife. Evidence also shows how similar symptoms are now becoming increasingly apparent in humans.

This book will help you figure out when and where you were exposed and discuss the many different ways chemicals can affect you and your loved ones. It tells you how to document your suspicions about possible harmful exposures and then the most important part–it tells you what you and your doctor, as a team, can do about it. You need to learn how to relieve your present symptoms, and equally important, how to prevent future medical problems. It will not help to pretend that it is not happening. Do not feel overwhelmed. Rather feel empowered and recognize that practical sensible answers do exist, and some of these are inexpensive, easy and effective. Prevention and avoidance are the keys. Detoxification or the elimination of chemicals from your body and surroundings, as much as sensibly possible, is a must. You can truly turn your life around. Your present and future health, as well as that of the animals and plants, and even the planet are at risk. The stakes are high but with a few sensible changes your present health can improve and your future well-being can be made much more secure.

CONTENTS

List of Tables

CHAPTER 1

Chemicals and Pesticides Can Hurt You and Those You Love

Overview

This book introduces you to some of the hazards of our modern world — chemicals and pesticides. You will learn which chemicals in your air, food, water and soil are the most hazardous to your health and how and where they are commonly used in such household basics as cleaning products, clothing, disposable diapers, cosmetics, plastic products, mattresses and even dog collars.

What chemicals and pesticides are we talking about? Industry data from the EPA indicates that 1.2 billion pounds of chemicals that potentially can be harmful to humans were released into the air and water nationwide in 1998. There are over 80,000 chemicals presently used in the United States. Less than 10% of these chemicals have even been partially evaluated for safety. Approximately 7,500 chemicals have only been studied in relation to healthy young males. They have not been properly studied for their effects on the human immune, nervous, endocrine and reproductive systems.[3a-d]

The facts are that chemicals can be a problem for anyone, at any age, and their safety has never been checked in the unborn, young children, females, pregnant women or older individuals who are the most apt to have adverse effects. Even more at risk is anyone who has a depressed immune system, such as a cancer patient undergoing chemotherapy. Almost any area of the body can be vulnerable and can be adversely affected from chemicals or other harmful environmental exposures. [1a, 2, 4, 8, 9, 13] Sensitivities to chemicals can begin at any time, so for those who think of themselves as not vulnerable, know it can happen to you.

About 50 different types of chemicals, such as herbicides, insecticides, termiticides or fungicides are collectively called pesticides. Of the 64 active pesticides used in schools, statistics show: 16 are probable causes of cancer; 24 are related to birth defects; 44 appear to cause reproduction problems; 49 can affect the central nervous system; 54 can damage the kidneys and 59 may cause eye and skin problems. Parents must ask why these chemicals continue to be used in schools or homes when safe alternatives are available.[22]

In many instances, allergic individuals also have sensitivities to multiple chemicals. This type of illness has become so prevalent that it can no longer be denied. Unfortunately, it is not uncommon for symptoms from allergenic substances, such as foods, dust and molds to begin very early in a child's life. It is also possible for symptoms from chemicals to occur at anytime, including while in the uterus and during infancy.[4] These types of exposures can cause much more than itchy skin (eczema or hives), hay fever and asthma. By not recognizing or diagnosing the chemical sensitivity part of an illness, it can remain untreated for many years. You can read about how chemicals seriously affected the entire life of one young lady, Alice, at the end of this chapter.

Is it necessary to be afraid? Maybe. But better than being afraid, let this book empower you by giving you the knowledge you need to help and protect yourself. This book will raise your level of awareness about your environment and enable you to decide what steps you can and want to take to provide yourself and your loved ones with a healthier, happier and safer, more fulfilling life.

What Exactly Is a Chemical Sensitivity?[7, 21]

A chemical sensitivity, unfortunately, is rarely due to a

single chemical. It is more apt to be characterized by a wide variety of bodily complaints related to many diverse odors. It typically occurs shortly after exposures to either an extremely minute or a large amount of one or more unrelated chemicals for either very brief or prolonged periods of time. Such exposures can cause illness from toxic levels of chemicals, but sensitivity reactions tend to commonly occur from extremely minute amounts of chemicals not typically considered to be toxic. Chemically sensitive patients often have some combined malfunction of their immune, nervous, endocrine and/or reproductive systems. Because fewer than 2% of practicing physicians or health providers have formal training in the recognition, diagnosis and treatment of sensitivities to multiple chemicals, many patients are unaware of the correct diagnosis or true cause of their medical complaints.[7] Once people become more aware, some practical changes in lifestyle can quickly be implemented to help them begin to regain their original level of health and wellness.

Do You Have Symptoms of Chemical Sensitivities?

Chemical sensitivities can affect any part of the body, and multiple areas are usually involved in both children and adults. Each person typically has a highly individualized or personal characteristic pattern of symptoms. For example, a few minutes before a chemical odor causes a child to become hyperactive or an adult to lose control (panic or rage attacks), you might notice changes in how someone appears. Certain common physical changes can provide typical clues to alert you to what is about to happen. Once adults and older children recognize the early warning signs, the more serious reactions and responses to chemical exposures can be aborted or lessened in intensity.[4a] Certain medical complaints are characteristic of chemical exposures but others are identical to those caused by the typical or the less frequently recognized forms of allergies. Most affected individuals have a combination of both. In Chapter 2, more aspects of the medical complaints are discussed in depth.

It must be recognized that the brain and nervous system can be damaged by exposure to some chemicals so the memory, physical actions and emotions, all can be affected. For example, after just a few minutes of smelling a marking pen, fingernail polish, typing correction fluid, a new carpet or fresh paint, some children and adults, temporarily, cannot even write their name or think clearly.[13]

Certain chemicals can cause cumulative and permanent effects in some individuals.[5] In fact, some children sniff toxic aerosol spray chemicals and damage their brains to such an extent that they are confined to institutions for the rest of their lives.[6] They simply can no longer think. *(Check your child's wastebaskets carefully for potentially toxic aerosol sprays.)*

How Often Does Exposure to Chemicals Cause Illness?[1a,b, 2]

It is estimated that 74 million Americans have some form of a chemical sensitivity. For some this might be something as simple as an occasional, temporary headache from the odor of a perfume or fresh paint, but about 10 million are so severely affected by chemicals that they must totally change their lifestyle and no longer can live in a normal manner.[40]

Pesticides and other chemicals in animals and/or humans have been reported to alter:

- The normal development of the unborn leading to miscarriages, stillbirths, birth anomalies and delays in normal development. (*At least two million children presently suffer from developmental, learning and behavioral difficulties.*)[34]

- The immune system causing an increased tendency to allergies and recurrent respiratory (nose, sinus or lung) or ear infections.

- The defense systems of both animal and human bodies making them more prone to cancer. (*Infants and young chil-*

*dren, as well as adults, are presently developing cancer at an alarming rate. See companion book, Can Chemicals Cause Epidemics?)**

- The brain and nervous system causing headaches, difficulty thinking or remembering, inexplicable emotional ups and downs, inconsolable depression, irritability, moodiness, aggression, hyperactivity or extreme fatigue. *(See Chapter 4.)*

- The endocrine system, contributing to illnesses such as diabetes, thyroid disease and weakened adrenal glands.

- The reproductive system causing a wide variety of sexual problems and infertility. *(See Chapter 5.)*

- The muscular system causing twitches, tics, muscle pains or weakness, in time possibly leading to fibromyalgia, multiple sclerosis, amyotrophic lateral sclerosis or Parkinson's disease.[1]

- The skeletal system causing chronic swelling and stiffness that eventually leads to pain and permanent joint deformities.

- The heart and circulatory system causing high blood pressure or irregular heart beats.[13]

- The blood vessels causing abnormal bleeding into the skin, joints, breasts, urine and elsewhere.

Of course, chemicals are not the only reason for such a diverse array of complaints, but many are not aware that they can be the major and critical factor in their own personal illness. In the companion book entitled *Can Chemicals Cause Epidemics?* many more aspects of our present day epidemic of unexplained illnesses are discussed in more detail.[4]

---

* *Can Chemicals Cause Epidemics?* Doris J. Rapp, M.D. ERF, P. O. Box 60, Buffalo, NY 14223-0060, 800.787.8780, www.drrapp.com.

What Are Some Common Causes of Chemical Sensitivities?[4]

How someone responds to a variety of chemical exposures is dependent upon the strength of a person's immune system, as well as the types, amounts and duration of chemical contacts.

Examples of chemical exposures causing illness are as follows:

- Watch for single and intermittent exposures including a gasoline or oil spill in your garage, pesticides used in or around your home or something as tiny as a whiff of someone's scented body lotion or an odorous cleaning disinfectant or deodorizer.

- Constant and prolonged chemical exposures can be caused by the installation of a new synthetic carpet, a tiny gas leak from a kitchen stove, a defective furnace or hot water tank, sleeping on a new synthetic mattress or "sanitizing" chemicals sprayed into your ventilation duct work.

- You can become ill from the adverse effects caused by living downwind from factory chemical pollution, working in a newly constructed or remodeled building, being exposed to an area that emits chemicals such as an underground parking garage or buying a new or different home with a foundation laden with known banned toxic termiticides. The chemicals used in beauty salons, printing, photograph-developing or dry cleaning stores routinely emit extremely toxic fumes. Children often become ill from riding a polluted bus to school, walking by a line of busses that are running their engines or simply attending a school located adjacent to an expressway.

Many also have unsuspected illness from an electromagnetic energy sensitivity caused by exposure to nearby high power electric wires.

- *And everyone's nightmare* — the possibility that the buildings in our lives, i.e. homes, schools, workplaces, churches, etc. are located above or too near a toxic dump or sludge site. *(Check with the health department for these locations in your city and you will be surprised about how many there are.)*

What Is One Theoretical Cause of Numerous Chemical Sensitivities?[35, 38]

A new biochemical theory of multiple chemical sensitivities proposes to explain why there is an obvious increased sensitivity to a wide range of chemicals causing symptoms related to many different areas of the brain after a single initial adverse chemical exposure. Some chemical initiates the problem by causing hypersensitivity in certain brain neurons. In response, the brain creates nitric oxide and peroxynitrite, which in turn makes the tissues even more sensitive. This can cause the nerve cells to become 100 to 1000 times more sensitive or reactive than normal. Ordinarily the system is highly regulated so that only specific brain areas are involved but because of the extent of the hypersensitivity that develops, expanded areas of the brain appear to be affected. The problem, therefore, theoretically appears to be a combination of more chemicals, more sensitivity and more brain involvement.

Are Reactions to Pesticides Due to Toxicity or a Chemical Sensitivity?[21]

To properly evaluate the role of pesticides in your health, you have to know the difference between a toxic chemical reaction and what is called a chemical sensitivity. Toxic chemical responses cause similar specific characteristic patterns of symptoms in the vast majority of exposed individuals. The symptoms typically become progressively more severe as the level of exposure increases. Physicians are trained to recognize these toxic types of cause and effect reactions.

In contrast, those who have chemical sensitivities, in time, tend to become progressively more ill from smaller and smaller levels of any chemical exposure. They can have some of the same medical complaints as those who have toxic reactions, but in addition, they typically also have a vast array of highly individualized medical symptoms. They often have a history of allergies such as hay fever, asthma or eczema in themselves or in their family suggesting that they have a weakened or compromised immune system. In addition, they tend to commonly complain of numb, burning or twitchy skin, headaches, muscle aches, a metallic taste in the mouth, creepy feelings under the skin, problems thinking clearly and extreme fatigue.

How Does the Medical Profession Perceive and Respond to Complaints of Multiple Sensitivities to Chemicals?

This type of illness is the stepchild sickness of the 20th century. The curriculum of most medical schools in the past, and even now, has not provided adequate training in the diagnosis and treatment of chemical sensitivities. Those who are most knowledgeable and successful with their patients (environmental medical physicians) are not routinely teaching doctors in training about this type of illness.[10] As a result, many individuals are chronically ill from unsuspected and unrecognized forms of this disease and their healthcare professionals often do not know why. The doctors and the patients can be perplexed because they are unaware or simply do not believe that some of the tiny, intermittent or constant chemical exposures of ordinary daily life might be the cause of a vast array of medical complaints. In fact, when family pets develop seizures and tremors after pesticide exposures, veterinarians are often the first to alert the families that their pets, as well as they themselves, may have been poisoned by a chemical used in or around their home.

The prolonged splatter effect of this illness can be immense. Unfortunately, when health professionals do not know why someone is ill, they tend to blame the patient for their illness. *(If your car continues to malfunction after a mechanic tries to fix it, do you blame the car?)* If you are not believed and are truly sick and in pain, this alone will most certainly cause an emotional impact that can only add to the stress of being ill. Though this additional emotional component is not the cause of your illness, it also often needs attention from a knowledgeable counselor or psychologist *after* the true causes of the chemical sensitivity has been found and treated. This is true for both children and adults afflicted with this type of illness.

Why Have Numerous Chemical Sensitivities Become So Common?

Immense numbers of individuals scattered over the United States are presently ill from the ever expanding number of chemicals in the foods we eat, the water we drink and the air we breathe inside or outside our homes, schools and workplaces. *(See Chapter 6.)* We are all being exposed to unrecognized aerial chemical pollution from factories, weed and insect-control measures and to surreptitious nighttime chemical spraying.

How Do Chemically Sensitive Patients and Others Perceive Their Illness?

Many who become ill have no idea why, where or when it happened and they do not know where to go for appropriate treatment.[4, 7, 8a, 9a,b] Some, such as teachers, can no longer work in their field of expertise because their polluted school is causing their illness. Some cannot work anyplace. It is not uncommon for some to be so sick they cannot begin to cope with any aspect of their illness.

Many, including spouses, relatives, friends and even some physicians, will not believe persons who react to many chemicals are physically ill. They refuse to recognize sensitivities to innumerable chemicals for what it is, namely a medical illness, and they attribute the patient's complaints to psychological problems or attempts to get more attention. They demonstrate their skepticism with varying degrees of non-support. Because of this, some who are ill with chemical sensitivities to many substances justifiably become very discouraged. Not only do they have physical pain but they also feel immense emotional deprivation and financial pressures. This happens especially when insurance coverage is denied in spite of obvious improvement after finally finding help with appropriate environmental medical therapy. This illness can be expensive to treat, and family funds can be depleted quickly. This book will help you treat this illness, sometimes inexpensively, and even better, it will help you learn how to prevent it.

Affected children are even more confused and bewildered than adults. Many are discouraged, depressed or even suicidal because they cannot keep up with their peers. Many feel alone and ostracized. Students who are ill find they are unable to learn, cannot engage in sports and many are forced to discontinue their education due to frequent illness, learning and behavior problems and physical limitations.

How Do Governmental Agencies Perceive This Illness?

Although there remains some disagreement about the diagnosis of chemical sensitivities to several chemicals, it is recognized by The Americans with Disabilities Act of 1990 and the Department of Housing and Urban Development. Some patients with multiple sensitivities to chemicals have won worker's compensation cases, though currently, it is not recognized by the Centers for Disease Control.[4b]

The Occupational Safety and Health Administration sets the chemical standards for industry but unfortunately they mainly target males in spite of the fact 80% of those with many chemical sensitivities are women. No studies have been conducted to ascertain how many children are affected but many are seen and helped, on a daily basis, in the offices of physicians who are knowledgeable about how to recognize this problem throughout the United States.[10]

How Worried Should You Be About Chemicals?

This book will help you become more aware of the profound, potentially harmful effects chemicals, especially pesticides, can have on our brains and nervous systems. It began during World War I, when chemicals were created to damage the brains and bodies of the enemy. These same chemicals, that have proven adverse effects on plants, birds, fish, waterfowl, whales, animals and humans, are now used in pesticides. Different groups of scientists predict about a quarter of the species of plants and wildlife will be extinct in about 25 to 50 years.[24, 38] There really is much more than suggestive evidence that this is happening. Chemicals appear to be hurting more than mankind.[24] If this is known, we must ask why proven toxic chemicals continue to be used routinely in our schools, homes, workplaces and on our foods.

Many are not aware that chemical exposures or unsuspected forms of allergy can play a role in the onset of inexplicable, sudden extreme anger, irritability, depression, aggression and violence, as is so evident in many of today's children and adults. Much too often, no one seems to know why certain medical and emotional problems arise, and surprisingly, sometimes even after they find out, they do not seem to care. It is hard to believe that when it is obvious that a chronically ill chemically sensitive person improves significantly, those caring for that person sometimes do not ask or even appear to want to know what was done to relieve the chronic illness or pain.

Traditional treatment includes one drug after another. Getting rid of the pain and discomfort seems to be the main priority. It is unusual for some busy health professionals not to take the time that is needed to determine the cause of an illness. In fact rarely are patients questioned in depth about possible common environmental factors that can cause their illness. This takes time and "clock-watch" medicine does not permit even caring doctors to take the hours it might require to find the answers that are needed to permanently resolve many of today's chronic, perplexing chemically-related illnesses.

Hopefully this book will provide some clues to tell you *exactly* why various forms of illness linger or keep reoccurring. The aim is to help you figure out *why* you or a loved one is not feeling up to par. Medications can temporarily relieve discomfort and pain but for many individuals the best answer is not drugs, but simple common sense. If someone can "find and take the nail out of the shoe", in other words, remove the cause of the illness, there is nothing to treat. You must try to eliminate the cause by "pulling out the nail". If your perfume or a smelly synthetic carpet causes asthma, stop wearing the perfume and get rid of the carpet.[40] The answer is not more or better asthma medication. Once you can pinpoint the cause — you often know exactly what you can do to get well. If the cause is gone, there is no need to take one medication after another because there is nothing left to treat — there is no more illness. Isn't that what you really want?

Can Multiple Chemical Symptoms Keep Recurring?

They certainly can. Chemically sensitive individuals typically find that as time passes a minimal amount of a vast number of unrelated chemical exposures can cause a sudden recurrence of their original complaints. For example, a new carpet can make you ill shortly after it is installed but later on, in a few weeks or months, you might find that you develop the same medical symptoms every time you put gas in your car or smell a whiff of perfume.[40] Chemicals that never bothered you before now cause obvious illness, and this is referred to as the "spreading phenomenon".[13a] As a result, the illness from chemicals tends to wax and wane flaring with each additional, unavoidable chemical, as well as from classical allergenic exposures, i.e. molds, dust, foods or pollen. *(Many typical aspects of this illness are clearly illustrated in the history of Alice, discussed at the end of this chapter.)*

Symptoms tend to improve when the causes are found and then eliminated or treated. This book was written to help you do exactly that. After a major chemical exposure, it is not unusual for affected individuals to initially suddenly develop prolonged flu-like symptoms. In time, allergies, especially to foods that were previously not a problem, can become evident. Along with unavoidable exposures to chemicals in homes, schools and work areas, contacts related to the many chemicals in our air, tap water, foods and clothing also must be critically evaluated. Any of these can cause some who are chemically ill to become sicker, and at times, totally incapacitated.

What Are the Major and Most Problematic Types of Hazardous Chemicals?

Below, a few of the major categories of chemicals known to be harmful are discussed. Clever chemists have created "designer" variants that are similar in chemical structure.[1a, 12a] Each new one can be even more toxic and dangerous than the original chemical product. Minute amounts of some of these newer designer chemicals can cause permanent damage to aquatic and animal wildlife, as well as to humans. A preliminary scientific report in April 2002 has shown that exposure for only one hour to one herbicide, Triphenyltin, is thought to potentially damage the human immune system permanently.[27] In addition, no one fully understands the combined effects when we are exposed to more than one chemical, and we are exposed to hundreds every single day.

One major critical concern related to the many synthetic pesticides is that some can mimic feminizing or estrogenic hormones. This means they can dramatically alter the sexuality of animals and humans. *(See Chapter 5.)* Natural forms of female hormones called phytoestrogens are less apt to cause these types of adverse effects in humans.

Organochlorides[11, 12b]

This large category of chemicals is known as chlorinated phenols or the organochloride pesticides. These can damage the skin, kidneys, liver and immune system. The most well known is DDT – then came chlordane used from the early forties to the mid eighties. Over 30 million homes were "treated" with chlordane for pest control, and this chemical can continue to cause symptoms in some homeowners. Heptachlor was the new designer chemical to replace it, and this too was also finally banned in 1978. Even though these pesticides were banned and eventually were supposed to be used no longer, there are newer varieties of other chemically-related chlorinated substances. Many of these are not only toxic but capable of causing chemical sensitivities. A few that can be potentially dangerous or toxic include:

- Aldrin, dieldrin, lindane, and endrin. *(These are other chemicals in the same basic category as chlordane.)*

- 2,4-D and 2,4,5-T are two herbicide chemicals that continue to be used on lawns and by many farmers in the United States. These chemicals also have been implicated in the increased incidence of cancer, especially lymphoma tumors. *(See Chapter 6.)* In Calgary, Canada they are no longer allowed to use this spray in the city because it is believed that this chemical can cause genetic changes and abnormalities, as well as cancer in mammals.[23] In addition, it is thought to be toxic for the unborn child and it can damage the liver and kidney, as well as the immune and central nervous systems. These specific chemicals are similar to the toxic ingredients such as dioxin in the infamous Agent Orange used to defoliate Vietnam. These appear to have caused innumerable health problems, typical of pesticide poisoning and chemical sensitivities, not only in the Vietnamese, but also in our Vietnam veterans, their wives and possibly even their offspring.

- An offshoot called PCP, or pentachlorophenol, is used as an outdoor wood or patio preservative. It was outlawed in Germany for indoor use after many individuals developed severe nervous system disease and psychological problems manifested by abnormal behavior.

- PCBs and PBBs, or polychlorinated or brominated biphenols, were available from about 1929 to 1975. Transformers and electrical equipment appear to be a major source for PCBs literally all over the world.[1b, 11a, 13b, 14] This chemical can cause cancer, damage the liver, skin and blood, and injure the immune, reproductive and nervous systems. Research has shown that the higher the concentration of PCBs in umbilical cords of children born to women who eat PCB-contaminated fish when they are pregnant, the more likely the child will have a lower birth weight, and a smaller than normal head size. In time, developmental delays and some learning problems are typically evident.[11b] In one study, exposed pregnant mothers had sons with smaller than normal penises.[11c] In the past, when minute amounts of PBBs in the form of a fire retardant accidentally contaminated some animal feed in Michigan in the early 1970s, the effects were devastating. They had to bury thousands of animals in landfills because they feared the meat and milk were contaminated and could make humans ill. *(See Chapters 5 and 6.)*

Today, for example, PCB products continue to be widely used in construction and recently, large amounts were released into the air during the World Trade Center tragedy. Almost a year later this chemical continues to pollute the air and potentially cause health problems in New York City.[1b, 11a, 13b, 14] *(See Chapter 8.)*

- Chloroform was initially used as an anesthetic and is formed when chlorine combines with organic material such as dead leaves, etc. It is routinely found in water treatment facilities and in the tap water in many cities. Some communities are now seriously and wisely considering an alternative to chlorine to decrease the germs in drinking water because chlorinated compounds, such as chloroform, are suspect causes of both bladder and bowel cancer.

- Carbon tetrachloride, trichloroethylene and perchloroethylene (perc) are cleaning products that, under certain circumstances, are known to cause confusion, sleepiness, anesthesia and even death. They can be found in paint, dry cleaning solutions and degreasing agents. These chemicals are thought to have contributed to the many health complaints of the Love Canal victims and those in Woburn, Massachusetts where it was found in one form in their water supply. [1b]

- Vinyl chloride (polyvinyl chloride) and ethylene chloride found in synthetic plastics and cosmetic sprays are similar in structure and effect. They can both cause liver, brain, intestinal and kidney damage, as well as cancer in humans and rats (at levels of 5 ppm).[37]

Even though most industrialized countries banned some of the above toxic chemicals more than 25 to 30 years ago, the concentrations in human tissues, especially fat, persist and for some, have remained essentially the same. DDT, for example, can be found in the blood or urine of human newborns, in breast milk and some adult human sperm. It is also found in penguins, polar bears, fish, whales and many other forms of wildlife on all parts of the planet.

Organophosphates

The organophosphates are another large category of pesticides. Examples of common organophosphates are Dursban®, diazinon, parathion and malathion. *(See Chapters 4, 6, 7, 8, 10.)*

This category of pesticide was originally designed as a nerve gas to damage the nervous system.[12b] This pesticide inhibits the proper function of the nervous system. At the end of each nerve cell there must be an enzyme called acetylcholinesterase which breaks down acetylcholine. If it is not broken down, acetylcholine accumulates and this in turn impairs normal nerve conduction so that nerve impulses cannot be transmitted properly throughout the body.

Organophosphates can extensively hurt the human body, potentially damaging the lungs, intestines, bladder, heart, muscles, nerves and brain. They also affect the behavior of both humans and animals.[11c, 15] *(See Chapter 4.)*

Examples:

- It has been reported that mothers who use an organophosphate flea shampoo (dichlorvos) on their pet during their pregnancy double the chance of a brain tumor developing in their unborn baby by the age of five years.[16] Prenatal or infant exposure to organophosphate pest strips unquestionably increases the risk of leukemia in young children.[16] Could this or other chemicals be related to the 30% increase of brain cancer and the 10% increase in leukemia that is unfortunately evident in today's children?[17, 18]

- TCDD (tetrachlorodibenzodioxin), a form of dioxin is an extremely harmful chemical that suppresses the immune system. *(See Chapter 5.)* This very toxic substance can be an impurity or by-product produced during the manufacture of chlorpyrifos or Dursban®. Dioxin is released into the air when plastics are incinerated or fossil fuels such as coal are burned. *(See Chapters 4, 6-8.)*

- Dursban® became the substitute for chlordane. It persists for at least two months after application in paper, wood and paint. It is one more chemical in the chlorpyrifos group of pesticides. Dursban® and Diazinon are direct descendants of the original nerve gas used in World War II. Many hundreds of gallons of Dursban® were routinely used in the foundations of homes constructed during the past 20 years to control termites. Vapors from this chemical can gradually seep up the walls into the indoor air and down into the soil contaminating the ground water. Surprisingly this chemical was only partially banned in 2001 in spite of its proven toxicity. *(See Chapters 4, 6, 7, 10.)*

- Diazinon is toxic to the nervous system. *(See Chapters 5, 6, 7.)* It can cause headaches, nausea, dizziness, tearing, sweating, blurred vision and memory problems. In animals, a decrease in coordination, birth defects, stillbirths and a delay in sexual development have been noted. In humans, it has been associated with an increased risk of brain cancer in children and non-Hodgkin's lymphoma in Minnesota and Nebraska farmers.[29] After 40 years of use, the EPA announced in December 2000 that its use would slowly be restricted. Sale of indoor products stopped in December 2002; lawn and garden use in 2003, *but 70% of agricultural uses can continue.*[19a-c] If it is potentially so harmful, why is its use not totally and immediately stopped?

- Parathion, known to disrupt fertility and reported to cause abnormal sperm, can be found in some of our foods. It has caused more deaths than any other organophosphate.

- Malathion is in this category. It was liberally sprayed over New York City, the East Coast, Florida and California in a misguided attempt to control insects during the past few years. *(See Chapter 8.)* It continues to be used in spite of safer and more efficient methods of insect control.[42]

Carbamates

The carbamates are another dangerous category of fungicide and herbicide. They are similar to the organophosphates but they are thought not to cause as much permanent damage. [13g] Common varieties are Ficam®, Sevin®, carbaryl and Aldicarb. This chemical is used in clothing, medicines and plastics. One granule can kill a bird. It kills bees resulting in decreased pollination of crops.

Symptoms tend to occur several hours after exposure. In humans, it can harm the lungs, intestines, eyes, brain and muscles, as well as the immune and nervous systems. Endocrine disturbances in the thyroid have also been reported. Blurred vision, twitches, convulsions, weakness, excessive perspiration, cataracts, memory loss, behavioral problems, cancer, defective sperm and damage to the unborn are only a few of the health problems this chemical appears to cause.[12b] It tends to cause excessive mucus or discharge in many forms of bodily secretions, such as perspiration, intestinal mucus, eye discharge, ear wax, bodily pore secretions etc. Like organophosphates it can sometimes be associated with sudden unprovoked extreme agitation, anger, rage and violence.

When this chemical was accidentally released in Bhopal, India, hundreds of thousands were hurt. It was then carried throughout the world on air currents. We are, indeed, one world. The sky and water have no borders.

Phthalates

These are found in industrial chemicals, inks, adhesives, vinyl floor tiles, paints and plastics. Phthalates make plastic more flexible. This chemical can cause the male offspring of rats to become more feminine and to have abnormal reproductive organs, while the female offspring have more miscarriages.[35a-c] This chemical causes precocious puberty in girls. It can be inhaled, ingested and absorbed through the skin. Certain types of plasticizers found in the most frequently used types of plastic wrap (not polyethylene) can enter foods, such as cheese and beef, from either direct contact or during microwave heating. Due to this, a European Scientific Committee for Food recommended that the safe amount of daily consumption of certain cheeses be less than one and a half ounces for a 40 pound child.[28b] Until we know how risky these released plasticizers or phthalates are in relation to the endocrine system, we should all be more careful. *(See Chapters 3, 5, 6, 8.)**

Solvents

One last large group of similarly toxic and sensitizing chemicals include solvents such as benzene, toluene and xylene. They are commonly used to dissolve the major ingredient in products and even though solvents may comprise 99% of an item, and are acknowledged registered toxic poisons, *they do not have to be specified on chemical information "Material Safety Data (MSD)" sheets. (See Chapters 5, 6, 7, 8.)* In fact, they frequently are inaccurately and deceptively lumped into a category referred to as "inert" even though they all have been shown to cause cancer or other serious illness.

- Benzene is a hydrocarbon and universal solvent used in engine fuels and in the plastic, paint and textile industries. It can damage bone marrow and, in particular, cause leukemia and tumors.

- Toluene is used to dissolve many common products, especially printer's ink. It damages the nervous system, liver, kidneys, lungs, skin and eyes and can cause delays in the normal development of children.

- Xylene is used in insecticides, plastics, spray paints and inks, as well as in the photography, leather and rubber industries. It can damage the brain, kidneys, eyes, skin and cause numbness of the extremities, as well as cause poor coordination, nausea and dizziness.

What Can You Do to Help Yourself Feel Better?

If you do not have chemical sensitivities and want to prevent this type of medical problem, these are the factors that need consideration. All of the following are discussed in detail in Chapter 3.

- Avoid all known offending chemicals in your air, water, food, clothing, home and work areas as much as possible.

- Strengthen your immune system with better nutrition.

- Eliminate as many of the stored chemicals in your body as possible by the use of various forms of detoxification.

- Receive treatment for typical allergies with allergy extracts after Provocation/Neutralization allergy testing.

Classic Sensitivities to Many Chemicals in an Allergic Child — Alice

Alice's parents and grandparents all had typical allergies. *(This would suggest that any child born in this family might be more apt to develop problems with allergies and chemicals early in life and that these problems would tend to worsen with age.)* Her parents stated that before birth Alice was not unusual. *(Unlike many who are destined to become ill with allergies and environmental illness, she was not hyperactive in the uterus.)* As is typical of many allergic children, she did have severe colic throughout most of the first year of life. This suggests a probable milk allergy. *(Allergy specialists often find that the cause of colic is the milk, soy or corn (dextrose) in formulas, but in today's world, the chemicals in and on these foods and phthalate chemicals released from microwave heated, plastic baby bottles are also of concern. The newest, serious, medical challenges are related to the immense potential problems that might arise from genetically engineered (GE) corn and soy and irradiated foods. See Chapter 9.)* [26] Alice slept very poorly, seemed to be overly hungry and tended to drool in excess during the infant period. *(Allergies at any age can cause excessive drooling from food, dust or mold. This is most common in very young children but certainly is also seen in adults who have excessive amounts of saliva.)*

Frequently Missed Forms of Allergy and Chemical Sensitivities[43]

Starting at age two years, Alice began with temper tantrums that could last from 20 minutes to two hours. She had severe episodes of itching and screaming. She would hit her mother and brother when she lost control. By the age of three, Alice's mother realized that her dark eye circles, bags under her eyes and wiggly legs were indications of an impending allergic reaction. She eventually figured out that orange juice caused Alice's intensely itchy skin and hives, and that this response was typically followed by temper tantrums.

In the next few years, Alice had periods of fatigue, depression, screaming, hyperactivity, aggression and poor concentration. *(Notice how many symptoms of allergy or chemical sensitivities she had already developed.)* She had an array of descriptive diagnoses, but very few helpful answers. As she grew older, intermittent evidence of classical Attention Deficit Disorder (ADD) with irritability and restlessness became more apparent. At times she acted obsessive-compulsive, inattentive, disorganized and overactive like those with Attention Deficit Hyperactivity Disorder (ADHD), Obsessive Compulsive Disorder (OCD) or bi-polar disorders. At other times, she had verbal outbursts like a child with Tourette's syndrome. She disliked being touched like autistics. She also had panic attacks, fears, phobias, insomnia, difficulty walking, lethargy and problems speaking clearly.

At six years, she was seen by an allergist and routine testing indicated sensitivities to molds, dust and pollen. Her mother noticed when she had touched old moldy books, she became ill.

As the years passed her mother realized her behavior was the most challenging aspect of her illness. One key to relieving these problems was the recognition of the cause of both her obvious and subtle forms of allergies. Her observant parents watched carefully to detect cause and effect relationships. They noticed what occurred just before she suddenly looked "allergic", became congested, developed a post-nasal drip or had itchy skin. It took a while, but after her mother tried an allergy evaluation diet *(See Appendix A)*, she was certain not only the typical allergic symptoms but many of the behavioral changes, including Alice's outbursts, were related to specific foods. In time, her mother determined that oranges caused severe itching, milk caused anger, sugar made her clear her throat and fructose caused her to have a disposition change and itchy skin. Her mother eliminated her bad breath by controlling her diet. *(This particular medical problem often represents undetected food allergies, especially to wheat, eggs or dairy.)* Her hyperactivity diminished after her diet no longer contained foods to which she was sensitive.

It was obvious, however, that other things were bothering their little girl. In time, her mother realized unrecognized chemical sensitivities had been present for years. Scented items, such as perfume in particular, unquestionably caused changes in her walk and ability to speak and think clearly. No one, including her doctors, ever mentioned chemical odors might be one more cause of her symptoms.

When she came to our clinic at the age of 10 years, we videotaped her responses to allergenic substances. When she was allergy tested for peas, she reacted so dramatically in a few minutes that she could not stand or walk normally.[4c,d] *(See video Environmentally Sick Schools 800.787.8780.)* Her voice became high-pitched and she babbled as she tried to say the alphabet and suddenly she could not speak so she could be understood. Similarly when she was allergy tested for garlic, at about age 13 years, she had difficulty walking, her head jerked backwards and she giggled uncontrollably.[4c,d] On both occasions one drop of the correct dilution of pea or garlic allergy extract stopped the reaction within eight minutes. *(See Chapter 3 about P/N allergy testing.)*

Once her parents learned how to check for chemical sensitivities, they wondered why they had not detected them for so long. On one occasion, she reacted when she was near a neighbor's outside vented clothes dryer that smelled of scented detergents and fabric softeners. Her neighbor told her mother Alice was not acting right. She was babbling and acting in a most bizarre manner, similar to the type of response when she was skin tested for peas.[4c,d] Her mother quickly recognized the chemical odor was the cause. It is difficult to relate to substances that have long chemical names. For this reason, Table 1 lists specific everyday exposures that caused Alice to have a variety of symptoms. These were characteristic for her, as well as for many others who suffer from multiple forms of chemical sensitivities. As you read this table, keep asking if this could be happening to your child or you.

At times, when her parents took her for a walk, she might collapse and be unable to walk home if a lawn truck sprayed pesticides in their vicinity. *(Could this be one reason for young, strong athletes to sometimes collapse or die in ballparks?) (See Chapter 6.)* For a long time it was routine for her to be irritable and difficult when her father arrived home wearing the clothes he had worn at work. In time they realized that he needed to change his clothes as soon as he walked through the door because the chemical solvents in the dry cleaning fluid had permeated his clothing and this odor caused a change in his daughter's behavior. Other chemicals that caused symptoms included the smell of ink and paper in new books or fresh newspapers, mimeo or copy paper, lighter fluid, soft plastic and fresh asphalt. Any of these could affect her so she could not walk or speak in a normal manner. She would act oddly, make strange noises or feel tired, depressed, angry, giddy and silly. In spite of a very high IQ, when she was reacting to some food or chemical exposure, she sometimes babbled or could barely speak. Some teachers thought she was a slow child.

Because of her chemical sensitivities and many allergies,

she was deprived of a regular education. For many years she could only receive home schooling. Her sensitivities to multiple chemicals, especially to perfume and many foods, interfered greatly with her ability to think or act normally.[40] If she ate organic food she seemed fine, but if she ate regular grocery store or restaurant foods she would repeatedly become ill from the pesticides on or in the foods. *(If she was ill from a food item, and not the chemical on or in it, it would be expected that she would become sick from both organic and regular grocery store forms of that food.)*

With comprehensive environmental and allergy medical care, she improved 85% in two weeks, and she remained much better but unanticipated chemical exposures continued to be a major challenge for many years.

When she was also treated using some of the newer chiropractic techniques *(See Appendix B.3 and D.5)* such as Total Body Modification *(TBM: 435.652.4340),* Neuro Emotional Training *(NET: 800.888.4638)* and Nambudripad's Allergy Elimination Technique *(NAET: 714.523.8900),* as well as interactive light therapy, she unquestionably could better tolerate chemicals and other problem exposures. For the first time she could attend school. The school administration would provide special education for her but they refused to provide an environmentally safe learning area. In spite of all her health challenges, she had an "A" average in high school and graduated with honors. She is presently on the Dean's list in college and is well enough to attend college and stay in a dormitory with other students most of the time. Typically she knows exactly what causes any flare of symptoms and she knows exactly what to do to prevent or treat a medical problem if one arises. The answer to relieve part of her health problems was simply increased awareness. She learned what made her ill and avoided it. This is the approach that will help many who have sensitivities to a spectrum of chemicals, as well as to many allergenic substances.[4]

Table 1
Examples of Alice's Specific Chemical Reactions

Duplicating Fluid: One hour after exposure to duplicating fluid, she became giddy, rolled on the floor, began to cough, talked like a baby and laughed for no apparent reason.

Ditto Copies: A dry piece of ditto paper caused Alice to change from calm and happy to tired and angry. She could not draw as well as previously and began to scribble. *Typical of patients with chemical sensitivities, she could easily smell chemicals on paper even though no odor was apparent to most people.*

Perfume:[40] A special education teacher decided to compare and evaluate Alice's academic performance when she was in a clean room without odors to an area that smelled of perfume. She found that on two different tests, her age performance dropped more than a year after simply smelling perfume. In addition, she had a dramatic mood change, began to whine, her voice became high pitched, she had difficulty moving normally and would no longer follow directions.

Floor Wax: After a hall in her school was waxed, she was found wandering about in a confused state. She had impaired judgment and memory loss and had no idea where she was supposed to go.

Laundry Detergents: She could walk a straight line but not after she dipped her hand into a common scented laundry detergent and smelled the aroma.[25] Moreover, she began to act inappropriately. She hugged herself and made high-pitched squeaks. On another occasion when she was exposed, her mood suddenly changed and she became irritable and upset. She spoke nonsense and laughed uncontrollably.[41]

Lawn Spray: She was walking with her parents when a nearby lawn truck began to spray. She became extremely upset and could barely stand up. She had to be supported in order to get home. In another incidence, when she walked near a recently pesticide laden lawn, she suddenly became angry and again, almost collapsed. She had to be supported and could not walk normally.

Diesel Fumes: When she was 13 and the family was on a long drive, they noticed if their car followed diesel trucks too closely, her mood became angry. This disappeared when they were again on the open road.[4] *(For this reason, those with sensitivities to multiple chemicals do best if they buy older cars with re-circulating air conditioners and heaters and use an air purifier attached to the cigarette lighter. 800.787.8780.)*

What Alice Taught Us

Alice's history clearly demonstrates how she began with typical childhood allergies which progressed to symptoms characteristic of ADD, OCD, bi-polar disorder, autism and Tourette's syndrome. Once chemical and food sensitivities were recognized and she either avoided offending substances or received Provocation/ Neutralization allergy extract treatment, she quickly improved. *(For testing AAEM: 316.684.5500.)* Her education remained in jeopardy, however, until she also received some newer creative forms of chiropractic therapy *(TBM, NET and NAET – See Appendix B.3)*. Because of her allergies and chemical sensitivities, her childhood was not normal and she was severely restricted scholastically, physically and socially. Her parents are to be commended for learning and understanding the true scope and role of allergies and chemical sensitivities in relation to her many health problems. Their persistence and eventual pinpointing of exactly which items caused most of her specific symptoms literally saved her life. Without the newer forms of Provocation/Neutralization allergy testing and treatment and chiropractic medicine, she would have been unable to begin to fulfill her most promising potential or to function effectively in today's world.

Summary

Chemicals presently permeate every aspect of our lives. They can significantly alter not only the physical health of your entire family, but also their actions, behavior and memory. Pesticides and chemicals are major missed considerations in relation to many forms of perplexing chronic illnesses from infancy through adulthood. The bad news is that as little as one exposure to a toxic chemical can sometimes ruin your health. The good news is that this book will unquestionably help you figure out if chemicals are a factor in relation to your family's health problems and guide you so you know what to do about it. It will hopefully enable you to determine if you have an unsuspected, undiagnosed or misdiagnosed medical problem due to some unrecognized chemical exposure. It contains information you will want to know and definitely need to know. If you are not aware of certain potentially harmful exposures, you cannot possibly prevent or resolve certain medical problems. You must repeatedly ask to what degree contacts with unsuspected factors might be contributing to your family's medical and emotional complaints. Consider if pesticides or other toxic chemical exposures are causing chronic illness or affecting some family members so they can't act responsibly, remember or learn at a level comparable to their ability.[18] We all need to recognize the full potential scope of physical, mental, emotional and sexual effects of chemicals in relation to our past, present and future generations. Once you become aware of possible harmful factors, you must be given practical, sensible information so you can make changes in your personal environment so you and your loved ones are better protected. By becoming more informed and by more fully appreciating the many health implications caused by the widespread use of chemicals, many have literally turned their lives around. Maybe you don't have to take one pill after another, or "learn to live with it". The bottom line is if the cause can be found and eliminated; there may be nothing left to treat.

It is my opinion that we should be gravely concerned about the scope of potentially harmful effects of chemicals, especially pesticides, on children. What we truly need are diagnostic, treatment, education and research centers and environmentally safe villages where the very best of traditional and alternative medicine can be provided. As funding becomes available, these will be created.[4] *(See Epilogue at end of this book.)*

CHAPTER 1 REFERENCES:

1a Sherman, Janette M., M.D., Chemical Exposure and Disease Diagnostic and Investigative Techniques, 1994, Princeton Scientific Publishing Co., P.O. Box 2155, Princeton, NJ 08543, 609.683.4750, Fax: 609.683.0838. www.janettesherman.com

1b pp. 124-126 Transformers and PCBs.

2 Caress, Stanley M., Ph.D., "MCS Prevalence, Symptomatology, and Etiology," Our Toxic Times: Chemical Injury Information Network, September 2001: 12 (9) Issue 135, pg. 16. P.O. Box 301, White Sulfur Springs, MT 59645. 406.547.2255.

3a Interview with Dr. Warren Porter by Carol Dansereau, Toxics Coalition, Washington, Fax: 206.632.8661.

3b Porter, W., M.D., et al., "Endocrine, Immune, and Behavioral Effects of Pesticides, Herbicides and Fertilizer Mixtures at Groundwater Concentrations," cdansereau@watoxics.org.

3c http://www.accessone.com/_~watoxics.

4 Rapp, Doris J., M.D., Is This Your Child's World? 1996, ERF (formerly PARF), Buffalo, NY 14223. 800.787.8780. Cost: $15.00 (plus S&H).

4a Chapters 1-5.

4b Chapters 16-17.

4c Environmentally Sick Schools Video, 800.787.8780, Cost: $25.00 (plus S& H). Spanish video available.

4d Chemical Reactions in Children and Adults Video. $25.00 (plus S&H).

5 Singer, Raymond, Ph.D., "Multiple Chemical Sensitivity and Neurotoxicity," Our Toxic Times, Chemical Injury Information Network, September 2001: 12 (9) Issue 135, pp. 4-25. P.O. Box 301, White Sulfur Springs, MT 59645. 406.547.2255.

6 Laseter, John L., Ph.D., "Solvent Abuse Monitoring in Juveniles," Accu-Chem Laboratories, Treatment Centers, April 1993. 972.234.5412, http://www.accuchem.com/solvent.html

7 Matthews, Bonnye L., Chemical Sensitivity, 1992, McFarland & Company, Inc., Box 611, Jefferson, NC 28640, pg. 10.

8 Rogers, Sherry, M.D., Prestige Press, P.O. Box 3068, 3500 Brewerton Rd., Syracuse, NY 13220. 800.846.6687; 315.468.4417, Fax: 315.468.8119.

8a Wellness Against All Odds, 1994. Cost: $17.95.

8b No More Heartburn, 2000. Cost: $15.00.

9 Krohn, Jacqueline, M.D. and Francis Taylor, 1991, Hartley & Marks, Inc., Box 147, Point Roberts, WA 98281.

9a The Whole Way To Allergy Relief And Prevention, 1991. Cost: $24.95.

9b Natural Detoxification: A Practical Encyclopedia: The Complete Guide to Clearing Your Body of Toxins, 2000. Cost: $24.95.
10 American Academy of Environmental Medicine [AAEM], 7701 E. Kellogg, Suite 625, Wichita, KS 67207. 316.684.5500.
11 Colborn, Theo, Dianne Dumanski and John Peterson Myers, Our Stolen Future: Are We Threatening Our Fertility, Intelligence, And Survival? 1996, Penguin Books, Inc. New York, NY. Cost: $15.95.

11a pg. 137.
11b pp. 24-27.
11c pp. 186-194 behavior.

12a Moses, Marion, M.D., Designer Poisons, 1995, Pesticide Education Center, P.O. Box 420870, San Francisco, CA 94142-0870. 415.391.8511. Cost $19.95.

12b pp. 41-47.

13 Rea, William J., M.D., Chemical Sensitivity, Vols. 1- 4,1992-1997. CRC Press Inc., 2000 Corporate Blvd., NW Boca Raton, FL 33431.

13a Vol.1, pp. 33-35.
13b Vol.1, pg. 192.
13c 214.368.4132.
13d Optimum Environment for Optimum Health and Creativity. 2002. Crown Press, Dallas, American Health Environmental Center. 800.428.2343. Cost: $39.95.
13e Vol. 2, pp. 800-802.
13f Vol. 2, pg. 879.
13g Vol. 2, pg. 865.

14 Rogan, W., et al., "Congenital Poisoning with PCB's and Their Contaminants in Taiwan," Science, 1988: 241, 334-36.
15 "Behavioral and Biochemical Effects of Malathion," Study No. 51-051-73/76, Department of Army US Environmental Hygiene Agency Document FY76.
16 Steinman, David and R. Michael Wisner, Living Healthy in a Toxic World, 1995. The Berkley Publishing Group, 200 Madison Ave., New York, NY 10016. Cost: $12.95 (plus S&H).
17 Seattle Post Intelligencer, March 3, 2001. www.seattlepi.nwsource.com (Archives)
18 Our Toxic Times: Chemical Injury Info Center, September 2001:12(9). P.O. Box 301, White Sulfur Springs, MT 59645. 406.547.2255.
19a Journal of Pesticide Reform, "Diazinon: Toxicology," Summer 2000:20(3)15-19.

19b Journal of Pesticide Reform, "EPA Takes Action on Diazinon, Too Little, Too Late," Winter 2000:20(4)8.
19c Journal of Pesticide Reform, "NCAP Members Sound Off About Diazinon," Fall 2000:20(3)4.

20 News on Earth, "New Studies Blame Plastics for Sexual Abnormalities," October 2000:3, 10. 101 West 23rd St., PMB 2245, New York, NY 20011.
21 Ashford, Nicholas and Claudia Miller, Chemical Exposures, Low Levels, High Stakes, 1998, Van Nostrand Reinhold, Chapter 2: "Definition," 115 Fifth Avenue, New York, NY 10003. Cost: $52.50.
22 Get Set, Inc., The Bug Stops Here, downloadable free book. Get Set, Inc., www.getipm.com 800.221.6188.
23 Carson, Rachel, Basic Guide to Pesticides: Their Characteristics and Hazards, 1992, Hemisphere Publishing, www.cehn.org
24 News on Earth, November 1998. http://www.earthscape.org/r3/grf01.html
25 Soapworks, 18911 Nordhoff St., Suite 37, Northridge, CA 91324, 800.699.9917.
26 Fagan, John, Ph.D., Genetic Engineering: The Hazards of Vedic Engineering: The Solutions, 1995, Maharishi International University, 1000 N. Fourth St., Fairfield, Iowa 52557. Cost: $12.00 (Amazon.com).
27 www.pestlaw.com/x/news/2002/20020407.html and www.foodsafetynetwork.com.
28a "Hormone Mimics Hit Home: Tests of plastic wraps, baby foods," www.consumerreports.org.
28b Fact Sheet: "Contents of Common Plastic Packaging Items." 888.ECO.INFO.
29 Cox, Caroline, "Carbaryl," Journal of Pesticide Reform, Spring 1993:13(1), Northwest Coalition for Alternatives to Pesticides, Eugene, OR. http://panna.igc.org/resources/pestis/PESTIS.1996.18.html.
30 Hayes, H.M., et al., "Case-control Study of Canine Malignant Lymphoma: Positive Association with Dog Owner's Use of 2,4-Dichlorophenoxyacetic Acid Herbicides," J. Natl. Cancer Inst., 1991:83, 1226-1231.
31 Epstein, Samuel, "Problems of Causality, Burdens of Proof and Restitution Agent Orange Diseases," Trial, 1983:91,138.
32 Schmidt, K.F., "Puzzling Over a Poison: On Closer Inspection, the Ubiquitous Pollutant Dioxin Appears More Dangerous Than Ever," U.S. News and World Report, April 6, 1992, p. 61.
33 "PBBs in Fire Retardant Associated with Early Menstruation in Michigan Girls Whose Mothers Were Exposed in 1973," NIEHS, Press Release, Emory University, December 8, 2000.
34 Goodman, Robin F., Ph.D. and Anita Gurian, Ph.D., "A Month of Mental Health Facts: Fact-of-the-day," http://www.aboutourkids.org/articles/mhfacts.html.
35 Pall, Martin, "Vicious Chemical Cycle May Cause Chemical Sensitivity," The Federation of American Societies of Experimental Biology Journal, September 2002.
36 Glanzing, A., "Native Vegetation. Australia Still in Top Ten Land Clearing Country Club," Life Lines: Bulletin of the Community Biodiversity Network, 1998:4(2):14.

37 Epstein, Samuel, M.D., The Politics of Cancer Revisited, 1998. East Ridge Press, USA, Freemont, NY. Cost: $17.00 (plus S&H).
38 Bell, I., et al., "Neural Sensitization and Physiological Markers in Multiple Chemical Sensitivity," Regulatory Toxicology and Pharmacology (1996c) 24:S47.
39 Randolph, T. and R. Moss, An Alternative Approach to Allergies, 1980, Lippincott & Crowell, New York.
40 Redemske Design, 413.773.5375. sandyr@shaysnet.com
41 Anderson Laboratories, P. O. Box 323, Hartford, VT 05084. 802.905.7344. www.anderson.
42 McKinney, Deanna, "Meeting the Challenge of West Nile Virus without Poisons," Journal of Pesticide Reform, Winter 2002: 22 (4).
43 http://www.turning-aboutface.com, PBS Interview by Bill Moyers with Philip J. Landrigan, M.D., Mount Sinai School of Medicine.

CHAPTER 2

How Can You Tell If Chemicals Hurt You?

What Are the Specific Clues of a Possible Chemical or Pesticide Sensitivity? [1a,f,g,i]

It can be easier than you think to find out if you or your child unknowingly has been hurt by an accidental or purposeful chemical exposure. It is often obvious. Look for changes in how you and your family members look, feel, act, behave, learn or write, as well as in your breathing and pulse, within seconds to minutes after a chemical exposure. In most individuals there are immediate changes. In contrast, most allergenic substances cause symptoms within 15 minutes to an hour. Depending on your degree of sensitivity and which area of your body is susceptible (each person is different), physical as well as emotional or mental changes can persist for hours, days or weeks after an initial contact. For example, if your heart is affected, the heartbeat can become irregular on an intermittent or regular basis from simply sleeping on linens that smell of a scented detergent or a mattress made of synthetic material. This intermittent daily exposure can cause your heart to function abnormally for years. The answer is to get rid of the cause or you may be on medications indefinitely.

The weak areas of the body in some people might cause them to wheeze or cough, have fatigue, headaches, chronic intestinal complaints, lung, ear or sinus infections, problems thinking clearly, joint pain or dizziness, etc.

Five Fast Ways to Recognize Reactions to Chemicals or Allergenic Substances[1b,g,i]

Look for the following changes after exposure and compare to what you consider to be "normal". Pay attention to the **"Big Five":**

1. How you look.
2. How you feel, act, behave and learn.
3. How you breathe.
4. Your pulse and blood pressure.
5. Your writing and drawing.

1.
How Can Chemicals Change How You Look?[1a,f,g,h,i]

When you or a family member suddenly feels unwell from exposure to chemicals or allergenic substances, look for changes in appearance. Many adults and children suddenly develop:

- Dark blue, black or pink eye circles.
- Wrinkles or abnormally puffy bags under the eyes.
- A spaced out or demonic look.
- Bright red cheeks, nose tips or earlobes.
- Wiggly legs.
- Nose rubbing.
- Throat clearing or coughing.
- Lip licking.
- A puffy look to face, hands and knuckles.

Adults also sometimes develop a blanched pale ring around the outer edge of their lips and slightly swollen lip edges.

The above changes provide clues to quickly warn family members, friends, teachers or co-workers that a reaction to a chemical or environmental exposure (i.e. dust, molds, pollen or foods) has begun.

Table 2
Symptoms of Chemical Sensitivities and Allergies

How many of the following characteristics do you have?

- Inordinate fatigue.
- Hyperactivity.
- Headaches.
- Fuzzy thinking, confusion, difficulty concentrating, thinking clearly or remembering.
- A peculiar metallic taste in the mouth.
- Sudden unexplained intermittent problems walking, reading, writing or drawing.
- Wiggly legs or tics, twitches, tremors, even seizures.
- Muscle aches, weakness or very tender painful skin areas.
- Joint or arthritic pains.
- Swelling or puffiness of the face, fingers, feet or joints.
- A runny nose or nasal congestion eventually causing recurrent ear, sinus and lung infections.
- Nose rubbing.
- Puffy eye bags or wrinkles below the eyes.
- Glassy, spaced-out look to the eyes.
- Dark blue, black or pink eye circles.
- Abnormally red cheeks and earlobes.
- Throat-clearing or coughing.
- Asthma, unexplained shortness of breath.
- Acting inappropriately, giddy, infantile, withdrawn, hiding in dark corners or not wanting to be touched.
- Burning or numb skin.
- Creepy crawly feelings under the skin.
- Easy bruising or black and blue marks on the skin.
- Itchy rashes, such as hives or eczema.
- Heartburn, nausea, bloating, intestinal gas or discomfort, constipation, diarrhea, bad breath.[8b]
- An irregular or very rapid heart beat or elevated blood pressure.
- Becoming irritable, agitated or manifesting atypical or unusual behavior such as sudden, inexplicable moodiness, uncontrollable crying, laughter or fear, depression, aggression and major control problems such as anxiety, rage or panic attacks.
- A heightened sense of taste, smell and hearing.
- Hoarseness or an inability to speak.
- Insomnia.

2. How Can Chemicals Change How You Feel, Act, Behave or Learn? [1a,f,g, 2a-c, 3a,b]

Chemicals can cause changes in many areas of your body affecting how you feel, act and think. Persons who have allergies or relatives with skin problems (eczema, hives), hay fever or asthma can be the "canaries in the coal mine". They appear to be particularly prone to develop chemical sensitivities and are often the first to become ill. Some of the signs are:

- Nose, sinus or lung congestion, a cough or wheeze, throat clearing, leg aches, stiff joints, bleeding into the nose, joints, skin or nipples.
- A metallic taste inside the mouth, sometimes after smelling some odor.
- Burning or numbness of the face, arms, legs or feet or a creepy crawly feeling under your skin.
- Prolonged flu or repeated ear, sinus or lung infections.
- Recurrent intestinal complaints such as abdominal pain, belching, gas or diarrhea.
- Extreme and total fatigue, even when arising in the morning.
- Headaches.
- Joint and muscle weakness, aches, pains or swelling, at times or all the time.
- Behavioral changes that include episodes of inappropriate hyperactivity, anger, crying, giggling, irritability, drastic mood swings, anxiety, panic, rage or sudden vulgarity. (*Yes, some Tourette's Syndrome are helped with treatment of*

chemical sensitivities and allergies[1f])[*]

- Difficulty learning and unclear thinking.
- Spasm in the bladder causing a sudden urge to urinate so the underwear or bed is wet.
- Sudden hoarseness, babbling and unclear speech. A few cannot speak at all.
- Ringing in their ears or a feeling of dizziness.
- Not wanting to be touched or recoiling from the slightest contact. Some scream if anyone dares to come near them.
- Hiding in dark places, under furniture or in tight, remote corners.

Each person responds in his/her own way though each follows an individualized, characteristic pattern. Different exposures will cause different patterns of response. Learn to recognize the patterns in yourself and your loved ones. You can do it. Remember that almost any area of the body can be affected. You can sometimes find answers that everyone else has missed for years by paying attention to when and why, you or someone you love, suddenly changes.

If specific parts of your brain are affected, there can be a wide range of different medical complaints.[1b,e] *(See Table 2.)* Depending on the brain area, it might cause difficulty remembering or learning, hyperactivity, extreme fatigue, irritability, moodiness, aggression, panic or vulgarity. Some children or adults become so agitated or overactive they simply cannot sit still. Others surprisingly tend to become too quiet, fall asleep, or do not want anyone to be near them. They want to be left totally alone. They crawl under chairs and tables and refuse to come out. When other parts of the brain or nervous system are altered it might not be possible to think clearly, do math, read, write,

[*] *Can Chemicals Cause Epidemics?*, Doris J. Rapp, M.D. ERF, P. O. Box 60, Buffalo, NY 14223-0060, 800.787.8780, www.drrapp.com.

speak or walk normally. Your skin can be affected so it tingles, twitches, burns, goes into spasm, hurts or feels numb. If a part of your body has been hurt or weakened in the past, this is often the body area that will be most vulnerable when you are exposed to the wrong thing. For example, if you hurt your right hip as a child, when you are exposed to chemicals or eat foods to which you have developed sensitivities, you will tend to have problems in your right hip when you are an adult.

3.
How Can Chemicals Change How You Breathe?[1b]

After chemical exposure some may experience wheezing, coughing or shortness in breath, which is alleviated with the use of asthma medicine. If you think that a chemical is causing this condition, you can use a Peak Flow Meter to check. This is simply a hollow plastic tube with a gauge on it that can record a decrease in your lung function after exposure to some chemical. If you blow 400 before exposure to a chemical odor and 300 in a few minutes, it suggests your lungs were affected. If you can pinpoint, avoid or eliminate the chemical that caused the drop, you might not cough, wheeze or need asthma medicine. This type of test is only necessary if breathing is a problem. Remember, similar decreases in your ability to breathe normally can occur within an hour after exposure to dust, molds, pollen or certain foods, but this only happens if these things affect your lungs.[1b] To find more answers, systematically check your breathing before and shortly after various everyday exposures. Then check with your doctor. Of course, infections in the lungs can also cause a similar drop in your ability to breathe.

4.
How Can Chemicals Change Your Heart or Circulation?[1b, 4, 10a]

If the cardiac system is affected, it is possible to develop an irregular pulse, called a cardiac arrhythmia. Others might suddenly develop a very rapid heartbeat (tachycardia) or high blood pressure (hypertension) from chemical exposures. Because some heart-related symptoms, such as high blood pressure, can go undetected for years, it is helpful if you try to protect yourself. Ask someone who knows medicine to show you how to take your pulse and blood pressure. By doing this, you can easily learn to detect if and when there are changes in your heart function, pulse or blood pressure. Then you can see if these changes are related to exposures to suspect chemicals or allergenic substances.[4] Again, the answers are often there. Be honest. Ask yourself how badly you want to get well. If you are willing to spend the time to find and eliminate the cause, you may not need to take numerous cardiac or other medicines for many years. Yes, you are right, you cannot always find the answers, but what is surprising is how often you can. It really is possible for you, alone, to turn your health around and find answers everyone else has missed, but always discuss everything with your doctor.

5.
How Can Chemicals Affect How You Write or Draw?

Changes in writing and drawing often reflect how an individual feels.[1a,f,g,i] Some will smell an odor and suddenly begin writing upside down, backwards or in mirror images. If hyperactivity is apparent after exposure to a chemical, the writing tends to become too large and sloppy. If chemicals cause someone to become withdrawn, the writing can become tiny or even pinpoint. Drawings by children often clearly reflect feelings of sadness, depression, anger or aggression in the form of tears, knives or physical violence. Any form of creativity can be affected such as poetry, paintings, music, literature, etc. Although these changes are most obvious in children, adults have similar responses that can be recognized easily once you are aware of what can happen. The key is to watch your own writing, drawing or other creative outlets. If there is a significant change, keep asking why. Notice if the changes occur after you smell chemicals, are exposed to dust, mold or pollen or have ingested certain foods or beverages. You can find the answers.

Four Ways to Pinpoint Possible Causes of a Chemical Sensitivity or an Allergy [1a,b,f,g]

Keep asking yourself over and over: What did I smell, eat or touch? Ask if a physical or emotional complaint or change in actions and behavior could possibly be due to:

A. Something inside
B. Outside
C. A food
D. A chemical.

You can pinpoint the cause by repeatedly considering these few factors:

A. Is it Something Inside?

Does some change in how you feel, act, behave or think occur when you go inside your home, school or work area? Did these changes occur when you moved into a different or new house, trailer or workplace?

If this is true, check each room or area for chemical smells, as well as for dust, molds, pets or the aroma from foods. Keep asking what is different in the exact area where there is a problem. The chemically sensitive can smell a gas leak or perfume when no one else can and their brains sometimes react to such tiny amounts of odors, that the offending chemical cannot even be smelled or identified by them or others.

Think about the following common chemical and other exposures:

- All routine disinfectants, deodorizers, laundry products or sprays used for oven or window cleaning materials, non-stick pans, starch, spot removers, etc.[6]

- Personal scented body products, scented candles, incense, etc.[7, 11b,c] Is anybody worse after using nice smelling items in a bathroom?

- Exposures to smelly items such as nail polish and remover, crayons, typing correction fluid, marking pens, auto exhaust or tobacco.[6,11b,c]

- New furniture with synthetic covers or stuffing, carpets, carpet pads and glue, synthetic pillows and mattresses, new synthetic clothing.

- Heating/air-conditioning system. Improper filter care or chemicals in the ventilation ducts commonly causes chronic, perplexing illness.[10b] Did your symptoms begin when you installed or repaired your furnace or cleaned the ventilation ducts? Do your medical complaints recur each fall when the heat goes on and subside when the weather is warmer?

- Molds from previous water damage or molds found in swamp coolers. Look for evidence of previous water leaks near pipes, on the ceilings, walls and under carpets. Molds can cause a greater variety of medical symptoms than most individuals would consider possible.[1f,g,h, 9]

- Toxic pesticide chemicals sprayed inside or around your home to control insects can make some or all family members ill. This should be a concern especially for toddlers or pets that play and move at ground level.

- Chemicals that are used for termite control are routinely poured under the foundation during construction. These can leak through basement floor holes or cracks and up the interior of the walls polluting the inside air throughout the house.

- Chemical spills in the basement or garage.[9] These types of exposures can cause illnesses making some houses and buildings totally uninhabitable for years.[10b]

- Intermittent or constant natural gas leaks from hot water tanks, kitchen stoves, furnaces or fireplaces.

- Insulation and building materials, such as paint, varnish, shellac, grout and formaldehyde in particleboard, etc. all can cause difficulty during construction or subsequent remodeling.[10b, 13]

- Soft, smelly plastics such as those found in artificial flowers, plastic containers, shower curtains, etc.

- Screens often emit chemical odors, particularly when exposed to the hot sun.

B.

Is it Something Outside?[1b,f,g,h, 3a]

If you tend to suddenly become ill when you are outside, look around. Some reactions might not occur for several minutes to an hour after you go outside, but many chemicals typically cause symptoms in seconds to minutes and they can last for hours or days. For example, when they were spraying the chemical malathion for mosquitos in New York City, some people came out of their office buildings in Manhattan and found they not only immediately developed a cough and asthma, but some could not even remember their home address. *(See Chapter 8.)* It can happen instantaneously because the olfactory nerve sends messages directly from the nose into the brain.

To find answers to illness due to the outside ask:

- Are you routinely worse or do your children act up mainly when you are outside or before you go inside? Pay very close attention.

- Do you not feel right when entering a certain polluted sector of your city? Some people regularly become ill within 10 to 20 blocks or miles from their home or an industrial area.

- Conversely, do you feel much better when you are away from home, on vacation or traveling and worse within minutes to hours after returning home? Notice if you are worse before or after you enter your home.

- Does your health change on certain days mainly when you are downwind from certain factories when they expel certain chemicals into the air?

- Is some family member routinely seen in emergency rooms because of sudden asthma attacks on the weekends, when factories emit noxious pollutants because there is less surveillance?

- Does your air smell of fresh asphalt, paint or scented fabric softeners from a laundry vent just before you change in some way?

- Are heavy traffic fumes a problem when you are near expressways or toll booths?

- Is your illness related to the same time of the year, each year? Think of pollen, for example, if your symptoms are related to cutting the grass.[1a] Maybe it is a herbicide used on some weeds?

- Could the cause be molds due to excess rain or dampness? Do you have a swamp or large body of water near by?

- Do you or a family member have a recurrence of certain symptoms whenever a weather inversion occurs? You may be more able to see, sense or smell certain factory pollution odors on foggy days or when the air is "heavy". Note if that is the time when you or certain family members routinely tend to become ill.

- Are you always better in a certain locale, city or vacation spot? If so, it is often easier, much better and less expensive in the long run to consider moving to the specific area where you feel better or well.

C.
Is it a Food or Beverage?[1b,f,g, 3a, 8, 11a,d]

If the cause of a sudden change in how you feel or act occurs after eating, it might be due to the specific item you ingested or to something on or in that food or beverage. For this reason you can easily be fooled when it comes to food sensitivities. If a grocery store apple causes some symptom but an organic apple does not, maybe the chemical on or in the food is at fault. If both the organic or grocery store apple causes symptoms, the apple is probably making you ill. For this reason, it is not uncommon for an apparent food problem not to be the food you suspect. For example, you might think you have a wheat problem because your favorite food is baked goods and you feel ill in a certain way after you eat them. The culprit could be yeast or some other item, such as egg, sugar or a dye, on or in the baked goods.

You will know if you have a food or beverage related allergy because you will typically have a reaction within a few minutes to an hour after ingesting a problem item.[1b,g, 2a-c, 3a] On occasion, symptoms from swallowing a food can begin in seconds or they can be delayed so that the reaction might not be evident for 8 to 12 hours (bedwetting, ear infections, cold sores, arthritis or colitis). Food reactions tend to last for about 30 to 120 minutes but it is possible for one meal of a problem food to cause symptoms that persist for eight days or longer. This means if you ate the problem food only once a week, it is possible to have symptoms every day for years and never know why.

Write down your five favorite food and beverages. If you have unsuspected food sensitivities, you probably have just written down the cause. To confirm if you have a food allergy, do not eat a speck of any of the items you wrote down for five days. After about four days of absolutely avoiding each possible suspect problem food or beverage, ingest each one separately when no other food has been eaten for four or more hours. See what happens. This can provide answers everyone else has missed for many years but check with your doctor first. *(See Chapter 3.)*

Determining a food or beverage allergy becomes more challenging now than ever before because we are presently confronted with genetically modified or irradiated foods.[8, 11a,d] Amazingly, these types of products do not need to be labeled. These foods can potentially create an unbelievable range of unsuspected, incapacitating and frightening symptoms. If this folly persists, the most astute physician or experienced environmental specialist will be challenged to try to figure out why people are ill. *(See Chapter 9.)*

D.
Is it a Chemical? [1b,f,g,i, 2a, 3a, 10a]

If the cause of some change in your health or behavior appears to be a chemical, the reaction will tend to occur within seconds to minutes after an exposure. For example, you can simply walk by someone who smells of perfume and immediately cough or wheeze, get stuffed up, develop a headache or feel dizzy. It is possible for the chemical to affect your brain so you cannot speak, walk normally or think clearly. Such reactions typically last for a few minutes, but at times the effect of one exposure can last for days or even weeks. If some toxic exposure is prolonged, the illness it causes can last for a lifetime. In general, whether you will react to some chemical or not is not related to how large the exposure is, but to how sensitive you are to it. Very minute whiffs of toxic substances can have devastating effects on some people.

Similar to those who absolutely can't resist certain foods, there are some people who crave unusual chemical aromas, such as the smell of fresh paint. If this is apparent, the most desired odors are often the ones to which you are most apt to be sensitive. If you do not notice or care one way or the other, chances are chemicals such as gasoline, perfume or formaldehyde in funeral parlors or furniture etc. are probably not a problem.[13]

In addition, those who have this problem can truly smell odors that others insist are not present. Most who complain are truly sick. They are not imagining the smell or the fact it makes them ill. They are ill!

More Tips to Find Answers Everyone's Missed[1b,f]

Here are some other obvious and more elusive tips to help you pinpoint if chemicals or common exposures might be the cause of medical, emotional or memory problems in yourself or your loved ones. The obvious clues are sudden headaches, congestion and asthma. More elusive clues are sudden light-switch changes in mood, behavior, activity or the ability to learn in children and adults. Many mothers have noted drastic, sudden changes in their child the day the house cleaning is done. Think dust, a leaky vacuum cleaner or cleaning materials. If a change occurs after a child drinks a colored, sweetened beverage, think food coloring, regular or artificial sugar or corn syrup. If it occurs when someone comes into a home smelling of hair spray or when the lawn trucks begin spraying in your area, think chemicals. If problems arise when a blower in a furnace clicks on, think dust, molds, natural gas or fumes from combustion. Defective heating units and ventilation systems can cause undetected recurrent seasonal chronic illness for many years.[6, 10a]

"The life of the party" child or adult may be reacting to something that was just ingested or smelled. Some develop hyperactivity, irritability, moodiness or they begin acting withdrawn, hostile, angry, aggressive or vulgar. It is easy to see who is affected. It is possible that adults might not be reacting to alcohol but to the grain from which it was made.[12] The challenge is to find out *why* and this can be simple once you realize you only have to think about what happened just before the change occurred.

> **To find out *why* you are sick simply recall what was new or different in your home, school or work area, or your diet, water or air immediately *prior to* the initial episode or any subsequent flare-up of your illness. Keep asking what was eaten, touched or smelled and write it down. The rewards can be immense.**

The answers are often easily recognized if you can recall exactly when an illness or behavioral change first began. Look at your old bills to help you recall if you made some major purchase or a significant change in your home before or after you became ill. In particular, consider when something different happened in your life in relation to when you began to feel unwell for the first time.

Here are some examples of more elusive causes. Ask yourself if the onset of your symptoms is related to:

- A change in the type, dosage or brand of medication or nutrient you are taking? Remember, even medicines you have taken for years without difficulty can suddenly make you ill. At any time you can become sensitive to a medicine or there can be a change in the formulation or preparation.

- A different car that smells new, moldy or of chemicals? The chemicals used to mask the odor of a moldy smelling air conditioner in a car, for example, can be toxic.[1]

- Some unavoidable or unexpected chemical exposures in a rented apartment, your school or dormitory, your work area or a nearby playground?

- It is possible for areas to be sprayed for insects or weeds without anyone being informed. Did flare-ups of the same types of symptoms occur in the past? Think about when similar patterns of symptoms occurred. For example, one 10 year old boy suddenly could no longer see clearly enough to read while in school. He stayed home and was fine in a couple of days. His mother checked and they had cleaned the carpets at school on the day he became ill. She was not told the next time they cleaned the carpets but she knew right way because again, her son suddenly could not read normally.

- Everyone who is exposed will not become ill in the same way. Some will remain well. In obviously contaminated schools or workplaces, for example, it is not unusual for about 30% of the children, teachers or workers to complain of some form of illness shortly after they re-enter a recently renovated or pesticided building. The same chemicals can cause similar or different symptoms in each person.[1a,f,g, 10a]

Here is one example that was discussed when I was a guest on Oprah: A vibrantly healthy adolescent girl became extremely ill, fatigued, weak and unable to attend school regularly because she was simply too sick and tired for over a year. No one knew why. Then one day she looked down and saw her blouse and bra were covered with blood. She later found out that several other girls at school had noticed the same problem. In addition, several teachers in her school had developed cancer and died. A newspaper report finally alerted her parents that there was something wrong in her school after it had been remodeled. Her illness began shortly after the changes in the building. She transferred to another school and soon was fine.

This sort of thing can happen and if it does, there are ways you can also find answers and resolve the problem. Check with others in your child's school, your apartment building, housing or work area. Check any health office records at school and at work, if that is possible. Talk to the PTA or union at work. Make lists of names, addresses, symptoms and other pertinent information. These may prove to be invaluable later on. There may be genuine reluctance on the part of employers or school officials to share salient information or to order laboratory tests that might provide definitive answers.[1d] This is especially true if there is a fear or concern about potential legitimate litigation. Those who are worried about a possible suit will sometimes provide "gag" money to those who are less ill if they will sign a statement saying they will tell no one that they became ill after some exposure. *(See Chapter 7.)*

Once a sensitivity exists, symptoms from future, unrelated chemicals can occur from many different minute exposures and these reactions can occur more quickly, be more severe and last longer than anyone thinks possible.

- Does some family member occasionally or regularly awaken in a rage, very angry or sick for no logical reason? Think about any chemicals, as well as late night foods or snacks, as possible suspects. If there were no recent changes in your bed, bedroom, bed partner or your own personal body care products, consider freshly dry cleaned clothes in the closet or the scent of toxic mothballs. These can be common, unrecognized causes of chronic serious perplexing illness.

- Are you worse when there is aerial crop or insect spraying in our area? Know that denial and evasive-run-around answers can be routine. Check with your city health department about aerial spraying during the night. Pinpointing exactly who knows what and who will share needed information, at times, can be an exasperating and lengthy challenge. Keep a paper trail with records of dates when symptoms occurred and who was called, when and why. In time, it may be easy to confirm cause and affect relationships when information is eventually released in news reports.

Can You Protect Yourself and Your Family from Chemicals and Pesticides? [1a,f, 2a-c, 3a,b]

The answer is yes. There is much that you can do to diminish or prevent future exposures but these too can be a bit of a challenge. Detailed, practical and sometimes inexpensive suggestions are discussed in Chapter 3. Remember, if you are suddenly accidentally exposed, move away from the source and run for cover. Hold your breath and get away from the offending chemical as soon as you can. Breathing cleaner outside air or oxygen often helps in a few minutes.

One example occurred when I was a guest on the Maury Povich talk show: One guest was a teacher who was describing how she would become ill with sudden laryngitis and breathing problems. These occurred mainly when school was in session or when she smelled chemicals.[1a,g,i] *She was speaking normally when another guest, who smelled of hair spray and perfume, came on stage and sat down next to her. In seconds her voice became hoarse and she could barely breathe. She was quickly taken outside and in a few minutes she was fine again.*

Is Everyone Made ill from Chemical or Pesticide Exposures?

No. Fortunately, everyone is certainly not obviously affected by pesticides or chemicals. Pollution will not affect those who have been blessed with genetically strong and undamaged immune systems. This is why one massive chemical exposure will typically affect only certain individuals. The same thing happens when the pollen count is high or an illness is spreading through a community. All those who are exposed do not become ill. The majority remain healthy in spite of the many toxins or poisons that cross their paths every day. This good health will continue, but only if the level of harmful exposures does not exceed an individual's personal level of tolerance. Potentially, however, anyone can be accidentally overexposed and can immediately be in medical jeopardy. The health and futures of entire families have been damaged by something as commonplace as a defective furnace or the installation of a new synthetic carpet.[1c,g]

In addition, a certain number will be ill and not recognize or admit they have an illness. *(Men are in the most denial)*. It is not uncommon for those who are affected with periods of extreme irritability or aggression to blame someone else and deny they have a short, uncontrollable wick. Problem spouses or children are typically blamed or accused of being bad or imagining they are ill, when the true cause is environmental, not psychological. Many have had years of counseling and tried a wide variety of mind or mood altering medications with only temporary or very little improvement because these forms of therapy will not eliminate illnesses caused by polluted environments, foods or a weakened immune system. When the causes are found and eliminated, it is certainly possible for some disposition problems to vanish. Many marriages have been saved after the cause – what brought on a child's or spouse's unacceptable or inappropriate behavior — is detected and eliminated. Once the problem sources are recognized and eliminated, psychological counseling, for the first time, can be most helpful and effective. In many, it is needed to help remove the anger, guilt, fear, resentment, depression and feelings of total inadequacy that they unfortunately have experienced.[2c] The ego suffers greatly when you hurt and no one believes you, particularly when these include those you trust, respect and turn to for solace, for example, your loved ones, physician, teacher and/or religious advisor.

Two Challenges Remain

The first major challenge in treating chemical sensitivities is to change the emphasis from drug treatment to prevention. The present epidemics of learning and behavior difficulties, cancer, serious bowel and cardiac problems and other chronic illnesses must be addressed.*

---

* *Can Chemicals Cause Epidemics?*, Doris J. Rapp, M.D. ERF, P. O. Box 60, Buffalo, NY 14223-0060, 800.787.8780, www.drrapp.com.

Prevention is not popular and rarely funded but it is the way we must go. In addition, in the long run it can be both health and cost-effective. We cannot continue to pollute every aspect of our world as we are doing at the present time without realizing that the consequences eventually can be monumental. The healthcare system, insurance, legal system and governmental agencies need to recognize environmental health problems and become part of the resolution.

The other challenge is to help the many chronically ill people who have been wrongly diagnosed or blamed for their illness and in some cases forced to live a life of partial or even total seclusion. Many have been to one doctor after another, and in time, naturally became discouraged, even suicidal.[2c] Their resources are depleted and they have no idea where to turn for help. Some eventually come to the conclusion that they must remain ill because it is assumed that no one can find and eliminate the cause. This attitude is often totally wrong. Chapter 3 provides a range of helpful suggestions some of which are both inexpensive and effective. Many who are presently ill can be helped if we can develop diagnostic, treatment, education and research centers that provide the best of both traditional and alternative medicine at a fee that most can afford. *(See Epilogue at end of book.)*

Summary

The simple types of observations discussed in this chapter will often quickly provide the answers to explain "the why" of many acute and chronic health, emotional, behavior or learning problems. Effective alternatives to drug therapy do exist. The key is to ask if the cause is due to something inside or outside— a food or beverage— or a chemical. Notice how someone looks, acts and behaves. Check the writing and drawing, as well as the pulse and breathing. Always think about how, when, where and why in relation to each of your own medical complaints, memory difficulties and/or activity or behavior problems. *The key question is: what did you eat, touch or smell?*

Make this your healing mantra. With the type of information provided in this chapter, all on your own, you can find answers everyone else has missed.

The more knowledge and awareness that you have and can teach your family members and friends, the more all of you can recognize and pinpoint causes. Once you have done that, you can take steps to prevent, eliminate or more effectively treat illness in your family. We are all one. We must help each other and all living things on this planet and we must do it now.

If you do find some unusual cause of some medical problem in your family, please write to P.O. Box 60, Buffalo, New York, 14223 or www.drrapp.com. Maybe you can provide fresh insight so others also can be helped.

CHAPTER 2 REFERENCES:

1 Environmental Medical Research Foundation: ERF (Formerly: PARF or Practical Allergy Research Foundation), P. O. Box 60, Buffalo, NY 14223-0060. 800.787.8780 (for Peak Flow Meters, air and water purifiers, books, videos and audio tapes), www.drrapp.com

1a Is This Your Child's World? 1996, Part 1, Chapters 1, 2, 4, 5, 6. Cost: $15.00 (plus S&H).
1b Chapter 3.
1c pp. 257-9.
1d Chapters 11 and 15.
1e Chapter 13.
1f Is This Your Child? 1991. Cost: $12.00 (plus S&H).
1g Video: Environmentally Sick Schools, 90 min. Cost: $25.00 (plus S&H).
1h Video: Mold Reactions in Children and Adults. Cost: $25.00 (plus S&H).
1i Video: Chemical Reactions in Children and Adults. Cost: $25.00 (plus S&H).

2 Rogers, Sherry, M.D., Prestige Press, P.O. Box 3068, 3500 Brewerton Rd., Syracuse, NY 13220. 800.846.6687, 315.468.4417. Fax: 315.468.8119. www.prestigepublishing.com

2a Wellness Against All Odds, 1994. Cost: $17.95 (plus S&H).
2b No More Heartburn, 2000. Cost: $15.00 (plus S&H).
2c Depression Cured at Last 1997. Cost $24.95 (plus S&H).
2d Detoxify or Die: The Ultimate Healing Plan, 2002. Cost: $22.95 (plus S&H).

3 Krohn, Jacqueline, M.D. and Frances Taylor, Hartley & Marks, Inc., Box 147, Point Roberts, WA 98281. 505.662.9620.

3a The Whole Way to Allergy And Prevention, 1991. Cost: $24.95 (plus S&H).
3b Natural Detoxification: A Practical Encyclopedia: The Complete Guide to Clearing Your Body of Toxins. Cost: $24.95 (plus S&H).

4 Omron® Portable Wrist Blood Pressure Monitor, Omron® 800.634.4350. www.costco.com or major retail stores.

5 www.sciencedaily.com/releases/2001/08/010818004941.htm

6 Soapworks, 18911 Nordhoff St. Ste. 37, Northridge, CA 91324. 800.699.9917, www.soapworks.com.

7 C.A.R.E.S. Foundation. 866.742.3310. www.lindachae.com.

8 Fagan, John, Ph.D., Genetic Engineering: The Hazards; Vedic Engineering: The Solutions, 1995, Maharishi International University, 1000 N. Fourth St., Fairfield, Iowa 52557. Cost: $12.00, Amazon.com.

9 EnviroGen Technologies, 131 Pitkin Street, East Hartford, CT 06108. 800.367.3634. Email: johnfantry2@hotmail.com

10a Rea, William J., M.D., Chemical Sensitivity, Vols. 1-4, 1992-1997, CRC Press, 2000 Corporate Blvd. NW, Boca Raton, FL. 214.368.4132.

10b Rea, William J., M.D., Optimum Environment for Optimum Health and Creativity, 2002, Crown Press in Dallas- American Health Environmental Center. 800.428.2343. Cost: $39.95.

11a Epstein, Samuel S., "Unlabeled Milk from Cows Treated with Biosynthetic Growth Hormones: A case of regulatory abdication," Int. J. Health Services, 1996:26(1)173-185.

11b Epstein, Samuel S., The Politics of Cancer Revisited, 1998, East Ridge Press, USA, Freemont, NY, $17.00 (plus S&H).

11c Epstein, Samuel S. and D. Grundy, eds. The Legislation Of Product Safety: Consumer Health and Product Hazards, Vol. II: Cosmetics and Drugs, Pesticides, Food Additives. 1976: Cambridge, Mass., and London, M.I.T. Press.

11d Epstein, Samuel S., M.D., Got Genetically Engineered Milk? Seven Stories Press, 2001. Cost: $7.00 Digital E-book.

12 Randolph, Theron and R. Moss, An Alternative Approach to Allergies, 1980, Lippincott and Crowell, NY.

13 Charles R. Bailey Cabinetmakers, 51 MD 7013, Highway 62 East, Flippin, AR 72634. 870.453.5433. www.southshore.com/~crbslf

CHAPTER 3

You Know What's Wrong, Now What Do You Do?

From the information in Chapter 2, you have probably gained some valuable and practical insight to help pinpoint the possible causes of illness in yourself or in your loved ones. Others will need some of the additional clues and details that are provided in this chapter to help them to understand more fully why they or others are ill. Just as important, it is critical for your well being to find out what you and your doctor can practically do about the diagnosis and treatment of chemical or allergy medical problems, once you figure out that these might be part of your personal health issues. [4c,f, 9a-f]

What Can You Do about a Chemical Sensitivity? [4c, 9a, 28a,b, 41]

Avoidance Is the Key

It does not matter if your problem is a chemical, your water, a food or something inside or outside your home. The best and easiest form of treatment is usually avoidance. Sometimes, if your sensitivity is mild, you need only to eliminate the source of a problem chemical (cleaning solution, perfume, pesticide, synthetic carpet or mattress) and you will be fine.[78] You must, however, also attempt to avoid all future chemical exposures, as much as sensibly possible. Those who have this illness must be aware of the potentially serious dangers that can be associated with a prolonged chemical exposure, even if it is miniscule. It is not how much, but how sensitive you are to a chemical that counts. The need for maximum and continued avoidance of chemicals to protect the health of your precious family cannot be underestimated. Avoidance can be the best, and by far the easiest, fastest and most inexpensive way to resolve certain chemically related health, emotional and memory problems. As you continue reading, you will learn many other things you can easily do so you can feel much better and remain well.

For Some

For some, the answer is simple; if the cause of your illness is obvious, simply move. If you live in your own little polluted "love canal" located near a toxic nearby factory, over a sludge and sewage dumpsite, or in an impossibly moldy or polluted home, it can be possible to regain your original health most quickly by moving. In the long run this can be the simplest and best answer for many.

The major clue is surprisingly simple. You feel better when you are away from your usual living, work or school area and sick shortly after you return. Sometimes it is easy to avoid known problem areas by simply moving to another home, to a different sector of town, to another school district or working in a different area of a factory, office or building. Because of the potential for debilitating illness from some short term and many long term chemical exposures and the possible need for prolonged expensive treatment, some individuals find they feel much better and regain their health most quickly if they simply abandon their present polluted environment. Trying to clean it up on your own can lead to more harmful exposure and potentially more debilitating illness. *(See Chapter 10.)*

For a Very Few

It is fortunately rare for individuals to be so seriously ill that they must entirely change their type of employment and way of life. However, at times, if the environmental problems are extreme, even those with specialized training and education, such as a teacher, painter, beautician, chemist, surgeon or nurse, might have to consider going into an entirely different aspect of their area of expertise or learning other skills. For a few exceptional families, sometimes it might even be necessary to cut their losses and move to a totally different city or area of the country and learn a different profession. As disruptive as this can be, at times, this can be the very best possible solution from both the health and economic viewpoint.

As discussed in detail later in this chapter, a few are so ill from chemicals that they cannot leave their house without realistic concerns about the minutest additional exposure. For such individuals, adequate avoidance can be a monumental challenge until detoxification measures are implemented to help diminish their total body load of stored chemicals. In addition, there is often a need to supply some digestive aids because of associated chronic intestinal malfunction and a variety of nutrients to build up the body's immune system.

For the Vast Majority[4a]

For most, the detailed information in this chapter will prove to be needed and most helpful to both prevent and treat the physical, emotional and memory problems of those who are chemically sensitive or environmentally ill. There will be no need to relocate, either locally or elsewhere, but you will need to make some significant but relatively simple changes in your ordinary lifestyle to regain or maintain your original or optimum level of health. The changes are more inconvenient than difficult. Look over the suggestions below. Start with what is practical, easy and inexpensive. Unless you quickly improve, work into the rest of the treatment options as rapidly as possible. You need only to do as much of the following as is necessary to regain your health. Throughout this chapter refer to Appendix B for locations and phone numbers of the various helpful resources.

Once you have developed an obvious chemical and pesticide sensitivity there is no doubt that this illness can sometimes become much more complicated than you originally anticipated. The development of multiple sensitivities to chemicals is not uncommon and reflects a definite weakness in the immune system. Because the body's defense systems are deficient, typically there are associated allergies to dust, mold, pollen and foods. The allergies can be present before or after the onset of the chemical aspect of this problem and without therapy, can become worse in time. These illnesses typically go hand in hand. Some degree of treatment of both of these conditions is usually required before you begin to feel well again. It is the total load or combination of chemicals and common allergens that typically determine how sick you are. If you can lighten the load by doing the things suggested below, this will help to decrease your total exposure below the level that makes you ill. You do not need to do everything that is suggested but you must do enough so you no longer are sick when you smell, eat or touch the wrong thing. Everything does not have to be perfect, but if you lower your level of exposure to things that bother you below your personal threshold, you should become much better.

In addition, you must try to eliminate the many chemicals that are already stored in your body because these have too great a potential to cause illness, both now and in the future. The elimination of these is called detoxification. This will be explained in detail later in this chapter.

Some of the changes just mentioned can appear to be challenging but sometimes they are exactly what are needed to help you restore your original good health. In the long run, avoidance can be much less expensive and much more effective than anything else you can do. Change is typically difficult but sometimes, by altering a very few aspects of your life, it is possible to feel better than you have in years. Admittedly, these might appear to be inconvenient but they are certainly not impossible. The rewards can be immense. Your aim should be to totally regain your health. One thing is sure. If you are ill from chemicals, you simply *must* stop your present and all future harmful exposures to toxic chemicals as soon and as completely as possible. Even a few extra days or weeks of contact can add years of illness to your life. See what happened to one child and family, as discussed in Chapter 10.

Let's Review the Basics

The following sections below will tell you how you personally can avoid chemicals and other offending substances in your water, food, air, indoors and outdoors, so you feel better.[76-78] Whenever possible more inexpensive choices will be suggested. *(Appendix C.3 will tell you where to purchase any of the items mentioned below.)*

How Can You Avoid Contaminated or Polluted Water?[77]

Try to drink water that is as pure and as free of chemicals as possible.

- Use a water purifier in your kitchen for drinking and cooking and also install a special water purifying showerhead in the bathroom. Use that water for showers and bathing but not for drinking.[1a-c, 2a,b] This approach is usually much less expensive than putting a purifier on the water intake of your home.[77]

- Avoid drinking or eating *anything* stored or served in plastic (water or food products), Styrofoam (coffee and tea) or aluminum, (soda pop and beer). Chemicals and toxic metals can leach or seep into the contents of such containers. As much as possible, use and buy food items *only* in glass containers.

Other Possible Water Options to Consider[83]

- Read the books by Dr. Batmanghelidj[2a,b] The Body's Many Cries for Water and ABC of Asthma, Allergies and Lupus.** His books provide fast, easy, inexpensive and helpful information that claim to help relieve chronic problems such as arthritis and asthma. His first book suggests that you drink at least six to eight glasses of water each day, along with your usual beverages.[2a] He suggests additional water before each meal, after eating or exercise and again before going to bed. Again, be sure to check with your physician before trying any medical program.

- Presently many new varieties of expensive, bottled, energized and alkalinized water are being sold. There is even a newer form called magnetized water.[67, 70] In general they all claim to enhance wellness, increase your energy level or relieve diverse symptoms.[3a, 77] *(Unfortunately the bottles are usually plastic and not glass. The latter is preferred because the phthalate chemicals found in plastic can spread or leach into the water and cause illness, such as precocious puberty in girls.) (See Chapters 1, 5 and companion book Can Chemicals Cause Epidemics?)**

- There is little doubt that the human body seems to have less of a tendency to allergies, for example, if it is slightly in the high normal alkaline rather than highly acidic range.[68a,b] You can easily check your morning saliva (less reliable) and urine with a bit of pH paper.[52] You can alter your body pH by your choice of foods and by drinking alkalinized water.[83]

- You can make your own alkalinized safer water if you purchase a machine that is easily attached to your faucet.[3c] If you tend to be too acid or the blood pH is too much below

---

* *Can Chemicals Cause Epidemics?*, Doris J. Rapp, M.D. ERF, P. O. Box 60, Buffalo, NY 14223-0060, 800.787.8780, www.drrapp.com.

** F. Batmanghelidj, M.D., Global Health Solutions, Inc., P.O. Box 3189, Falls Church, VA 22043, www.watercure.com.

7.365, you might have headaches, fatigue and muscle aches because of accumulated lactic acid. If your blood and urine are somewhat more ideally alkaline, or above 7.4, the tissues will have more oxygen and this, for example, is claimed by some to diminish infection, allergies, yeast problems and decrease the tendency to disease, even cancer.[52, 83]

Some will disagree with the above and want more critical scientific evaluation to more fully and properly evaluate both the effectiveness and safety of what is claimed. Check with your physician. If there is no objection, try to make your body a bit more alkaline and judge for yourself.[52,83]

- You might want to test your tap water for chemicals.[114] For a mini-free or a relatively inexpensive and accurate water evaluation, check out www.AquaMD.com. There are "do it yourself kits" that will enable you to check for many of the common contaminants, trace metals and pollutants.[114] It might be helpful to know exactly which chemicals are in the water your family drinks. Routine laboratories no longer do this test but if you prefer you can call the EPA for companies that do a certified water analysis in your area. Don't depend on anyone else's assurance. Check out your own water source, especially if you use well water. Even if your tap water tastes and looks all right, it can be toxic.

- Your water is one potential major source of chemicals and your blood, urine and hair will typically reflect exactly how serious your own personal body level of pollution is. To find out how contaminated you personally are, you can have a blood and/or urine examination for chemicals. *(See Appendix D.1a and Table 3B).*

If these tests show some reasons for concern, check with your physician and consider detoxifying your body to eliminate the overload of chemicals or toxic metals as discussed later in this chapter.

How Can You Avoid Problem Foods?

You can be allergic to what you eat and/or sensitive to the chemicals in the form of pesticides or fungicides on or in your foods and beverages. You have several options to help you diagnose and treat a food problem and some are both effective and inexpensive. *(See Appendix A.)*

How Can You Change What You Are Eating?

- First, notice if a grocery store product, such as an apple, causes symptoms repeatedly while that same item from an organic food store is well-tolerated. This would suggest that a pesticide or chemical, on or in the grocery store variety, is probably at fault. This would mean you should try to ingest only non-pesticided or organic foods or beverages, as much as possible. *(See Appendix D.5a,b for an unproven way to possibly provide some inexpensive insight.)*

- Organic food is relatively expensive. To cut costs you can raise your own organic food or join an organic co-op if there is one in your city. Sometimes you can find some nearby organic farmers who sell directly to customers or there are farmer's markets that sell organic foods. Their produce tends to be less expensive than organic foods purchased at grocery stores. There are also places to buy organic foods that can be shipped directly to your home but they tend to be quite expensive.[61a-d] Once the public is more aware of the extent and health concerns caused by chemical pollution of our foods, organic produce should become more available and less expensive. *(See Chapter 6.)*

- You can eat mainly organic whole grains, brown rice and fresh fruits and vegetables, if you are not allergic to them. *(Do the "Big Five" in Chapter 2 to help you determine if any of these might be a problem. (Also see Appendix D.5a,b.)* Limit or totally avoid all "white foods," such as flour, sugar, and dairy products, especially cheese. Soda pop, coffee, tea and caffeine are definitely unsuspected problems for many. The chemicals in decaffeinated beverages cause chronic unrecognized illness in some. Fish can be a concern because the water in which they live can be heavily polluted.

- The above dietary advice alone will help many who have chronic unexplained food-related illness in less than one week. If only the so called "white" foods are your problem, you can feel worse for the first three or four days but much better in about five to seven days after these are totally eliminated from your diet.

- If your body is too acidic, a few simple dietary changes are claimed to help.[52, 83] More fruits and vegetables will help keep the body more alkaline. It also helps if you chew your food longer and more completely.

- It is important to totally avoid use of all artificial sweeteners. You can try liquid Stevia, a natural sweetener, which is sold in health food stores;[1] Splenda or sucralose, which is quite expensive, is available in many regular stores. Another possibility is xylitol. There are, also, some kiwi fruit natural sweet substitutes that are supposedly better than sugar.[119] (*I personally would avoid any artificial sweeteners, especially aspartame, at all times.*)[48, 85]

- You can try to drink large amounts of pure water and organic juices and organic herbal teas, in glass, as much as possible. In addition some believe it helps if more fluids are ingested between meals, rather than with meals. Stop all coffee and carbonated beverages.

- You should try to stringently avoid genetically engineered or irradiated foods until much more is known about them.[14] This can be an immense challenge because our government, unlike the countries in most of Europe, does not regulate them so there are no required labels to tell you what is or is not altered. *(See Chapter 9 and cry.)* Certain food companies (for example, organic baby foods) are attempting to provide only non-genetically engineered products but because of no labeling and cross contamination of farm produce, this may be impossible to accomplish. Whole Foods and Wild Oats food chains want to provide safer forms of foods but they too have little control over what is put into combination foods. Read the fine print on all labels of everything and try to buy single fresh products as much as possible.

Diets and Tips that Help You Quickly Detect Problem Foods[4a,b, 6a,b 124b]

Start by making a list of your five favorite foods and two favorite beverages. *If* you have a food allergy, you may have just written down the most likely causes. If you crave or cannot "live without" a specific food or beverage, such as coffee, chocolate, cheese or bread, that item is a major suspect in relation to any of your health problems until proven otherwise.

As mentioned earlier, chemical sensitivities are often associated with or followed by the appearance of obvious food allergies. If you want to feel really well, you must address both issues. One of the following three diets typically helps.

I. A simple **Single Food Allergy Elimination Diet**, in a week or less, will often quickly and easily relieve a vast array of diverse symptoms. Particularly check out each of the few major suspect foods and beverages that you crave.

II. If more than one food is a problem, you need the **Multiple Food Allergy Elimination Diet**.

III. If you want a little or no expense diet, there is a third one that enables you to eat most foods in moderation, every four days, but not more frequently. It is called a **Four Day Rotation Diet**.

I
Single Food Allergy Elimination Diet
(See Appendix A for more details.)

Merely totally eliminating one single suspect food, in *all* forms, for four to seven days can sometimes resolve perplexing acute or chronic health problems in just a few days.[4] Of course, if a food has nothing to do with your illness, or you have not excluded your personal major problem foods from your diet, this form of treatment will be of little value.

The major problematic foods for most people include one or more of the following: white sugar, white flour, white rice, milk and dairy, chocolate, corn, eggs, food dyes, aspartame or artificial sweeteners, fruit juices, coffee, regular tea, alcohol and tobacco. If you have food sensitivities you will probably find that one or more of these will be a factor related to your personal health problems. Remember, *any* area of the body can be affected. Each item can cause single or multiple health complaints. If you have one major suspect, the single food diet can be most helpful.

II
Multiple Food Allergy Elimination Diet

If you are sensitive to more than one food item, which is extremely common, the following simple two-part Multiple Food Allergy Elimination Diet can provide even more answers, quickly and relatively inexpensively.[7a] Below is a brief overview, but see Appendix A for more details because this diet can help pinpoint exactly why you are ill and quickly reveal most major food or beverage sensitivities. If your entire family does this diet, it typically clears up a large variety of acute and chronic medical, behavior, activity and memory complaints in several family members, all at one time.[4a]

Like many of the solutions suggested in this book, these two diets are fast, easy to do and relatively inexpensive. If you cannot afford organic foods or they are not available, do the diet with grocery store foods, but keep in mind that you might not see improvement if the pesticides on or in your foods are significant causes of your health problems. Be prepared to be pleased in four to seven days if you have typical food allergies. You can feel and look better than you have in years.

(After reading my previous books and before patients came to my office, this simple diet helped more children and families than I ever believed possible. By simply reading the books, many found answers they never dreamed could possibly be related to foods and over twenty years later I am still receiving letters of gratitude because someone, who never saw me, found and tried this diet in the 1980s.)[4]

Be sure to check with your regular doctor before you try this diet to be certain you have no medical problems that need special consideration. If you want a doctor who knows how and when to test and treat food allergies, call the American Academy of Environmental Medicine.[5] Although some well-trained doctors will disagree, most food allergies that do not cause frightening reactions certainly can be effectively treated with allergy extracts. *(Like most board-certified allergists, I was trained to believe you could not treat food or chemical sensitivities with an allergy extract. It took over 20 years in practice before I realized I was wrong and this, indeed, was possible.)*

Under no circumstances should you consider testing for any foods or beverages you already know cause severe or extreme reactions. The aim is to detect unrecognized problem foods or beverages, not to confirm a known sensitivity by creating another bad reaction.

Part 1 of Multiple Food Allergy Elimination Diet [4a]

During the first week of this diet, stop eating the major foods that commonly cause allergies. *(In Appendix A there are lists of the many foods you can or cannot eat.)* During this diet you cannot eat or drink, in any form, milk and dairy, wheat (flour), eggs, corn, chocolate, sugar, orange juice or food coloring. Adults should also stop all coffee (especially decaffeinated), tea (except organic herbal), alcohol and tobacco, as well as any "unusual" craved or frequently eaten items, such as mushrooms, sunflower seeds or carbonated beverages such as cola.[4a]

This diet typically causes symptoms to worsen in some way (fatigue, headaches, muscle aches, bowel problems, etc.) during the first few days but by the end of the first week, many feel better and some are much better. The aim of this part of the diet is to show you that foods can cause your medical complaints because you definitely feel better within a few days after you stop eating them.

Part 2 of Multiple Food Allergy Elimination Diet

The aim of the second part or week of the diet is to make you suddenly feel unwell again when you resume eating each of the foods that make you ill. For the first time you will be able to clearly see which food does what to your body. This diet provides many answers that you need to know but don't be surprised if you do not like what you find out. You may have to choose between what you like and what will make you feel better.

During the second week you will begin ingesting each of the foods that you have not eaten for the previous week. To lessen the confusion about which foods do what, start each day of the second week by eating only one of the previously omitted foods all by itself. You may find that each food item causes the same or different symptoms in each family member because food allergies, in general, tend to run in families. The vast majority of food reactions will occur within an hour, but some might not become apparent for 8 to 24 hours. The harder to detect common delayed reactions include those foods causing bed-wetting, arthritis, colitis, ear infections and canker sores.

III
Four Day Rotation Diet

This diet can be diagnostic and therapeutic, as well as effective and relatively inexpensive. In time you should be able to eat most, but not all foods, every four days. You will not be able to eat those that cause extreme reactions. Most food sensitive individuals can begin to gradually eat certain mildly to moderately problematic foods, but only at a four day interval, for example, Monday and Friday, Tuesday and Saturday, etc. In time, this alone helps to relieve many food allergies.[4b,6a,b] If you have a flare of your symptoms every fourth day, it is certainly possible that one of the foods you are eating repeatedly, on that particular day, is causing you to become sick.[4a-c] With a little thought and effort, you can easily find and eliminate that specific culprit.[4] Although this diet enables you to eat most foods every four days, by trial and error you must determine how much of each food or beverage you can safely ingest each time. If you eat or drink too much, too often or too soon, your symptoms will recur at a regular four-day interval. In general you start with a very small amount of suspect food and then gradually increase it to tolerance, every few hours on one day and then you increase the amount again every four days to tolerance.[4, 6a,b] If you have difficulty finding out which foods cause only mild, moderate or severe symptoms, check with an environmental medical doctor or a nutritional consultant.[5, 6a,b]

One Example of a Rotation Diet for One Beverage:

Suppose you drink large amounts of coffee (tea, cola etc.) every day and have determined it gives you a headache. *(These beverages are common unsuspected causes of many chronic medical complaints. Coffee, especially, tends to cause headaches and high blood pressure and many other symptoms.)* You start by stopping all coffee for four full days. *(This is a challenge but you can do it—if you realize this might give you the answers to why you never feel well.)* Then you can begin by drinking a teaspoon. If you remain all right, in three to four hours, try two teaspoons. Keep doubling the amount all day every three hours or so to see how much you can tolerate without developing a headache. Then, drink no coffee for the next four days. Resume coffee again, but this time, start with the maximum amount of coffee you tolerated *without* getting a headache, four days previously. Remember, you can have a delayed reaction so you must have been well for 24 hours after the previous day's ingestion of coffee. Then again, continue to double the amount every three to four hours all that day. At some point you will determine how much coffee will cause you to develop your headache. Stop all coffee again for four days and then ingest *less than the amount that made you ill*. For example, if a cup caused a headache but a half-cup was all right, go back to a half-cup. You should be fine drinking that amount every four days and in a few weeks you can again try gradually increasing the amount again at four-day intervals. If questions arise, check with an environmental medical physician or a rotation diet specialist.[5, 6a,b]

Options Once You Know You Have Food Allergies

Once you know which foods are problems, you have a number of choices or ways to control the food sensitivities. You can continue to eat the problem foods, and remain ill—or you can consider the following:

First Way: Stop Ingesting Foods that Obviously Make You Ill

This is easy if it is liver but it can be most difficult if it is a basic food such as milk, wheat, sugar, corn or eggs. You often have to stop eating *all* forms of all the foods that make you ill. Children, however, cannot grow properly on a diet that is too restricted. You have other choices and nutrition consultants are available to help with your personal concerns.[124a] Their fees are sometimes entirely covered by your health insurance so you might want to see if this choice can be practical for you.[6a,b]

A Second Way: Eat Most Allergenic Foods, But Only Every Four Days.[6a,b]

The previously discussed Rotation Diet requires no skin tests or allergy injection therapy or additional costs to treat many food allergies. It helps to prevent future allergies and helps you detect food sensitivities if, for some reason, they suddenly recur. It can provide answers you never suspected. In time, it enables many food sensitive patients to eat a wide variety of previously problematic foods without difficulty. You must, however, be very organized because it can be a challenge to eat only the allowed foods no more frequently than every four days.

If a food is a known significant problem but does *not* cause emergency medical complaints, sometimes you can ease it into your diet gingerly. For example, with medical guidance you can start by eating a tiny, tiny amount once every two or three weeks (not every four days), and then gradually increase the amount and frequency of ingestion, very slowly. You will need the help of a knowledgeable environmental medical doctor or dietician to do this but it can be done for some foods. Eventually, it might be possible to eat normal-sized portions, but usually no more often than every four days.[5, 6a,b]

Once again, it must be repeated. This diet will *not* help frightening life-threatening food allergies. If you are apt to need to go to the hospital if you smell or eat a certain food, obviously those foods should not be smelled or eaten, or even allowed in your home. In that situation the answer is typically total elimination of any contact with that food.

Again, do *not* ever purposely eat any item that you suspect or know causes a severe reaction unless you have been treated and advised to do so by your doctor.

A Third Way: Receive Provocation/Neutralization (P/N) Food Allergy Extract Treatment[5]

This method can be effective in treating most uncomplicated food allergies. *(Details are later in this chapter.)* If you have a major medical emergency after exposure to some food, such as incapacitating asthma or collapse, it is typically not possible to treat for that substance using P/N testing. *(On rare occasions however, it might be possible to treat such extreme forms of food allergy with allergy extracts after Provocation/Neutralization testing but this would require a most experienced, environmentally-trained medical physician.)*[5]

A Fourth Way: You Can Try Chiropractic Muscle/Energy Techniques to Treat Allergy[21, 108, 109]

There are also some newer unproven energy, muscle testing and acupuncture approaches to treat food, chemical and other allergies discussed below that might provide some degree of protection when you are faced with unavoidable sudden exposures and have no idea what to do or when you have a medical problem that simply won't go away.[5] *(I personally have not tried to treat serious allergic reactions with these methods but some of these methods have certainly quickly relieved mild to moderate symptoms without drugs. I cannot provide more information at this time and it is obvious we need more research. See Epilogue.)*

- There are some chiropractors who claim that some newer muscle testing methods are helpful to diagnose and relieve both food allergy and chemical sensitivities. (*See Appendix B.3 and D.5a.*) One such technique is called Total Body Modification TBM. Courses of different types are available for the public and for health professionals. TBM is not the typical "snap and crack" type of chiropractic treatment, but a practical course on the application of muscle testing in relation to allergy and other medical problems. *(For more information call Dr. Victor Frank. TBM: 435.652.4340. Read books by Dr. John Diamond and those about energy)*[21, 54a,b, 84, 106, 108, 109, 122, 123]

- A most simplified example of muscle testing that appears to show how you can possibly detect an offending substance and relieve some symptoms in less than a minute is discussed briefly later in this chapter. *(See Appendix D.5a,b.)* I must admit it is not scientifically documented but that does not mean it cannot help. It might only mean there is much we do not know and cannot fully understand at this time. Check with a chiropractor or doctor who knows TBM so you can be shown this one simple test and then you can try it yourself and see what you think.

- Of course, these newer chiropractic techniques will not help everyone or every medical problem. The amazing thing to me, however, is how often they appear to provide insight and relief. These techniques are certainly not presently scientifically or adequately documented, but in my personal experience, they appear to be helpful to stop some mild to moderate allergic reactions. We urgently need to do impartial, unbiased investigations to verify or negate their effectiveness. The bottom line in medicine, however, is a well patient. If this method helps without hurting, what is wrong with using it even though we presently do not understand the basic physiology that is needed to explain why? The human body is much wiser than we are, and in time, some academic physicians will surely figure out why certain methods appear to be effective or not.

On a personal note:
How I Was Exposed to TBM Chiropractic Energy Medicine:

A patient of mine was 85% improved using my environmental medical treatment but claimed to be 95% better after TBM

(Total Body Modification) chiropractic treatment. I simply did not believe this was possible. (Many physicians unfortunately have this attitude about chiropractors.) I most reluctantly went to see this chiropractor (Steel Center) and his patients. [109] *I was bewildered and amazed by what I saw. Still with an immense amount of skepticism, I decided to take courses in TBM and Neuro Emotional Training (NET). What I saw at these courses made absolutely no medical sense but, amazingly, I found that it appeared to help some people when traditional medical, allergy or environmental medical therapy had failed. The TBM course was so impressive that I gave up my medical practice in Buffalo, NY in 1996 and moved to Phoenix, AZ to try to build integrative diagnostic, treatment, research and education medical centers. As funding becomes available, I hope to help develop the first of many such impartial scientific clinics in Scottsdale, AZ to properly evaluate the above-mentioned alternative treatment methods and other potentially helpful but unproven newer methods of treatment. These centers will emphasize finding out why you are ill and will evaluate to find out if newer, faster, easier, safer, more effective and less expensive approaches do, indeed, help. (See Epilogue at end of book and check www.drrapp.com for updated information.)*

How to Stop More Chemicals from Accumulating In Your Body

- You must make every sensible effort to stop any further contamination of your body with more chemicals. Organic foods, which are more devoid of pesticides in or on them, would be most beneficial to prevent any additional toxic load. *(See Appendix C.4.)*

- Maharishi University has an organic food rejuvenation program that they claim decreases toxic substances in the blood by 50% in two weeks. Then they urge five day treatments twice a year to keep the blood levels of toxins considerably reduced.[36]

What Can You Personally Do to Avoid Indoor Chemical and Other Pollution? [4, 9a-f, 10a, 28a,b, 33a-c, 110]

(See Appendix C.3 for general information about safe products.)

You can easily tell if something indoors is a problem because you will become ill shortly after you enter your home or some building and you are well when you are outside, someplace else or traveling. If there are fewer allergenic exposures in your home, your chemical sensitivities will be diminished. The following are some basic suggestions that would help prevent environmental illness if you tend to be worse when indoors and better when outdoors:

- As much as possible, replace everything from clothing to furniture with all natural products.[76] These include bedding, mattresses and pillows. The box springs and mattress (or futon) ideally should be organic cotton and have dust covers. Use hard tile, cotton throw rugs or expensive non-synthetic natural carpets.

- For general home maintenance, use only all natural everything. Avoid all plastics, especially soft varieties. Use metal and solid wood furniture, not formaldehyde-laden particleboard, plywood or fiberboard. Use water-based adhesives, caulks and the least odorous paints for maintenance.

- Use a quality air purifier to remove as much dust, mold and pollen as possible from your home, work and study areas.[1b] Some varieties claim to remove more chemicals than others.[110] The molds, germs or chemicals found in ordinary dust can cause much illness, including learning and behavior problems.[1c] If possible, also use an air purifier in your child's classroom and your personal work area. It is not unusual for these machines to provide obvious health benefits to everyone who is exposed in a classroom or a work area.[110] *(In time, hopefully, we shall have air purifiers in the ductwork of schools. This one simply relatively inex-*

pensive change will raise academic performance and attendance while decreasing illness, behavior problems, and hyperactivity. Try an Austin Air Purifier. 800.787.8780) *

- Thorough regular cleaning is essential.[38] Be sure to include the drapes, upholstered items such as furniture and plants (both synthetic and real). Use a quality, non-leaking vacuum. *(Check it out in a dark room using a flashlight.)*[4d, 37]

- Be certain that your furnace filters fit correctly and are routinely replaced or cleaned when soiled with dust, molds or chemicals. Clean the ductwork in your home at regular intervals or at a minimum, about once every six months.

- Never allow any chemicals to be placed in your ventilation heating or air-conditioning ductwork. Some chemicals are so toxic they never can be completely removed and they can make a home or building permanently uninhabitable.[28a, 46, 47]

- If you are in contact with molds, much more can happen than hay fever, asthma or rashes. Molds can affect almost any area of your body and this includes changes in behavior, activity and memory, as well as depression, fatigue, muscle aches, arthritis, intestinal pain and much more.[1d, 4] *(A special video is available that shows some of the many surprising ways that allergic children and adults can react to a drop of a mold during an allergy skin test or after exposure to an environment that is moldy. Similar videos are available to show the many surprising ways that dust, pollen, foods and chemicals can cause all these same types of illnesses. See Appendix E.4.)*[1d]

---

* Aerotech Laboratories, 800.651.4802, evaluates buildings for dust, mold and chemicals.

What Can You Do to Avoid Indoor Mold Problems?

You can try to do as much of the following as is needed to resolve the odor and the numerous, pervasive, and obvious or unrecognized health problems related to mold exposures. *(See Appendix C.1 and C.3 for mold resources, consults and web sites)*[1c,d, 7a-c, 13, 15, 17, 28a,b, 79]

a. Eliminate any obvious water or plumbing leaks. Typically insurance coverage in the past provided payment for repair of water damage that led directly to a mold problem. A broken pipe, for example, was a common cause of serious illness, such as asthma, that eventually developed after the subsequent excessive mold growth. This form of mold damage unfortunately is often presently excluded in many original or renewed insurance policies. Insurance companies are presently revising their policies and have capped the amount of their coverage or totally excluded certain forms of mold remediation. You have some legal recourse, however, because there apparently is a ruling that your policy cannot be changed without prior notification. You might want to check the fine print of your policy at the time of your annual review to see if you have been issued a new policy that excludes this form of water damage repair.[69]

b. If you have a sudden water leak, immediately look in the yellow pages under water damage and control. You need to suck up the water and place fans in the wet area to dry it out. Some firms are on call 24 hours a day. Fast action might make it possible to save wet carpets providing they were wet for less than 48 hours. Of course, a plumber should be called to repair any leak.

c. Use dehumidifiers, mold absorbers and fans. These are helpful but dehumidifiers must be cleaned very frequently. These measures are not adequate to resolve serious mold problems in buildings.[1]

d. Illness related to mold spores or toxins, also, will not be resolved by painting over a wall that has mold growing on the other side.

e. Certain air purifiers, such as the Alpine, produce ozone. They appear to reduce both mold and germ contamination and although many have used these machines and claimed to feel better, certain health concerns keep arising.[82] Because of ozone sensitivities at low levels and possible lung irritation from the smell of ozone, some recommend that ozone-generating machines be used only in areas where there are no humans, pets or plants. After several hours of use, the windows and doors can be opened, and this should prevent or diminish mold or ozone-related health issues.[81, 82]

   Some believe there are no safe levels for ozone above certain acceptable normal outside air levels.[82] Minuscule amounts, that cannot be smelled, unquestionably can cause some sensitive people to have definite respiratory distress. In addition, reports indicate that while ozone generators diminish certain airborne pollutants, they also can possibly raise the levels of certain air contaminants, such as formaldehyde. Negative ion generators also are not recommended by the American Lung Association because they are similar to ozone generators and can make some asthmatics worse.[82]

f. Wash all moldy items with bleach (one cup per gallon of water). The concentration to eliminate mold varies from one part bleach to anywhere from five to 20 parts of water but pay close attention if you seem to become ill in anyway after being exposed to the odor. It is possible to be sensitive to the smell of bleach. Hydrogen peroxide has no odor but it is not as effective.

g. Do not use kerosene, formaldehyde, phenol or pentachlorophenol to eliminate molds because they all can be too toxic.

h. Whatever you use must eliminate and kill the mold, not just stop the mold from growing.[15] There is a new product, FEN-X™PRO-TEC, that appears to be most promising.[15] This product is thought to effectively eliminate molds in the air and inside the walls, including the toxic mold called Stachybotrys atra. This product is a purely organic enzyme-based substance that is forced through the walls into mold-contaminated areas. With this treatment, walls, ceilings or insulation should not have to be removed and replaced. Potentially this product might provide some major cost-effective applications in relation to the remediation of certain heavily mold-contaminated homes, schools and work places. Moldy buildings are presently being condemned when they might be salvageable.

   With this product, significant mold spore reduction is apparently possible and its effect can last for prolonged periods after only one application. Some mold sensitive patients appear to improve very quickly, within a few days.[15] Only preliminary research is presently available but these reports suggest this product can be most helpful.[15]

i. A common challenge is what to do if you happen to be ill from living in a very moldy house. *(See Appendix C.3.)* The bottom line is, is it necessary to move or not? It is probably best to try, from the health and financial viewpoint, to find a drier place to live that has no evidence of water leaks if your apartment or home has a serious mold problem.[9a-c] Exposure to a damp moldy environment appears to make chemical sensitivities, as well as the typical and less common forms of allergies, much worse. *(See Chapter 2.)* If several family members are already sick, move as soon as possible so the mold symptoms do not become more severe. This is especially true if you have infants or young children

j. If you suspect a very toxic mold, such as Stachybotrys atra, you might need advice from someone who has vast expertise in this field. Try to contact experts in mold remediation in Appendix C3. [7a-c, 25]

k. Congressman John Conyers, Jr., of Michigan, has proposed a toxic mold safety and protection bill that also may prove to be of benefit if it is passed into law.[44]

Special Mold Contamination Challenges

a. If you have mold sensitivities, the problem can be due to both the mold spores and/or mold toxins (mycotoxins). These sensitivities usually can be detected by blood, nose mucus, saliva and lung secretions.[5a] (*ImmunoScience: 800.950.4686.*) The specific effects of mold spore exposure usually can be confirmed and treated rather easily by special allergy skin testing called Provocation/ Neutralization.[1d] Traditional allergy treatments also certainly can help some mold-related seasonal or year round hay fever or asthma.[5a]

b. Mold toxin or mycotoxin detection and confirmation, however, presents a challenge because there are presently few available methods for testing patients for this.[39]

c. In addition, a new trichothecene mycotoxin urine or patch test has recently become available. This test might help to confirm the presence of a mold-related illness and the need for mold remediation and treatment.[31]

d. One other possible helpful tip for mold treatment is the use of an inexpensive homeopathic remedy sold in health stores or by homeopathic suppliers called Mucosa compositum (*800.621.7644*). This remedy and a product called Opsin II have been found to help some mold allergic patients, especially asthmatics, but again, the best answer is to stop the mold exposure if that is possible.[80] *(See Appendix D.4.)*

e. The Mold Source is a website which can provide some important information.[17] *(www.themoldsource.com.)*
f. You can contact the American Industrial Hygiene Association to find the nearest hygienist who specializes in mold remediation. *(www.aiha.org.)*

Other Home Indoor Air Suggestions Regarding Chemical Exposures

- If possible, eliminate natural gas heat in kitchen stoves, hot water heaters and furnaces. (*See Chapter 2.*) Electric, radiant and solar heat, are preferred in contrast to natural gas, oil, kerosene or coal. Swamp coolers are not recommended because they are typically moldy. It may be necessary to use a heat pump on some furnaces.[4, 28a]

  (*A Peak Flow Meter, as mentioned in Chapter 2 and Appendix C.3, will help you to detect if asthma is due to an intermittent gas leak or some other chemical or allergenic exposures.*[1g] *I have been repeatedly impressed with how damaging natural gas leaks can be in relation to so many human health problems including some chronic arthritis, learning problems, headaches, heart irregularities and inappropriate activity and behavior.)*[1c-e, 4]

- Contact an engineering firm that does evaluations for harmful environmental organophosphate pesticide exposures.[46, 47] The standard proposed by NIOSH (National Institute of Safety and Health) is method 5600. Samples can be obtained from the air in OVS 2 filter/solid sorbent tubes which can be analyzed by gas chromatography for chemicals by Data Chem. Labs. (*960 West Levoy Drive, Salt Lake City, UT 84123, 801.266.7700.)* The nanograms per cubic meter of toxic chemicals inside homes is often much higher than found outside.[49] For example, in Chapter 10, a family is discussed who were all poisoned in a new home which contained 660 to 2000 nanagrams/cubic meter of organophosphates, mainly from Dursban®.

- A new sophisticated small portable chemical sensor hopefully will be available soon. It is said to be able to detect chemical vapors in parts per billion.[13]

- Learn about safe, effective and less expensive pest control or IPM (Integrated Pest Management).[16a,b]

- Use only natural cleaning products, disinfectants and deodorants. *(See Appendix C.3.)*

- Use only natural personal cosmetics and body preparations.[78] *(See Appendix C.3.) (The toxic chemicals in many cosmetics are not controlled in any way or checked for safety because they are a trade secret.)*[111]

- Women should use only natural sanitary products and tampons. Try "Essentials" available at Health Food Stores. *(See Appendix C.3.)*

- Use natural cotton or disposable diapers (Tushies) for infants. *(See Appendix C.3.)*

- Do not microwave any food or beverage. This includes baby formulas in plastic bottles, in particular. Use a small electric oven for routine food re-heating.[45a,b]

Also see Table 6A in Chapter 6 for a list of common, unsuspected indoor chemicals that cause illness.

How Can You Avoid Outdoor Chemicals and Other Pollution?[4, 28a, 33c]

The outdoor exposures that typically cause symptoms are listed on Table 6C in Chapter 6. You can easily spot if there is something outdoors that causes your illness. You will notice you tend to feel worse in some way when you are outside and better when you are inside. If that is what happens, try to determine why. A neighbor's laundry vent expelling scented cleaning products is one common unsuspected cause of difficulty. *(See Chapter 1.)* Keep asking yourself: What is in the outside air at the time when you are outside and suddenly become ill?

- Is it damp and swampy in your area? Is there a stream or a lake nearby? This would suggest a possible mold problem. Asthmatics are often worse outside, if the area near their home is damp.

- Is the pollen count high? This would cause repeated yearly, seasonal flare-ups for only a few days or weeks in most areas of the country. Each year, at almost the same time, airborne tree, grass and weed pollen can cause symptoms.[4]

- Do you live downwind from air polluted with chemicals from factories, roof tarring, asphalt and lawn maintenance, etc? Look around. Do you repeatedly smell a certain odor from some factory in the air at the time when you become ill? Are others from your area in the emergency room at the same time?

- Do automobile, bus or truck gasoline or diesel exhaust fumes from nearby highways, expressways, toll booths or traffic jams make you ill? Try an air purifier in your car.[1b]

There may be little you can do about some of these types of exposures. Moving to a less polluted area might be the very best answer if there is a significant health problem and the cause is permanent and cannot be eliminated.

How Can You Avoid Indoor and Outdoor Electromagnetic Exposures? [28a, 57, 6]

Think about how you feel when you are near high power electrical lines, television sets and transmitters, cable dishes, radio towers and microwave ovens. Exposure to electromagnetic energy (EM) can cause a surprising range of symptoms. Some are as minor as tingling in the extremities; others as major as epilepsy.[4g] Those who are very sensitive notice changes in how their bodies feel or how they can think when they get in front of a television or ride under or are in the vicinity of high power lines. Again, the answer is avoidance.

- If your home is very near electric power lines, think seriously about moving. Long-term exposure can be dangerous for some. Symptoms, also, can suddenly occur when there are major repairs or changes in the power lines near your home.

- Indoor exposure to electrical energy in the bedroom should be kept at the very minimum. Everything electrical should be as far from your bed as practical. Even better, if possible, all electricity in your bedroom should be unplugged and totally disconnected during the night.[4g]

- Some upright computers, in particular, tend to cause symptoms such as chest pain, headaches or fatigue. Laptops tend to be better-tolerated. Protective chest shields or medallions worn over the chest are thought to help protect against EM emissions. (*See Appendix C.3.)*

- Keep your children at least three feet from television sets at all times.[4g]

- The use of electric blankets or heating pads (especially if pregnant) is strongly discouraged.

- Buy a set of earphone adapters so there is no need to hold a cellular phone directly over your ears or on your head. Stickers also can be applied to your cellular phone as shields.

- Tesla Watches are thought to help protect against the harmful effects of electromagnetic energy.[24a,b, 122]

How Can You Find a Chemically Safe Home?[28a, 33a-c]

This is not always easy to do. Each person is different and you must determine the location in which you personally feel best. Review the "Big Five" in Chapter 2 and check each family member before and again about one hour after exposure to a different location, apartment or house. If there is no change, and everyone looks and feels fine, it is a good sign.

There are also some safe houses and mobile homes available and advertised in the newsletter provided by NEEDS. *(See Appendix C.3.)* At times, available remodeled safer mobile homes can be found scattered throughout the USA. In time we hope to create environmentally safe villages so the most chemically sensitive people can live in a truly healthy area. *(See Epilogue.)*

Things to Consider:

Location[33c]

- Your home should be located as far away as possible from factory air pollution, gas stations, dry cleaners, airports, expressways, damp swampy areas or bodies of water, printing presses, beauty salons, paint shops, high tension wires and cables, pulp paper plants, nuclear plant sites and underground superfund dump sites.

- If land is available near a national forest, it is probably cleaner and safer. Payson, Prescott, Cottonwood and Sedona, Arizona, as well as isolated parts of Colorado and New Mexico for example appear to be well-tolerated by some. (*For example, some sick children who could not play outside in polluted Eastern cities can play outdoors for hours without illness in Sedona, AZ.)*

- Living near the least polluted outskirts of a city is typically one good way to avoid much of the typical urban pollution. Check with your health department.

- You should not live downwind from industrial areas or over or near a toxic dump site.

Construction:

- The best house is often one that is neither very new nor very old.[4, 18, 28a] About 15 to 20 year old homes seem to be tolerated best. While older homes tend to have dust and molds, many newer homes built in the past 20 years are contaminated with chemicals in construction materials and furnishings, as well as toxic pesticides and termiticides. Some of these can continue to emit multiple potentially harmful chemicals for many years.

- An environmental home evaluation would be helpful before any move to a new or different house. [7a,b,c, 25] (*See Table 3A.)* In time this should become mandatory for the safety of the buyer.

- Because of present-day "tight home" construction, newer homes have poor air exchange so there is relatively little contact with the outside air. As a result, both chemical pollutants and indoor air allergens, such as dust and molds, tend to be at higher levels inside, rather than outside most homes. Quality room or furnace air purifiers and proper ventilation duct maintenance can significantly reduce some of these types of exposures.[1b]

- A major challenge can be related to termite control within new or other buildings. There appears to be no laws about which chemicals can or cannot be used if termites are a problem. If a sale requires a loan, the bankers or mortgage companies who handle FHA or VA transactions insist on building inspections and certification in relation to termites or other wood-destroying pests. Some even insist on pretreatment of the ground before a building is erected. A termite appraiser decides if pest control is needed. The seller is supposed to be given a choice of different methods of termite or wood control and then the seller sees that termite control measures are taken if that is indicated. At some point the buyer is given a certificate stating there are either no termites or that termite control measures have been conducted and the banker is also informed.

There appear to be no laws, however, in relation to which substances are safe to be used and some are unquestionably toxic to humans. In the warmer states, for example in Arizona, it is routine to put hundreds of gallons of toxic chemicals, *such as the recently partially banned Dursban®,* below the foundation of newly constructed homes to control termites. *(See Chapter 10.)* These chemicals can gradually seep up the walls and into every part of a house potentially harming the health of inhabitants, especially pregnant women and unborn infants.

Alternatively, homes in other areas of the country, such as Florida, are "tented" for insect control. These also can be totally permeated with toxic chemicals that are potentially dangerous to human health. While this method can kill pests in the house *at that time*, the effect is transient and does not last. When the tent is removed, the toxic chemical is released so it contaminates the air in the nearby vicinity. Pregnant women could be in possible danger. If such a house is not properly aired out before a human enters, it is possible to become very sick.

When you move, purchase or rent a home, consider checking the amount and type of chemicals that have been or are being used inside and around the building.[50] *(See Chapter 10.)* If you look at a new home or building and it smells of a perfumed deodorizer, be very suspicious. Is the pleasant aroma hiding mold or chemical pesticide odors? There is no doubt that some of the chemicals presently used in homes can endanger the health of the occupants and possibly damage the brains of unborn babies. These same chemicals can seep into the soil and contaminate food crops and water. Some are believed to be causes of cancer, heart, liver and kidney disease, birth defects and serious emotional and psychological problems.

- For better pest and mold control contact Get Set *(800.221.6188)* or use a safer less expensive products such as Tim-bor or Bora-Care which uses sodium borate to permeate wood used for construction. This is said to permanently protect against wood-destroying organisms such as termites and also make wood fire-retardant without any odor.[87] Another product TTR (Trap-Treat-Release) is a sulfluramid that is considered to be relatively safe for both people and pets. It has low toxicity. Its progressively slow action can gradually wipe out 90% of termite colonies in two years, and 98% in three years.[118]

- If you want a safer home, consider building a new one or attempt to retrofit your present one using a safe "green" company that knows about chemical, mold, pest and electromagnetic pollution sources in buildings.[18, 28a]

- Newly constructed, more pest and mold-free environmentally-safe homes are now available that cost as little as 10% to 15% above usual construction fees.[18] Prefab safe houses eventually should be available. (*See Appendix C.2.)* [6]

- Try not to live in a trailer if you are chemically sensitive because they tend to be constructed with materials that outgas or emit toxic chemicals such as formaldehyde (*in particleboard and plywood*) and phthalates (*in plastic*). Many who live in trailers have been ill for years and have no idea the cause is the chemicals inside their home. Safer porcelain trailers are available. (*Christopher Rea: 214.368.4132.*)

- Log cabins are also not recommended because they tend to contain wood treated with toxic chemicals to control insects. [51a-d] These can include various extremely toxic wood preservatives such as creosote, pentachlorophenol and a chromated form of arsenic. These also can be found in pressure-treated wood used for decks and patios, fences and children's outside wooden play furniture and toys.[86] Exposed children are presently thought to be in increased jeopardy because of their greater sensitivity to chemicals compared to adults.

How Do You Find an Expert to Do a Home Evaluation? [7a, 25, 64]

Many who read this book will be suspicious that something inside of their home or workplace might be causing their illness. They know that they need help from someone who has in depth knowledge about the chemicals found in construction materials, furnishings, upholstery, carpets, drapes, mattresses, screens, household cleaners or scented personal products but the challenge is to find someone who is capable.[64] It can be difficult to find a qualified informed company that is reputable and knows how to properly do a comprehensive environmental inspection. The company hired to evaluate a home or building must be able to test for many types and levels of allergenic substances, toxic molds and bacteria. These levels of various indoor air substances must be compared to those found outside. The examination must analyze the size, number and types of particles in the indoor air and check for innumerable chemicals. If the check does not include the right or enough chemicals, or is not sensitive enough to detect those present, you can erroneously be told chemicals are not a problem. You easily can be fooled by advertisements so be careful to check thoroughly to be certain you have a proper and thorough evaluation. Nearby environmental medical specialists often can advise you concerning who is best qualified to do these types of evaluations in your city. *(AAEM: 316.684.5500.)* Some consultants will travel to your home to do a thorough quality environmental evaluation. *(Appendix C.1.)* [7a, 25, 64]

For building evaluations specifically in relation to mold consultations and remediation, see mold discussion earlier in this chapter and see resources in Appendices C.1 and F.3. Videos are available that show exactly how children and adults can react during Provocation/Neutralization allergy testing for chemicals or mold allergies. *(See Appendix E.4.)*

Table 3A
Environmental Home Evaluations

Should include a check for:

Dust	Many Chemicals
Bacteria or Germs	Pollen
Many Molds	Toxic Metals, Lead, Asbestos
Pet Dandruff/Hair	Electromagnetic Exposures

In General, What Else Can You Personally Do? *(See Appendix E.1)*

Before the discussion of what a doctor can do for you, here are a few other ideas about what else you can do to help yourself if you have chemical sensitivities.

- Check the internet for current information in the web sites of environmental medical specialists. Some have constant updated information to help keep you up to date. (*See Appendix B.1c.)*

- Join some knowledgeable advocacy organizations that are interested in protecting your food, air, water, soil and environment. (*See Appendix F.3.*)

- Subscribe to newsletters or journals to keep updated about alternative natural ways to help yourself and others. These publications (*Townsend Newsletter, Total Wellness, E-Healthy News and Alternative Medicine*) will keep you abreast of what is new, what appears to be helpful, what is possibly inexpensive or what is of little value or potentially harmful. (*See Appendix F.1.)*

- Look at the videos that clearly demonstrate how some children and adults react when exposed to chemicals, and common allergens such as molds, dust and pollen. *(See Appen-*

dix E.4.) This may enable you to help many others who do not know they have this problem.

- Read other basic "how to" books for the public, physicians, psychologists and lawyers to explain what is known, practical and proven in relation to helping those with environmental illness.[84] *(See Appendices E.1-3.)*

You Know What You Can Do, Now What Can the Right Doctor Do?

You know what you can personally do to change your water, diet and the inside and outside of your home, school or workplace. You know some of the choices you have concerning treatment of possible health-damaging exposures. You also have a better idea of how and where to find a different and better place to live. Now you need to know where you can find a doctor knowledgeable about environmental medicine and exactly what such a physician can do if you have questions or have not resolved your health issues to your satisfaction.

How Do You Find a Qualified Physician to Help You? *(See Appendix B.1.)*

You can call the American Academy of Environmental Medicine, AAEM, *(316.684.5500)* in Kansas City for the nearest qualified environmental medical specialist. Many of these physicians are board-certified in one or more specialties, and they are knowledgeable about chemicals, allergies, nutrition, digestion and methods of detoxification or elimination of chemicals from the body.[9f, 10] They typically have experience using several newer more informative methods to diagnose and treat allergies such as Provocation/Neutralization (P/N) and Serial Endpoint Titration.[4c,e] Although some medical authorities have called these methods controversial, for over 50 years these methods have effectively helped many patients.[4c,f] Their methods are sometimes beneficial when more traditional forms of therapy have failed.[4e] Check out some of the websites of these specialists for more specific information. *(See Appendix B.1c and B.3-B.6 for other health professionals who are knowledgeable, well-trained and claim to be successful in their treatment of patients who are sick from chemical exposures.)*

Surprisingly most insurance policies will not cover environmental medical care in spite of its obvious benefit. This is in sharp contrast to the many patients who are routinely reimbursed for more traditional allergy care, regardless of the therapeutic response.[4e] Thousands of positive responses in infants, children and adults to P/N allergy skin testing were observed and videotaped in my former Buffalo clinic for over 20 years. *(See Appendix E.4.)* These same types of responses are seen on a daily basis in the offices of environmental medical physicians throughout the United States. It seems strange that insurance reimbursement is not a problem for treatment that does not help, but refused for what not only relieves the patient's symptoms, but saves the insurance company money. We must all reflect about why this would happen.[1c-e, 4e]

How Do Environmental Medical Physicians Make A Diagnosis? (*See Appendix B.1.)*

Qualified environmental medical specialists do somewhat different specialized tests to diagnose and treat a wide range of sensitivities and regular allergies. Environmental medical therapy can effectively treat many dust, mold, pollen and yeast allergies, as well as many food and some chemical sensitivities.[4c,e,f, 5] They can also recognize and treat the less-readily recognized forms of allergy as discussed in Chapter 2. Some use under the tongue or sublingual allergy extract therapy, which certainly has been found to be effective, especially for respiratory allergies.[115]

Comprehensive environmental medical (EM) care typically includes much of the following:

- Environmental medical doctors typically will take the time to review your past records thoroughly and do an initial, comprehensive medical history and physical that can require from one to three hours. This is not the "clock watch" HMO medicine of today. Their aim is to find out why you are ill and eliminate the cause, if that is possible. This type of medicine requires time, dedication, genuine interest and a larger overhead because of the need for numerous employees with specialized expertise.

- They perform routine laboratory tests if indicated and order specialized diagnostic tests.[4j] *(See Tables 3B, 3C and Appendices D.1 and D.2.)*

Table 3B
Preliminary Diagnostic Laboratory Tests

Basic Routine Tests to Detect General Illnesses
Complete blood count (CBC).
Routine urine test.
Routine blood screening tests for lung, liver, kidney and heart function.
Special blood and hair tests for lead and other heavy metal poisoning.
Tests for function of metabolic pathways.

Basic Immune System Tests for Allergies and Immune Weaknesses
Total IgE and IgE RAST test for general and specific allergies.
Secretory IgA test for intestinal allergies.
Select IgG RAST tests for non-life-threatening food allergies.
Immune complex levels.
B and T cells, Helper/Suppressor ratios.

Special Immune System Tests for Chemical Sensitivities
Ta1 (or CD26) test for activated T-lymphocytes.
Trimellitic Anhydride (TMA) chemical test.
Natural killer cell counts and function tests.
Acetylcholinesterase tests.
Autoimmune or autoantibody assay tests.

What Laboratory Tests for a Chemical Sensitivity Can Doctors Order?

The following includes the basic initial tests your physician can order plus certain special tests that provide more insight concerning a possible chemical sensitivity. *(See Tables 3B, 3C and 3D and Appendices D.1and D.2.)* If you find your test results indicate a significant probable chemical exposure, you or your physician can consult with an environmental medical specialist. *(AAEM: 316.684.5500.)* You might also need an occupational medical doctor if an illness is directly related to your work area. Laboratories that do a variety of tests for chemicals or other toxins on blood, urine, fat, feces, breast milk, semen, hair, etc. are discussed below and are listed in Resources. *(Appendices D.2a to D.2f.)*

Major Basic Routine Diagnostic Laboratory Tests [4c,f, 28c]

(See Appendix D.1, D.2 and Tables 3C)

Many laboratories do routine blood and urine tests to evaluate the function of various organs. Some also do hair tests for heavy metal poisoning.[28c]

- A complete blood count can show if you have a lower than normal level of white blood cells. These are the cells that normally fight infection. Forty years ago the normal white count was 7000. Now the accepted normal is in the range of 5000 or lower. (*Can chemical exposures be one reason why this has happened?)* Chemically sensitive individuals tend to have white counts in the range of 2500 to 5000. Some with normal white blood counts have a decrease in the white blood cells called lymphocytes. After these patients have responded favorably to treatment, their white counts typically increase. In some women this count can drop precipitously just prior to each menstrual period, and at that time, they tend to develop a monthly bacterial or viral infection, such as cold sores (herpes). *(This is typi-*

cally rather easily treated with a combination of flu vaccine and progesterone allergy extracts treatment.[35]) (AAEM: 316.684.5500.)

- Select EM patients will be advised to have a blood or hair analysis to help detect excessive heavy metals such as lead, aluminum, mercury, cadmium, copper and arsenic, which can interfere with normal brain function.[8a-d] *(Lawrence Wilson, M.D.: 800.296.7053; Great Smokies Diagnostic Laboratory: 800.522.4762; Doctor's Data: 800.323.278.*

Your water, along with your air, food, dental fillings, toothpaste, underarm deodorant, pots, mouth mints etc., can contain some of these metals. Medical insurance tends to cover payment for hair studies in some states, but only if they are done to rule out possible lead poisoning.

- Some special laboratory tests can evaluate the basic metabolism in the body.[116, 117] They can tell if the function of the liver or intestines, for example, is normal and they can do a number of tests to determine if the sequence in the so called metabolic pathways are in some way not functioning up to par. Your body has pathways to make what the body needs from what is supplied to it. Very simply if you have too much A and not enough B, there is a block between A and B that can interfere any normal body function that requires B. These tests figure out why this happens and which specific nutrients or enzymes might be helpful so more A goes onto B. As a result from these types of studies, certain organs or tissues will be able to function more normally. Once again, the insurance companies do not always reimburse a patient even though these tests can determine exactly why someone is ill and provide insight as to specifically what is needed to correct a problem and make someone feel better.

Basic Immune System Tests for Allergies and Immune Weaknesses

- A total IgE (Immunoglobulin E) test is used to detect general allergies but this is elevated in only 10% of those with chemical problems.[28c]

- The specific IgE RAST tests help gauge the degree of sensitivity to specific allergens such as to pollen, molds or dust, etc. These tests are elevated in 50% of those with chemically sensitivities and the food RAST tests are elevated in 20% of these patients. [28c]

- IgG RAST (Immunoglobulin G) tests can particularly aid in the identifying some less severe types of food allergies.[28c]

- B and T lymphocyte counts or Helper/Suppressor lymphocyte ratios are helpful in the evaluation of the immune system. Dr. William Rea in Dallas found the T cells were low in 55% chemically sensitive hospitalized patients; the B cells were low in about 5%.[28c]

- The measurement of the number and activity of the natural killer cells provides more insight about the state of the immune system. This latter test helps to evaluate how well someone might be able to cope, for example, with an infection.

Special Immune System Laboratory Tests for Chemically Sensitivities[4]

Tests suggesting chemical sensitivities *(see Table 3B)* include:

- The Ta1 or CD26 for activated T lymphocytes and the TMA (trimellitic anhydride) tests are useful in confirming possible chemical exposures or sensitivities. The CD26 was elevated in 90% of 200 of Dr. Rea's chemically sensitive patients.

- The levels of natural killer cells and phagocytic index were depressed in 95% of Dr. Rea's patients who had recurrent infections.[28c]

- The acetylcholinesterase test can help confirm an organophosphate or carbamate pesticide poisoning. The plasma (pseudo) cholinesterase test is the first to decrease after an organophosphate exposure and within a month the red blood cell cholinesterase levels will also decline. Then the level of this enzyme in cholinesterase panels will gradually return to normal and this can be monitored over a period of several weeks.[107] *(See Chapters 1, 8, 10.)*

- Autoantibody tests can detect if you have developed antibodies that can harm certain tissues or organs in your body. The antinuclear antibody tests tend to be positive in 17% of outpatients versus about 70% of hospitalized chemically sensitive patients.[28c] Those who have damaged nervous systems, for example, can have antibodies against the myelin sheaths or tissue that cover their nerves. Of Dr. Rea's hospitalized patients, 15% had antibodies related to specific organs.[28,c] When the chemical exposure and body load is reduced, these abnormal test results often return to normal.

Special Detection Tests for Chemicals in Your Body

If you tell a laboratory, Accu-Chem or ImmunoScience, the name of a suspect chemical, pesticide, or an item that bothers you *(synthetic carpet, deodorizer or mattress, ink, dry cleaning fluid, mothballs, perfume, etc.)*, they can tell you which specific test might be most helpful to detect certain substances, or break down products, in your blood or urine. *(See Table 3D and Appendices D.1 and D.2.)* They also test for hydrocarbons, which are common chemicals derived from natural gas, oil or coal. Table 3D lists the major general categories of chemicals that can be tested.

Table 3C
Diagnostic Laboratory Tests

Special Detection Tests for Chemicals in Your Body
Tests to find which specific chemicals are in your blood or urine.

Special Detection Tests for Chemicals in Suspect Items
Tests for carpets, mattresses, etc.

Major Diagnostic and Treatment Methods Include:
1. Routine Provocation /Neutralization (P/N) Allergy Testing
a. Tests for common chemicals and allergic substances.
b. Allergy tests from suspect items, carpets, room air, etc.

2. Serial End-point Titration (SET) for molds, dust, pollen, etc.

3. Nasal Challenge Tests for Chemical Odors
a. By directly breathing specific chemical odors in room air.
b. By breathing controlled amounts of chemicals in glass booths.

Nervous System Tests
1. Romberg Test.
2. Nerve Conduction Tests.

Brain Tests
1. Single Photon Emission Computerized Tomography (SPECT) brain image tests.
2. Electroencephalogram with evoked potentials (QEEG).

Bioassay or Mouse Tests
Tests with mice to show effects of exposure to chemicals.

Special Detection Tests for Chemicals in Suspect Items

Matrix Analytical Laboratory will examine specific items such as a synthetic carpet or mattress and tell you exactly which chemicals are in them.[64] If the same chemical is in your blood and/or urine, you may have found the cause of your illness.

Major Diagnostic and Treatment Methods Include:

1. Provocation/Neutralization Allergy Testing

a. The following routine testing method has helped to verify and treat dust, mold and pollen allergies, and food or chemical sensitivities for over 40 years. Most environmental medical doctors do Provocation/ Neutralization (P/N) allergy testing and treatment. *(See Table 3C)* For example, tests for hydrocarbons (gas, oil, coal, etc.), chlorine, fluoride, phenol, formaldehyde and glycerine sensitivities are routine in many environmental medical offices. The baseline before testing, the response to the skin testing and then the response after allergy extract treatment all can be videotaped for medical, scientific and legal documentation. These videos typically show patients stating how they feel before and during testing, while receiving various dilutions of an allergy extract. It is possible to clearly demonstrate changes in their appearance, actions, behavior, writing and drawing, as well as changes in the pulse, blood pressure, breathing and hearing.[1c, e] The responses can be duplicated. Repeated blood studies before and after testing typically show distinct changes in the levels of specific chemical mediators and immune factors in the blood.[4a, 28b]

The P/N testing procedure entails skin testing every eight minutes with different items or dilutions of a substance, for about six hours a day, with extremely tiny needles. (No, it really does not hurt very much) The testing over a period of several days can easily require 20 to 30 hours or longer and cost at least $3000. If only one item is causing symptoms, it can be tested and treated quite inexpensively but this would be a rarity. The number of sensitivities is typically much larger than most anticipate.

The specifics and pros and cons of this type of testing is discussed in great detail in Chapters 13 and 15 of the book entitled, Is This Your Child's World? *(800.787.8780)*.

b. In addition, special allergy extracts can be prepared from the air in a room or a piece of synthetic carpet or mattress etc. and P/N allergy testing with these can reveal exactly what they can do to the health of an individual.

The above treatment usually include detailed instruction about how to self-administer an allergy extract therapy by injection or sublingually (under the tongue) for common allergenic substances, as well as for some chemicals.[115] The good news is that children tend to take less time and respond more quickly to treatment than adults. Infants respond even faster. Some youngsters and adults can dramatically improve in only a few hours, while others appear to be better after three or four days of testing and treatment.

(In our Buffalo clinic, it was not unusual for parents to cry with relief when they saw their child being tested. It was clearly evident that a drop of an allergy extract caused their child to become ill or suddenly change in activity or behavior and a drop of a weaker solution suddenly relieved the exact type of symptoms that had distressed both the child and parent so often in the past. For the first time they realized they were not bad parents with a bad child, but caring parents who had been unable, on their own, to determine the cause of their child's unrecognized medical illness. No, this is not the answer for everyone or everything, but this type of testing and treatment is surprisingly helpful for many who could not find help elsewhere.)

2. Serial End-point Titration (SET)

Another alternative method of testing, such as Serial End-point Titration, is also used by some environmental physicians to test and treat for pollen, molds and dust allergies.

3. Nasal Challenge Tests for Chemical Odors

Most chemical allergy tests are done with injections of extracts of chemicals such as phenol and fluoride. Some, however, are direct nose challenge tests. For example, a patient might be asked to purposely breathe a perfume or to smell gasoline or a cleaning solution to see the effect it has on how that person feels, acts, writes, etc.

A few environmental medical specialists also have glass booths in which they can purposely expose patients to miniscule quantities of specific chemicals and document on videotape exactly what happens.[30a-c] *(See Table 3E)* The levels of exposure can be quantified and sometimes the amount is so minute that the item being tested cannot be smelled or recognized. Of course, appropriate control tests are necessary. When someone is skeptical, or legal issues are present, this type of testing can be essential .[4k, 28b, 32] *(See Appendix B.1b.)*

Nervous System Tests

For nervous system problems, various tests are typically suggested.

1. The first is the Romberg Test. You should have someone else present when you do this test. Stand very close to a bed because you can suddenly fall over and might need a soft landing. With your feet close together and when your eyes are closed, go up on your toes. Those with severe chemical sensitivities will be unable to stand for even a second. They will *immediately* fall over. If this happens, you may need the help of an environmental medical physician and neurologist.[60]

2. Your doctor also can request special nerve conduction tests. Although these can be most informative, they are very painful.

Brain Tests

1. Some patient's symptoms can be explained by various brain changes noted during certain forms of brain imaging such as the SPECT or Single Photon Emission Computerized Tomography Test which uses a "triple camera". *(See Table 3C.)* This particular test can demonstrate changes in the blood flow and function of specific portions of the brain. It can correlate a person's symptoms directly to specific malfunctioning brain areas. For example, if you cannot walk normally, brain changes

Table 3D
Major Categories of Chemicals

1. Organochlorides for DDT, dieldrin, chlordane, lindane and endosulfans.
2. Organophosphates for diazanon, malathion and parathion. Mevinphos, Dursban® (chlorpyrifos).
3. Volatile or Gaseous Aromatic Solvents for benzene, toluene, xylene, styrene or ketone solvents.
4. Aliphatic Volatile Solvents for pentane, hexane and butane.
5. Chlorinated compounds, for phenoxy herbicides such as 2,4-D, 2,4,5- T.
6. Polychlorinated biphenols or PCB's.
7. Pentachlorophenol or PCP.
8. Paradichlorobenzene for mothballs.
9. Triazine herbicides for atrazine in fertilizer and herbicides.
10. Permethrins in flea and tick insecticides and in termiticides in wood and on fruits and vegetables.
11. Phthalates in soft plastics and polyvinyl chloride in hard plastics and often in perfumes.

related to chemical exposures probably would be evident in the motor area of the brain image. If your behavior or personality were altered, one would expect changes in the frontal or forehead area of the brain. There is also some preliminary evidence that some mold exposures can cause brain changes similar to those found after chemical exposures. This brain image test appears to be informative, fast and safe, even for young children. It can be expensive because insurance reimbursement is often denied unless, for example, your major symptom is a chronic headache and there is a need to rule out a possible brain tumor. *(See Appendix D.2b.)*

2. It is also possible to show quantitative EEG brain changes in some chemically-sensitive patients.[4, 28b]

Bioassay or Mouse Tests[1c, 12]

Bioassay tests using mice can clearly demonstrate the extreme toxicity of some chemicals. *(Anderson Laboratory: 802.295.7344, See Appendix D.2c.)* Many are so toxic that it would be better and safer to do a bioassay test by purposely exposing a mouse to a suspect chemical than by observing what happens, for example, to a child who is exposed in a classroom or an adult who breathes certain chemicals at work or home.[12] This laboratory conducts a variety of tests as indicated below:

a. As a baseline control, the mice are closely monitored in a glass cage while they are exposed to pure air. This same air is then blown over a test item, such as a piece of synthetic carpet or an open jar containing some suspect chemical. The mice inhale the chemical vapors, just like humans do, as they leave or out-gas from test items.[1c,f] In this manner the effects of various chemicals emitted from test items can be evaluated. Even though you may not be able to smell any chemical odor, the dramatic responses in mice to such emissions can be most surprising and easily documented on videotapes.

b. They also can conduct bioassay tests to evaluate outdoor or indoor air samples collected from schools, homes or work areas. In this situation, a sample of air is collected in a special bag from a specific area where someone repeatedly becomes ill and this air sample is shipped to Anderson laboratory. After proper controls, the mice breathe the air collected in the bag from the problem area and then they are carefully watched, examined and can be videotaped.

The results can be quite dramatic. In the above types of tests, some mice develop congestion, breathing problems, rashes, swellings, skin hemorrhages, muscle weakness, twitches, paralysis and even death. These responses can occur within one to four hours after exposure to chemicals or items used everyday in many

Table 3E
Detoxification Medically-Supervised Centers:

CENTER FOR ENVIRONMENTAL.MEDICINE 803.572.1600
Allan D. Lieberman, M.D., 7510 Northforest Drive, North Charleston, SC 29420 www.coem.com. *He has a glass booth for chemical testing.*

ENVIRONMENTAL HEALTH CENTER 214.368.4132 FAX: 214.691.8432
William Rea, M.D., 8345 Walnut Lane, Suite 220, Dallas, TX 75231-4262 www.ehcd.com. *He has a glass booth for chemical testing.*

DETOX MEDICAL CLINIC 916.387.6929 FAX: 916.387.6977
David Root, M.D., Medical Director, 5501 Power Inn Road, Suite 130, Sacramento, CA 95820 .
www.healthmeddetox.com (For Non-Drug Abuse Chemical Exposures).
www.getoffdrugsnow.com (For Drug Abuse Cases).

DOWNTOWN MEDICAL CENTER 212.587.3961 FAX: 212.587.3960
Apryl McNeil, M.D., Medical Director, 139 Fulton Street Suite 515, New York, NY 10038, www.healthmeddetox.com, www.getoffdrugsnow.com.

RANDOLPH-SHAMBAUGH CLINIC 847.519.7772 FAX: 847.519.7787
Marsha L. Vetter, M.D., Ph.D., Director, 2500 W. Higgins Road, Suite 1170, Hoffman Estates, Chicago, IL 60195, www.randolphclinic.com.

KALPANA PATEL, M.D. 716.833.2213 FAX: 716.833.2244
65 Wehrle Drive, Buffalo, NY 14225, www.medicallibrary.net/doctors/patel *She has a glass booth for chemical testing.*

ALFRED JOHNSON, D.O. 972.479.0400 FAX: 972.479.9435
101 S. Coit Rd., Suite 317, Richardson, TX 75080. *He has a glass booth for chemical testing.*

LOS ALAMOS MEDICALCENTER 505.662.0960
Jacqueline Krohn, M.D., 3917 West Road, Suite 136, Los Alamos, NM 87544.

homes, schools and work places.[1c] In one study, the mice died in 15 minutes after breathing the air from a school in the northeast. A mouse is not a child but should school children be breathing air that is so contaminated and toxic that it paralyzes or kills a mouse in a few minutes? *(See Appendix D.2c.)*

The previous sector of this chapter outlined some of the diagnostic tests your doctor can order to help confirm you have a chemical sensitivity. Now let us examine some suggestions your doctor can advise for treatment.

Common Modalities of Treatment Used by Environmental Physicians Include

Suggestions for Detoxification or the Elimination of Stored Chemicals[28b,70]

A major consideration for all chemically sensitive individuals is detoxification or instruction about what can be done to help eliminate the many chemicals that are already stored in the body.[4c,e,f] *(I personally believe that our bodies are truly toxic dump sites and everyone needs to eliminate as many chemicals as possible before they accumulate to such a degree that serious or incapacitating illnesses become evident.)* Many respond to simple inexpensive methods but those who have severe chemical sensitivities should try to find a doctor's office that provides a detoxification unit. *(See Table 3E and Appendix B.1a.)* If money is not a factor, some of the more expensive forms of detoxing can easily be done in your own home but professional supervision is usually required, at least initially.[73a,b]

It is possible to document the level of pollution in a person's body before and after treatment by measuring the levels of chemicals stored in the blood, urine or fat.[28b] Decreased levels should correlate roughly with the time when a person shows improvement.[56] When the chemical levels fall in your body fluids and fat, you should feel better.

1. Suggestions for Eliminating Chemicals with Water

- Drink, drink and drink— plain water, preferably only in glass. This would be well-tolerated and beneficial for many. This alone appears to relieve some types of chronic illness.

Check with your doctor, however, if you have kidney, heart or other serious medical problems prior to doing this. Liquids are needed to enhance the excretion of chemicals in your breath, perspiration, urine and feces. It is best if you drink no beverages from aluminum cans or styrene, no coffee, no tea (except herbal and organic) and use absolutely no artificial sweeteners. The tap water in many cities needs more purification so consider putting a water-cleansing unit on the kitchen faucet. This is much better than water in plastic containers and more economical.[4]

- How much water do you need to flush out the wastes? One estimate is you should drink half your body weight in ounces each day. If you weigh 100 pounds, you need 50 ounces or at least six full 8 ounce glasses a day. In addition, it is suggested you drink two cups of pure water for each cup of coffee or other beverage.[70]

2. Suggestions for Detoxing with Improved Lymphatic Drainage

- Many patients will need to be advised about how to improve their lymphatic drainage since movement or circulation of lymph fluid is an essential necessary adjunct for detoxification or elimination of stored chemicals in the body. [1f, 73a,b, 75a,b] This should also help to prevent and control some infections. This can help those with chronic ear, sinus or lung infections, intestinal problems or headaches, in particular. [62] *(Lymphatic drainage specialists are in the phone book under massage, or check with a nearby environmental medical physician for a referral.)* For example, there are some simple things you can do to open or drain the lymphatic system in specific problem body areas. A video demonstrating how to do sinus drainage is available and observing this might be most beneficial for some who have chronic sinus complaints.[41] *(See Appendix E.4.)*

- Here is one inexpensive way to stimulate the movement of lymph, all on your own. Walk in such a way that you rock up on your toes with each step. Do this for ten to twenty minutes a day.

- Some massage specialists also believe that regular lymphatic drainage of the breast and prostate areas will help to diminish the tendency to cancer in these areas. We need research to determine how much this might help. Tight brassieres, for example, should be discouraged because they can block proper lymphatic drainage in the breast area and possibly make females more prone to cancer.[55] Regular prostate massage needs to be evaluated to determine if it might be helpful to diminish the prostate cancer epidemic in males. A larger part of medical therapy for these and other serious medical problems needs to be a greater emphasis on prevention.

- There are also some relatively expensive machines that in essence shake up your lymphatic system so lymph movement and drainage is promoted.[73a,b, 75a,b] One such devise tends to vibrate the entire body so it moves the lymph and reduces stress while it supposedly also stabilizes the skeletal and autonomic nervous system. This also is thought to improve the function of internal organs, such as the muscles, stomach and intestines. This is called The Evergain or Stressbuster/ Aerobic Exerciser.[73b]

- Another uses an expensive electrical device over specific lymph centers to restore and improve lymph flow. In addition, it also provides super oxygenated oxygen to enhance the healing potential of targeted areas. This is called the ST8 or the Scalar Transmitter Tissue Detoxification System.[73a, 75a,b] *(One side benefit of interest to women is the observation by some that these machines supposedly reduce cellulite, which some believe is due to faulty lymph drainage.)*

3.
Suggestions for Detoxing with Homeopathics or Herbal Remedies

- Single homeopathic items or mixtures of oral herbal or homeopathic detoxification preparations are believed to be helpful and inexpensive forms for treatment to help eliminate toxins from your body. One relatively inexpensive product by Heel is called the Detox-Kit.[41] *(See Appendix D.4 for other individual homeopathic and herbal remedies.)*

- Some EM specialists suggest herbal or single or mixed homeopathic preparations routinely to treat chemical sensitivities. Some of the companies who sell these remedies have studies to help document the effectiveness of their preparations. You can check for their claims and research on their web sites. See detailed information in Appendix D.4 for suggested homeopathic remedies for illnesses related to chemicals, as well as for ADHD, allergies, infection, heavy metals, immunity and diseases in various organs.

(As a traditionally-trained allergist, I was amazed to find how easily, effectively and inexpensively some homeopathic remedies helped certain illnesses, especially chronic ear and flu infections and sprains or joint injuries. If these remedies, however, do not quickly relieve an infection, antibiotics should be prescribed. Again we have to use common sense. See qualified physicians and in time more unbiased research will help us to better evaluate what helps and what does not appear to be effective. Many scientific studies, some double-blinded, show the efficacy of homeopathy and others are in progress. Some of my patients, as well as myself, certainly found some of these preparations to be most effective.)

4.
Suggestion for Detoxing Muscles

- Everyone needs regular exercise to help muscles contract so wastes can be eliminated. The minimum is walking 20 minutes every other day. (*If your leg muscles tend to cramp, check your magnesium red blood cell level.)*[9a] *For exercise book/video: Jack Nirenstein, www.amazon.com.*

5.
Suggestion for Detoxing Lungs

- Deeper breathing, with or without exercise, is one simple excellent way to help eliminate some gaseous or volatile unwanted body wastes via the lungs.

6.
Suggestions for Detoxing by Increasing Perspiration in Saunas

- Infrared or other saunas are claimed to help detoxify or eliminate chemicals and heavy metals, but these are quite expensive.[3c,d, 27a,b, 29] A two-person unit will cost about $3000 to $4000. Two excellent new books are available that explain more about what saunas do, and how and why they work.[27a,b] *(See Appendix E.1.)* Dr. Lawrence Wilson also has information on a "how to make your own" inexpensive sauna.[27b]

Three cautions in relation to saunas:

1. You should be careful if you decide to use the less expensive plastic sauna versions. They can emit harmful phthalate chemicals when they heat up. These can definitely cause illness for some who are very chemically sensitive.

2. If you have major chemical sensitivities, detoxify very

slowly in a sauna or you can become sicker. Do not attempt to do it yourself without experienced supervised environmental medical care. (*AAEM: 316.684.5500.*)

3. This form of therapy is sometimes used in conjunction with machines that make compressed oxygen at 6 liters per minute. This will enable you to increase the oxygen level in your body cells, including the brain. The sauna, however, enables chemicals to leave the body and if you are breathing oxygen, this might enable these to go directly into the brain, along with the oxygen. It might be best to use these forms of therapy at different times. Also, be most careful of electrical sparks and oxygen! Check with your doctor before using saunas or oxygen.

Other Methods Recommended or Used by Environmental Physicians

Suggestions for Nutrition

- A quality, comprehensive, natural (*not synthetic)* nutrition program is often needed because those who have chemical sensitivities typically have a weak immune system.[19, 105, 112]

- Nutritional weaknesses can lead to repeated infections at first, then later on to allergies. In time, if not corrected, the result can possibly be some form of chronic illness or even cancer. Most people will need a number of quality nutrients to strengthen their immune systems.[19, 112] In particular, most need antioxidants such as Vitamins A, C, E, the B's, glutathione, taurine and CoQ10, as well as the omega 3, 6, and 9 essential fatty acids. When indicated the present levels of nutrients in your body should be examined prior to the creation of your individualized nutrient program, but this can be expensive.[4] Check with an environmental medical specialist.[5]

- EM doctors might suggest a new anti-aging test called the OxiData Test™. It measures the free radicals in your urine that are caused by chemical exposures and is thought to help to monitor the effectiveness of your nutrient program at a cellular level.[34]

Suggestions for Digestion and Intestinal Care

- Intestinal or bowel problems such as abdominal discomfort or pain, belching, burping, a "leaky gut", diarrhea, constipation, colitis, irritable bowel, reflux, etc. often need to be addressed because these complaints are extremely common in so many who have chemical sensitivities, as well as those who have typical food or mold allergies. Many people appear to need digestive enzymes, healing intestinal nutrients and a number of other enzymes or metabolic factors, as suggested in Dr. Sherry Roger's excellent book, No More Heartburn.[9d, 116, 117] Liver, gall bladder and bowel cleanses, organic coffee enemas and colonic irrigation also might be indicated.[9a,b,d, 10, 52] *(For liver cleansing with coffee enemas use three to four empty Fleet Enema bottles filled with organic coffee to make it easy and less messy.)*[9a] The answer again is to find the cause, not merely to treat symptoms repeatedly with one pill after another.

- Many need to chew their food more thoroughly and to use digestive enzymes and lactobacillus to help improve their digestion, absorption and gut flora.[116, 117] This alone will help eliminate some food allergies and improve the absorption of necessary nutrients. These measures will also help release chemicals from contaminated food products so they can be excreted more easily.

- EM doctors can determine if you need treatment to control a yeast overgrowth. This can happen, particularly, if antibiotics have been taken repeatedly in the past. The physical clues that suggest this treatment might be beneficial are as follows: a white coated tongue, a red sore rash around the anus, a bloated abdomen, persistent smelly hair and feet, itchy genitals and/or a chronic, barely visible, itchy rash that has responded poorly to many previous medications.[4c]

- Regular sized and shaped bowel movements should occur one to three times a day and the feces should be excreted easily and appear normal.[70, 71] Colonics are sometimes helpful initially to clean out any retained residual bowel contents.

- Some also need treatment because they have unrecognized parasites in their intestines or other areas of their body.

Suggestions to Reduce Excessive Infections

- If indicated, EM doctors often suggest bacterial and flu vaccine treatments to control and prevent recurrent infection and allergies.[35] Not all doctors will agree, but if properly done, this form of treatment appears to be surprisingly helpful for some children and adults.

- Homeopathic remedies to prevent or treat various types of infection are available. (*See Appendix D.4.)*

- There is a new well-studied egg product made from chickens inoculated with various bacteria that transfers immunity that is thought to both prevent and treat infection. In time it may be used more extensively.[113]

Suggestions for Female Hormone Problems

- In some women, testing and treatment with hormone vaccines (mainly progesterone) are required to relieve menses-related illnesses, such as PMS and endometriosis.[35] In addition, the stress associated with a menses appears to decrease the tolerance level in some women in such a way that recurrent viral or bacterial infections tend to occur at that time and some also notice more reactions from chemicals and cravings for allergenic foods.[35]

- Anti-aging natural hormone replacement with homeopathic remedies is another well-studied alternative used by environmentally-trained physicians and naturopaths.[121]

Suggestion for Acupuncture

- Some EM specialists recommend Chinese diagnosis and treatment with acupuncture. These doctors open blocked internal pathways called body meridians so all the organs on each pathway can function more normally. For example, an unsuspected infected tooth on the same meridian as the gall bladder and shoulder can cause chronic recurrent symptoms in any of these areas. Sometimes, it is possible to treat a tooth infection and find this totally relieves chronic gall bladder or shoulder pain.

Suggestions for Biofeedback, Hypnotherapy and Psychotherapy

- A few too many hypnotherapy sessions are claimed to totally eliminate food and chemical sensitivities in some children and adults.[72, 84] *(I did not believe this was possible but was absolutely amazed to see how effective and fast this form of treatment sometimes can be.)*

- Some patients, especially those with ADD or ADHD, respond well to many sessions of biofeedback.[65a,b]

- Some patients need an expert who can conduct psychological tests to help differentiate if there are major critical psychological and emotional components in those who have environmentally or chemically-related illness.[26] There are very few experts in this area. (*Nancy Didriksen, Ph.D.*:

972.889.9933.)

Suggestions for Dental Considerations

- Unrecognized dental problems are sometimes key unsuspected factors in relation to the health of some individuals. It is also difficult to remain healthy if you have chronically infected root canals, tooth abscesses or an infected jawbone cavity. Any of these infections should be eliminated because distant body areas on any specific acupuncture meridian can be adversely affected.

- If all else fails, consider removal of *all* metal fillings or other forms of metal (braces, posts etc.) from your mouth. The good news is that for some individuals, this form of treatment sometimes totally and quickly eliminates chronic symptoms, such as headaches, arthritis or depression, even though these symptoms do not appear to be directly related to dental disease. More good news, depending on the dentist, is that removal of metals from the mouth, including caps covering "mercury or silver" fillings, can be totally painless.[11a,b] In addition, it is also possible for chronic tooth indentations on swollen tongues to totally disappear in a few days after dental metals in your teeth are removed. The bad news is that this most expensive procedure is sometimes of no help at all. It therefore can be a financial gamble, but the reward, if your chronic symptoms subside in a few days, truly can appear to be almost a medical miracle. [11a,b] (*Appendix B.2a.)* It is best to see only the nearest holistic dentist because adjustments are typically required.

There are other more sophisticated, expensive and exotic types of blood, urine, brain and nervous system tests, but an environmental specialist and neurologist should help make these decisions.[4f]

Nothing Has Helped? Consider Some Unproven Alternative Methods *(For details about how to muscle test or the*

use of a pendulum, see Appendix D.5a-c.)

(Some in the medical profession will be very upset that the following information is included in this book. Others in the medical profession, however, are as discouraged as I am because too many patients remain ill and on drugs, in spite of everything that has been tried to earnestly help them. The physicians and the public want better answers. While I wholeheartedly agree that it is indeed difficult to differentiate a genuine medical advance from a new idea without merit, we must keep an open mind. If we always do what we have always done, medicine will never change for the better. Too many at this time have no routine medical care or insurance. They cannot afford needed nutrients or medications. To help the masses of sick and uninsured people, we must actively seek to find ways that teach people how to figure out some answers on their own. We need faster, easier, less expensive, safer and more effective ways to approach uncomplicated medical illnesses. Increased awareness is the first step. It is my hope that those who disagree with the following will do some unbiased research and determine why some of these methods appear to be effective. Many facets of the human body remain so complex that the most erudite medical scientists cannot begin to explain or comprehend what they observe. When I first heard about homeopathy and muscle testing, I thought it was too ridiculous to even consider. Then my patients taught me. Some were helped by some of the methods described below, not a little, but more than I thought possible. In fact, the newer creative chiropractic approaches, TBM and NET, proved to be so effective I gave up my medical practice in Buffalo and moved to Phoenix. What I did in Buffalo helped many, but I learned there were different methods that appeared to be easier and better. In time, this led to the ideas formulated in the Epilogue at the end of this book. We simply must try to find ways to help more people.)[92, 106]

- There are a variety of machines that use probes on acupuncture points to find causes of illness and various types of therapy. (*Enterro II, III Best, QX1.,Bi-Com, Bio-Tracker)*

In general, these machines register if an acupuncture meridian is blocked. You can put various vials into the circuitry of a patient and the machine will register if the contents of the vial appear to open or close certain energy pathways in the body. For example, there is an allergy point on a finger. If a doctor touches that allergy point, that energy acupuncture circuit will register an abnormality in that pathway. If dust is a problem for that person and the right dust antidote remedy is put directly in the circuit, the machine will register that the pathway is no longer blocked. The patient can take a few drops of this remedy under the tongue at various intervals and, surprisingly, this treatment appears to relieve many types of illness.

- If your doctor has *not* been able to help you and is open to use newer chiropractic techniques such as TBM, NAET (Nambudripad's Allergy Elimination Technique) and/or NET, it is possible that these methods can sometimes quickly provide insight and meaningful relief.[21,22,23] In spite of the apparent and repeated successes with these methods, however, like other approaches that are newer and novel, they urgently need more scientific evaluation and validation. They also need insurance coverage.

- There is also a basic chiropractic course designed specifically for parents called Stress Management. *(Victor Frank D.C.: 435.652.4340.)* It provides a simple, fast, muscle-testing method that appears to be helpful in relation to some allergies and other sensitivities. (*See Appendix D.5a.)*

- There is also a new treatment that uses the "Life Vessel". You merely lie down and relax in a large chamber while your body is exposed to various sound, light and vibration energies. It appears to balance the autonomic nervous system by relaxing the body. It supposedly enhances self-regulation and healing within the body. The chamber often smells strongly of chemicals after someone with chemical sensitivities has been in it for about an hour suggesting that chemicals are being released during the procedure. Preliminary research is in progress but much more solid scientific evidence is needed to ascertain and document the possible beneficial effects of this form of energy therapy as a treatment for chemical sensitivities.[42]

- A number of progressive alterative independent health healers are now engaged in the new field of energy psychology.[84, 88-98.] More critical research is again needed before we can fairly evaluate the claimed benefits of these types of therapies but some of their methods appear to be fast, easy to use, safe, effective and inexpensive. We need funding to fairly evaluate and explain their observations, successes and also the failures.

1. Some tend to use mainly sound, light and/or aroma energy to help and heal both children and adults with problems, for example, as challenging as OCD (obsessive compulsive disorders).[98] These energies are thought to "balance and tune up" the heart, mind and spirit creating a calming relaxing effect within the body. Inexpensive audio and videotapes are available concerning this form of therapy for a variety of other emotional or physical illnesses.[43, 74, 84, 89, 92, 98]

2. Other promising muscle testing techniques are said to provide insight to the tester and the body of the person being tested.[84, 89, 97a,b] One is called the Jaffe-Mellor Technique (JMT™).[97a,b] This checks the energy of the body by muscle testing and then uses verbal and breathing patterns, along with acupuncture pressure, tapping and laser stimulation along the spine to correct various imbalances.

3. Another variation of the above energy psychology techniques uses muscle testing with vials which contain the energy of various allergens and other substances. Once the

tester determines the effect of the item being tested, the treatment consists of some form of specific acupuncture stimulation using tapping or lasers. The methods of Dr. Sandi Radomski appear to provide antidotes for some allergy-like reactions, including chemical sensitivities.[84]

4. There are some other scientifically unproven ways claimed to help you differentiate if a food, beverage, vitamin etc., for example, are good or bad for you. *(See Appendix D.5a,b.)* These methods possibly can be applied, for example, to determine whether a food is organic or not. One previously discussed method is called muscle testing and this is utilized by the many chiropractors who use muscle strength energy to evaluate patients.

5. Another way is to buy a pendulum to check out everything you intend to buy in a manner similar to that used when someone is dowsing for water or oil under the ground. These methods are detailed in Appendix D.5a-c [53, 66a,b] (*ERF: 800.787.8780.*) See what you think. No, it is hardly scientific but energy medicine is a definite reality.[58a,b] Food and beverage contacts affect the energy of our bodies and although these are not seen, their effects unquestionably can be measured.[53, 58a,b, 59, 62, 66a,b] If these methods provide any insight above the placebo effect, it is better than simply blindly guessing to determine what is good or not good. In time we shall know more because rigid research in relation to energy medicine is in progress at the present time in many areas of the world.[58a,b, 88-92, 99-104,108,109]

6. Spiritual energy healers from China, Korea and Japan sometimes resolve chronic medical problems when all else has failed using ancient methods of energy transfer. These can include Qi Gong exercises, acupuncture, and herbs that

---

* Master John 775.323.4455, Master Hong 626.445.4284, Ruth Scott 623.551.9073.

have been helpful for centuries.[122, 123] * *(See Appendix D5.)*

How Do You Verify a Chemical Sensitivity Medically and Legally?[4k, 32]

There are times when you must prove a cause and effect response in relation to a chemical for health or legal reasons. The following suggestions will help you document if chemicals in an item, i.e., a mattress, carpet, shower curtain, screen, etc. might be making you ill.

- Send any suspect item to a laboratory that can determine exactly which chemical is in a particular product. (*See Appendix D.1a, Matrix Lab: 972.818.8155.*)

- Check your blood, urine and fat levels for that same specific chemical. *(See Appendices D.1, D.2.)* To detect most chemicals, the blood sample must be taken in a matter of minutes, although specific breakdown products from a chemical can be detected later on. If you think you might be exposed and become ill, call Accu-Chem or ImmunoScience for advice and have the blood kit on hand.

- If the vapors from the suspect product could be in the room air, check the air for the same chemicals found in your blood and the suspect item to which you were exposed using special badges or tubes for individual or groups of common chemicals. Labs that do environmental evaluations have the badges and tubes so they can do this type of testing. *(See Appendix D.1, D.2.)*[7a,b, 25]

- Make an allergy extract of the air in a suspect room.[5, 7a] This is done by bubbling the room air through a solution of normal saline for several hours, as is routinely done in fish tanks. Whatever is in the air (molds, dust, chemicals, etc.) can gradually accumulate in the saline. Then the saline sample is filtered and checked for sterility and used for P/N allergy testing.[5] Again, video the response.

- Have an allergy extract made of a suspect item. One merely soaks a bit of the carpet, mattress or clothing in just enough of a normal saline (salt) solution to cover it. Refrigerate the mix and shake it repeatedly over a period of several days. Then pour off the saline, filter it and check it for sterility before it is used for Provocation/Neutralization allergy testing. (*ERF: 800.787.8780.)*

- Using appropriate controls, video the response to Provocation/Neutralization allergy testing from an allergy extract made from a possible problem item or the air from a suspect room or area.[1c] This can be done in the office of most environmental medical specialists.[5]

- Send a sample of the suspect item or the room air to Anderson Laboratory for a mouse bioassay test.[12] *(See Appendix D.2c.)* Find out how long it takes before exposure to a suspect item or the air collected from a certain room makes a mouse sick and video the response showing the exact ways that a mouse becomes ill.

One Example of Practical Application of the Above

If specific tests determine that the same chemical is in a suspect item and also in your room air and in your blood, urine or fat, it is more likely there is a connection. If a properly controlled allergy skin test with an extract made from chemicals, a suspect item and/or room air also reproduces your symptoms, and if a mouse bioassay test produces similar symptoms when the mouse is exposed to that same item or air, these findings again strengthen the possibility that there is a connection. The aim is to find and confirm that something that is harmful in your environment is also within you and that it could be causing your illness.

Several videos of responses of test mice to various common items or chemicals, such as disinfectants, are also available directly through Anderson Laboratory.[12]

(See the video, Environmentally Sick Schools, which shows the reaction of mice to a piece of school carpet and the video, Chemical Reactions In Children and Adults that shows typical responses to chemical exposures as listed in Appendix E.4.)[1c, e]

You Do Not Have to Do It All

Remember you do not have to do everything suggested in this chapter. You should feel better as soon as your level or amount of exposure is below your personal tolerance level. When your symptoms diminish, this means you have done enough to help *at that time*. It may not be enough, however, if you are faced with unusual stress, such as an infection, incapacitating illness, loss of a job, separation, divorce, money problems, a car accident or the death of a loved one.

Whenever you are stressed, it will typically take less exposure to chemicals or common allergenic substances (mold, dust, pollen or problem foods) to make you ill. At that time, you must do more to remain well because your previous level of tolerance will no longer be adequate to protect you. You can lower your exposures by using any of the above suggestions but that level must not be higher than the level your body can tolerate. When your level of tolerance is down and your exposure levels are up, you will tend to be sick. At times, this can be reversed quite easily.

Why Would the Above Suggestions Not Help?

There are many reasons why people do not get well. Treatment success depends on the right diagnosis, plus a number of other factors. If you are checking for chemicals and the problem is something totally unrelated to this type of exposure, you will not get better by eliminating chemicals. The treatment must fit the disease. Below are some down to earth reasons why an individual can remain sick, in spite of being given the correct diagnosis and advice.

- There is also a tendency to blame the doctor if you do not improve, but sometimes the reason is that you simply could or would not completely follow your doctor's advice. Communication and compliance can be a problem.

- You must completely understand what is needed on your part to get well. If an illness or suggested treatment is too complicated or overwhelming, an environmental specialist might be essential to guide you slowly through all that needs to be done. It is certainly possible to be so ill that it is impossible to handle any of the above suggestions without supervised professional and personal help, and most will also need a solid family or friend support system.[5] *(See Appendix B.1 to B.6.)*

- Financial limitations are a common justifiable reason why some people do not do what needs to be done to make themselves or their children well. It certainly can require a minimum amount of financial resources to do what is expected and needed to begin to get well. Many single mothers must work two jobs and when they have sick or hyperactive children at home, they can barely handle all that is required to get through an ordinary day. Purchasing air and water purifiers, making significant home changes, buying nutrients, doing special diets, monitoring meals and exposures at school and reading more "how to" books are simply not feasible due to realistic cost and time restraints.

- Others simply do not want to be bothered trying to figure out why they are ill and what they can do about it. They have their own busy lives and want to do the things they have always done and eat whatever they like. They simply want a fast, effective "fix it" drug covered by their insurance policy. Those who have this type of attitude should not even try to see an environmental physician. These individuals require a physician with a totally different approach to medicine.

- Some patients want the responsibility of finding out what is wrong with them to be totally up to the doctor. They are right. It is the doctor's job to find the answers but sometimes an adult, a parent of a sick child or an older child can do it more quickly and better than anyone else. No one knows his/her own body as well as the person who has lived in it for years. No one knows a child, as well as a parent.

- Some patients, especially men, firmly deny their illness in spite of obvious signs and symptoms. If they believe it does not exist, there is no need to change anything. A caring articulate doctor can often change such attitudes by explaining all the specific pros and cons in relation to improved compliance. Many men have found their marriages have been saved after they received treatment. It would not be unusual for them to have more stamina, energy, mental alertness, athletic ability and sexual prowess after treatment. *(The desire for these types of changes convinced some fathers in my former practice to follow through with their treatment.)*

- Some are simply not ill enough to accept the degree to which they will have to change their life style to regain their health. Some must wait until they or some family members are more ill before they are willing to reconsider their choices and seriously do what they can to reverse or diminish their illness.

- Sometimes divorced parents purposely create major illnesses and upsets in their children. Most parents typically cooperate, but there are unfortunately a few "weekend" parents who do everything possible to cause havoc in the estranged spouse's life — even if this means using their child as a pawn. For example, they will not keep the weekend home or bedroom environmentally clean and they purposely feed foods or expose their child to chemicals that are known to make their child ill. If problem exposures are timed, it is also possible to regularly cause a child to become ill shortly after a child returns home from a weekend spousal visit. This type of behavior creates both physical and emotional illness and stress, in both the estranged spouse and the child. Such purposeful actions should be recorded and documented for both medical and legal purposes. The child should be videotaped before and after visits so an uncooperative spouse can more fully realize that a change in attitude is required.

(To confuse the situation, if a food that causes an allergy is not eaten for several weeks, it is sometimes possible to eat it, on a few occasions, without any apparent difficulty. In this type of situation, on a temporary basis, no reaction will occur from eating a problem food. If such a food continues to be ingested, however, a reaction will surely reoccur, in time, if a true sensitivity exists. If this is not understood a child will believe there is no sensitivity and a disgruntled parent will feel justified in his/her action.)

- Some simply give up because they feel it is impossible to clean up their home, food, water and environment. It can be discouraging, but if they will gradually follow the easy suggestions in this chapter, they will find it helps. It can be inconvenient, but many can certainly make enough changes so they will see and feel a difference that will be evident to themselves and everyone else. This can and does happen in a few days in some individuals. The answer is to be informed. The more a person knows, the easier it is to determine why someone is ill and take realistic approaches to avoid harmful exposures.

- And lastly, there are some who have much more to gain from being sick than being well. *(For a long time I doubted this was possible, but I was wrong.)* If someone gets more attention, lots of sympathy, help from relatives and friends, does not have to work or gets money from the government or some other source, at some level they may not truly want to lose their symptoms. They too need the help and expertise of a trained counselor, psychologist or hypnotherapist. Sometimes they can be helped quickly.

Summary

This chapter gives you practical answers to document why you are ill, tell you what you can do to confirm your suspicions and then correct the situation. It explains which tests your personal doctor can order to document a toxic exposure and where you can find experienced environmental physicians with specialized expertise to help you substantiate your personal diagnosis and initiate meaningful treatment. It explains what is beneficial to maintain your health and protect yourself and loved ones from future exposures to major toxic pollutants and allergenic substances in your environment. By choosing safer products to use inside and outside your home, school and workplace and for use on and inside your body, you can tremendously enhance your health and ability to stay well and feel exuberant.

Many of you, on your own, can improve the quality of your family's life by making a few simple changes. Those who are more seriously ill will need to do much more to regain and maintain their health, but with the right help and a positive attitude, you certainly can improve.

Hopefully, as funding becomes available, truly integrative medical eco-centers can be created that will combine the very best of traditional and alternative medical care. These environmentally-safer urban eco-centers will not only diagnose and treat, they will educate patients and open-minded physicians, osteopaths, dentists and psychologists, as well as other health professionals, about various traditional and alternative methods of healing. Because this type of medicine impacts the fields of education, architecture and jurisprudence so directly, teachers, builders and lawyers will have the opportunity to learn about these newer and different medical approaches in special seminars. The centers will conduct extensive impartial research to find out which treatment methods or products are practical, cost effective and truly helpful. *(See Epilogue at end of this book and www.drrapp.com for more information.)*

CHAPTER 3 REFERENCES:

1 Environmental Medical Research Foundation: ERF [Formerly: Practical Allergy Research Foundation], P.O. Box 60, Buffalo, NY 14223-0060. 800.787.8780. www.drrapp.com.

1a Water purifiers and water filters.

1b Air purifiers.

1c Video: Environmentally Sick Schools. Cost: $25.00 (plus S&H).

1d Video: Mold Reactions in Children and Adults. Cost: $25.00 (plus S&H).

1e Video: Chemical Reactions in Children and Adults. Cost: $25.00 (plus S&H).

1f Video: Sinus Drainage. Cost: $25.00 (plus S&H).

1g Peak Flow Meters to detect asthma, $25.00 (plus S&H). 800.787.8780.

2 Batmanghelidj, F., M.D., Global Health Solutions, Inc., P.O. Box 3189, Falls Church, VA 22043, www.watercure.com.

2a The Body's Many Cries For Water, 1995. Cost: $14.95.

2b ABC Of Asthma, Allergies And Lupus: Eradicate Asthma Now, 2000. Amazon.com. Cost: $12.

3a Revitalized Structured Water, 1204 Avenue U, Suite 1292, Brooklyn, NY 11229. 888.897.8030 or 10573 West Pico, Suite 283, Los Angeles, CA 90064. www.revitalizedwater.com.

3b Bio-Hydration Research Lab, Inc., (Penta water) 6370 Nancy Ridge Drive, Suite 104, San Diego, CA 92121; 858.452.8868. Fax: 858.452.8890, www.hydrateforlife.com.

3c Whang, Sang, Reverse Aging, High Tech Health Inc., Water Ionizers and Infrared Therapy, 800.794.5355, www.hightechhealth.com. $11.95

3d Thermal Life Far Infrared Therapy, High Tech Health, Inc. 800.794.5355

4 Rapp, Doris J., M.D., Is This Your Child's World? P.O. Box 60, Buffalo, NY 14223-0060. 800.787.8780. Cost: $12.00 (plus S&H).

4a Chapter 3, pp. 52-62.

4b Chapter 3, pp. 62-64.

4c Chapter 15.

4d Chapter 6, pp. 157-158.

4e Chapter 17.

4f Chapter 13.

4g pp. 229-234.

4h Chapter 2 & 4.

4i pp. 195-6.

4j pg. 322.

4k Chapter 16.

4l pg. 359.

5 American Academy of Environmental Medicine (AAEM), 7701 E. Kellogg, Suite 625, Wichita, KS 67207. 316.684.5500, www.aaem.com.
6 Rockwell, Sally J., CCN, Ph.D., P.O. Box 31065, Seattle, WA 98013. 206.547.1814. Fax: 206.547.7696. www.drsallyrockwell.com.

6a A Rotation Diet, 1998. Cost: $ 12.95 (plus S&H),

6b Rotation Diet Game. Cost: $18.95 (plus S&H).

7a Olinsky, Russell, M.S., Enviro-Health: Environmental Engineering, Mold Remediation, Environmental Investigations and Consultations. 3421 N. Paiute Way #4, Scottsdale, AZ 85251. 602.432.1449.

7b Vance, Paula, microbiologist, 8911 Interchange Dr., Houston, TX 77054, 713.663.6888. pv@microbiologyspecialist.com, www.microbiologyspecialist.com

7c Straus, David, Ph.D., Texas Tech University, Microbiology. david.straus@ttmc.ttusc.edu.

8a Analytical Research Labs, 2225 W. Alice Avenue, Phoenix, AZ 85021. website: arltma.com.

8b Great Smokies Diagnostic Laboratory, 63 Zillicoa St., Asheville, NC 28801-9801. 800.522.4762.

8c Doctor's Data, 3755 Illinois Ave., St. Charles, IL 60174-2420. 800.323.2784 or 630.377.8139.

8d Wilson, Lawrence, M.D., The Hair Analysis Handbook, P.O. Box 54, Prescott, AZ 86302. 800.296.7053; 928.445.7690.

9 Rogers, Sherry, M.D., Prestige Press, P.O. Box 3068, 3500 Brewerton Rd., Syracuse, NY 13220. 800.846.6687; 315.468.4417. Fax: 315.468.8119. www.prestigepublishing.com.

9a Wellness Against All Odds, 1994, Cost: $17.95 (plus S&H).

9b Newsletter: Total Wellness, March 2000. Annual Fee: $39.95 (plus S&H).

9c Wellness Mold Plates, NE Center for Environmental Medicine, P.O. Box 2716, Syracuse, NY 13220. 315.488.2857. One per room, Cost $40.00/each.

9d No More Heartburn. 2000. Cost: $15.00 (plus S&H).

9e Depression Cured At Last, 1997. Cost: $24.95 (plus S&H).

9f Detoxify or Die, The Ultimate Healing Plan, 2002. Cost: $22.95 (plus S&H).

10 Krohn, Jacqueline, M.D. and Francis Taylor, M.A., Natural Detoxification: A Practical Encyclopedia: The Complete Guide to Cleaning Your Body of Toxins, Hartley & Marks Publishers, Inc., October 2000, P.O. Box 147, Pt. Roberts, WA 98281. Cost: $24.95.

11a Cook, Douglas, DDS, www.dentistryhealth.com.

11b Margolis, Michael D., DDS, P.C. mydentist4@aol.com

12 Anderson Laboratories: P.O. Box 323, 4967 Route 14, West Hartford VT 05084, 802.295.7344, www.andersonlaboratories.com

13 Knight, Will, "Breakthrough Patches Detect Dangerous Chemicals," New Scientist Journal: Science, Vol. 293, pg. 1296. www.mindfully.org/Health/Chemical-Sensor-New.htm.

14 Fagan, John, Ph.D., Genetic Engineering: The Hazards; Vedic Engineering: The Solutions, 1995, Maharishi International University, 1000 N. Fourth St., Fairfield, Iowa 52557. Cost: $12.00 Amazon.com.
15 EnviroGen Technologies, Stephen.Gorton@verizon.net. 214.244.4192.
16a Steven Tvedten, 800.221.6188. www.getset.com.
16b The Bug Stops Here, downloadable free book, www.getipm.com
17 The Mold Source, P. O. Box 2421, Forney, TX 75126. 972.564.4245. www.themoldsource.com.
18 Dale Bates and Associates, Living Architecture, 671 First Ave. N. Box 2012, Ketchum, Idaho 83340. 208.726.3691. Fax: 208.726.3694.
19 Sahley, Billie, Ph.D., Pain and Stress Clinic, 5282 Medical Drive, #160, San Antonio, TX 78229-6043. 800.669.2256. www.painstresscenter.com.
20 "Not All Nutrition Products are Created Equally," Chase Swift, www.nutriadvisor.com/44.5billion.htm.
21 Frank, Victor, D.C., N.M.D., D.O., Total Body Modification [TBM], 1907 East Foxmoor Circle, Sandy, UT 84092. 435.652.4340. Fax: 435.652.4339. email: health@tbmseminars.com, www.tbmseminars.com.
22 Nambudripad, Devi, D.C., Nambudripad's Allergy Elimination Treatment, [NAET]. naet@earthlink.net, 714.523.8900.
23 Walker, Scott, D.C., Neuro-Emotional Training [NET], 524 Second St., Encinitas, CA 92024. 800.888.4638. email: scottwalker@earthlink.net, www.netmindbody.com.
24a terri@onepost.net. Cost: 2 phone stickers for $18.00.
24b Lowery, John, http://www.energyworks123.com/indexSwf.html
25 Rea, Christopher, 8345 Walnut Lane, Suite 220, Dallas, TX 75231-4262. 214.368.4132.
26 Didriksen, Nancy, Ph.D., 972.889.9933.
27a Silver, Nina, The Complete Guide to Sauna Therapy, 2002. 845.687.0963. www.healingheart-harmonics.com.
27b Wilson, Lawrence, M.D., Manual of Sauna Therapy, 2003, L.D. Wilson Consultants, Inc., P. O. Box 54, Prescott, AZ 86302-0054, 928-445-7690. Larry@drlwilson.com.
28a Rea, William J., M.D., Optimum Environment for Optimum Health and Creativity, 2002, Crown Press, Boca Raton. Call: American Health Environmental Center, 800.428.2343. Cost: $39.95 (plus S&H).
28b Rea, William J., M.D., Chemical Sensitivities, Vol. 3, CRC Press, Inc., 2000 Corporate Blvd., N.W., Boca Raton, FL. 214.368.4132.
28c Rea, William J., M.D., Chemical Sensitivities, Vol. 4, CRC Press, Inc., 2000 Corporate Blvd., N.W., Boca Raton, FL. 214.368.4132.

29 Heavenly Heat, 1106 2nd St., Encinitas, CA 92024, 800.697.2862.
30a Allergy and Environmental Health Center, Kalpana Patel, M.D., 65 Wehrle Drive, Buffalo, NY 14225. 716.833.2213.

> **30b** Environmental Health Center, Christopher Rea, 8345 Walnut Lane, Suite 220, Dallas, TX 75231-4262. 214.368.4132. Fax 214.691.8432.
>
> **30c** Johnson Medical Associates, Alfred Johnson, D.O., 101 Coit Rd., Suite 317, Richardson, TX 75080. 972.479.0400; Fax: 972.479.9435.

31a Croft, Dr. William, et al., "Clinical Confirmation of Trichothecene Mycotoxicosis in Urine," Journal of Environmental Biology, 2002: 23(3) 301.320.

> **31b** Environmental Pathology, Toxicology and Biochemistry, 715.757.3756.

32 King, Linda Price, Chemical Injury and The Courts: A Litigation Guide for Clients and Their Attorneys, The Environmental Health Network, P. O. Box 16267, Chesapeake, VA 23328-6267. 757.546.0663.
33a The homestore.com.

> **33b** OMB Watch. http://www.ombwatch.org/.
>
> **33c** EPA: Air quality where you live. http://www.epa.gov/airnow/where/.

34 The OxiData Test, 800.736.4381 www.oxidata.com
35 Miller, Joseph B., Relief at Last: Neutralization for Food Allergy and Other Illness. 1987. This book is out of print—limited availability. Cost: $47.50 Springfield, IL.
36 Sheffield, Billy, Research Shows Treatment Greatly Reduces Toxins, The Review, Maharishi University of Management, February 2000:15 (8). http://www.mum.edu/TheReview.
37 N.E.E.D.S, 527 Charles Avenue, 12A, Syracuse, NY 13209. 800.634.1380.
38 Soapworks, 18911 Nordhoff St., Suite 37, Northridge, CA 91324. 800.699.9917.
39 Constantini, Dr. Anthony, JFOVERLAG@aol.com.
40 Our Toxic Times, September 1998, pp. 8-9.
41 Detox Kit, Heel, 11600 Cochiti SE, Albuquerque, NM 87123. www.HeelUSA.com. 800/621-7644 ; 505.293.3843.
42 Thomason, Randall, "Overview of Biochemical Changes Induced by "The Life Vessel," Women's International Pharmacy, Youngstown, AZ.
43 Culin, Lenore, M.A., Tools for Color and Music Therapy and Energy Balancing, Attunements Unlimited, PO Box 32711, Phoenix, AZ 85064, or www.IMowerTV.com.
44 "Congressman John Conyers, Jr. Introduces H.R. 5040: The United States Toxic Mold Safety and Protection Act ("The Melina Bill")," Michigan's 14th Congressional District, 2426 Rayburn House Office Bldg., Washington, DC 20515. 202.225.5125.

45a Minnesota Extension Service of the University of Minnesota, 1989, "Microwave Heating of Milk."

45b Lee, Dr. Lita, "Microwaving Baby Formulas Converted Certain Amino Acids Into Synthetic – Non Biologically Active' – cis- isomers," Lancet, December 9, 1989.

46 Ott, Wayne R. and John W. Roberts, "Everyday Exposure to Toxic Pollutants," Scientific American, February 1998.

47 Immerman, F. and J. Schaum, Final Report of the Non-Occupational Pesticide Exposure Study, U.S. EPA, Research Triangle Park, January 23, 1990.

48 Murray, Rich, "How Aspartame Became Legal – The Timeline." www.rense.com/general33/legal.htm.

49 Ashford, Nicholas and Claudia Miller, Chemical Exposures: Low Levels and High Stakes, Chapter 2: "Definition," 1998, Van Nostrand Reinhold, 115 Fifth Avenue, New York, NY 10003. Cost: $52.50.

50 http://poisonedinparadise.com/poison16.pdf., pg. 15.

51a Memo To: Public Information and Records Integrity Branch (PIRIB), Information Resources and Services Division (7502C), Office of Pesticide Programs (OPP), EPA, Pennsylvania Ave., NW, Washington, DC 20460 USA, August 19, 2002, on CCA-treated wood; docket ID OPP-2002-0147, by Laurette Janak, 7185 Liebler Rd., Colden, NY 14033. 716.941.4622.

51b http://www.epa.gov.pesticides/citizens/1file.htm

51c http://www.preservedwood.com.

51d www.www.beyondpesticides.org.

52 Force, Mark, D.C., Choosing Health, 2003. 7500 E. Pinnacle Peak Road, Scottsdale, AZ 85255. 480.563.4256 FAX: 480.563.4269. www.theelementsofhealth.com Cost: $24.95.

53 http://www.elementofharmonv.net/dowsing.htm

54a Diamond, John, M.D., Life Energy: Using the Meridians to Unlock the Hidden Power of Your Emotions. 1998, Paragon House. Cost: $12.95.

54b The Clinical Practice of Complementary, Alternative, and Western Medicine, 2000, CRC Press. Cost: $99.95.

55 Stoddard, Darrell J., "Could Bra-Wearing Increase the Incidence of Breast Cancer and Also Painful, Lumpy Breasts?" Pain Research Institute, 266 E. 3200 North, Provo, UT 84604. 801.377.6900. www.healpain.net

56 Loes, Michael, David Steinman and Megan Shields, Arthritis: The Doctor's Cure, 1999, McGraw-Hill/Contemporary Books.

57 Reuters. "Sophisticated New Type of Chemical Sensor Created." August 16, 2001. http://www.mindfully.org/Health/Chemical-Sensor-New.htm

58a Tiller, W. A., et al., Conscious Acts of Creation, 2001, Pavior Publishing, CA. Cost: $29.95.

58b Tiller, W. A., Ph.D., Science and Human Transformation, Subtle Energies, Intentionality and Consciousness, 1997, Pavior Publishing, CA. Cost: $24.95.

59 Gerber, Richard, A Practical Guide to Vibrational Medicine: Energy Healing and Spiritual Transformation, 2001, Quill Publishing. Cost: $15.00 (amazon.com).
60 Ishikawa, S., et al., "Abnormal Standing Ability in Patients with Organophosphate Pesticide Intoxication (Chronic Cases)," Agressologie 24(2):143-144.
61a "Second Helpings: Farm Stands and Farmer's Markets," The Austin Chronicle. www.austinchronicle.com/issues/dispatch/2001-10-12/food_second_all.html

61b Boggy Creek Farms, www.bogycreekfarms.com
61c Diamond Organics, 888.ORGANIC (888.674.2642) www.diamondorganics.ocm
61d Boxed Greens, www.boxedgreens.com

62 Healing Touch International, 12477 W. Cedar Drive, Suite 202, Lakewood, CO 80228. 303.989.7982. www.healingtouch.net.
63 Harezi, Ilonka, The Resonance in Residence: An Inner and Outer Quantum Journey, 2002. www.ilonkaharezi.com. 618.948.2393.
64 Matrix Analytical Laboratories, Inc., 4501 Sunbelt Drive, Suite B, Addison, TX 75001. 972.818.8155. FAX: 972.381.0348. www.matrixlabs.cc, mail@matrixlabs.cc
65a Bates, Phil, Ph.D., ADD/ADHD Biofeedback Home Training, http://www.ADHD-biofeedback.com.

65b drvonh@mindspring.com.

66a Greg Nielsen, Pendulum Power, 1987, Inner Traditions Intl Ltd. Cost: $8.95 (amazon.com).

66b Sig Lonegren, The Pendulum Kit, 1990, Fireside; Book and Access Edition, Cost: $21.95 (amazon.com).

67 Explore, November 2001:10 (5). www.ohno.org
68a Health Treasures, 265 SW Port Saint Lucie Blvd., #146, Port Saint Lucie, FL 34984. www.healthtreasures.com/ph-paper.html

68b Make your own pH paper: http://www.miamisci.org/ph/phydrion.html

69 George, Stephen, "Toxic Mold, Menace or Myth," Better Home and Gardens, April 2003.
70 Fitzgerald, Patricia DHM, CCN, L. Ac, The Detox Solution: The Missing Link to Radiant Health, Abundant Energy, Ideal Weight, and Peace of Mind, 1137 Second Street, Suite 116 Santa Monica, CA 90403. 800.DETOX NOW. www.detoxsolution.com. Cost: $19.95 (plus S&H).
71 Slagel, Dr. Kirk, "Pleo Muc Eye Drops: A Product Worthy of a Second Look," Explore! 2001:10 (5).
72 O'Connor, Robert, Certified Hypnotherapist. Current President of ASHPH.
73a ELF International, State Route 1, Box 21, St. Francisville, IL 62460.

73b The Stressbuster Circulation/Lymphatic Stimulator, CAC Inc., 3801 Pineoakyo Court, Rescue, CA 95672. 877.867.2477. Cost: $350-$500

74 House of San Dan Yi, 2675 West Highway 89A, #1252, Sedona, AZ 86336. 928.204.5885. www.houseofsandanyi.com
75a Harezi, Ilonka, The Resonance in Residence: An Inner and Outer Quantum Journey, 2002. To order: 618.948.2393. Cost: $28.00/Set.
75b Harezi, Ilonka, The Resonance in Residence: An Inner and Outer Quantum Journey, Science Edition, 2002. To order: 618.948.2393. Cost: $28.00/Set, Quantum Book.
76 Charles R. Bailey Cabinetmakers, 51 MD 7013, Highway 62 East, Flippin, AR 72634. 870.453.5433. www.southshore.com/~crbslf
77 The Pure Water Place, Inc., 3347 Longview Blvd., Longmont, CO 80504. 888.776.0056. www.purewaterplace.com
78 Redemske Design. 413.773.5375. sandyr@shaysnet.com
79 ImmunoScience Labs, Inc., 8693 Wilshire Blvd., Suite 200, Beverly Hills, CA 90211. 800.950.4686. www.immuno-sci-lab.com
80 Nielsen, Dr. Joan, 919.467.5770. amtoft@aol.com
81 Voorhees, Bruce, "The Dangers of Ozone Generators." http://www.birdsnways.com/wisdom/ww23ev.htm
82 "Ozone is dangerous for People with Asthma and other Respiratory Problems," Blueair, http://www.airfilterstore.com/blueair/ozone.htm
83 Young, Robert O., Ph.D. and Shelley Redford Young, The pH Miracle: Balance Your Diet, Reclaim Your Health, 2002. Warner Books, Inc., 1271 Avenue of the Americas, New York, NY 10020. www.twbookmark.com. Cost: $24.95 (plus S&H).
84 Radomski, Sandi, Allergy Antidotes™: The Energy Psychology Treatment of Allergy-Like Reactions, 2000, 1051 Township Line Road, Jenkintown, PA 19046. 215.885.7917, FAX: 215.572.1175. Email: SandiRadom@aol.com or emofree.com/randomski. www.emofree.com
85 Martini, Betty, "Former FDA Investigator Exposes Aspartame as Deadly Neurotoxin that Never Should Have Been Approved," April 22, 2003. http://www.rense.com/general37/ddly.htm
86 "New Research Indicates Toxic Playgrounds in the Capital Region," New York Coalition for Alternatives to Pesticides (NYCAP). 518.426.8246. http://www.crisny.org
87 Tim-bor, http://www.bugspray.com
88 Shealy, C. Norman, M.D., Ph.D., The Methuselah Potential for Health and Longevity, 2002, Brindabella® Books, 5607 S. 222nd Road, Fair Grove, MO 65648. www.shelfhealthsystems.com. 888.242.6105.
89 Namka, Lynne, Ed. D., Good Bye Ouchies and Grouchies, Hello Happy Feelings: EFT for Kids of All Ages, 2003, Talk, Trust & Feel Therapeutics, 5398 Golder Ranch Road, Tucson, AZ 85739. www.AngriesOut.com
90 Hover – Kramer, Dorothea, Creative Energies: Integrative Energy Psychotherapy for Self-Expression and Healing, 2002, W. W. Norton & Company, 500 Fifth Avenue, New York, NY 10110. www.wwnorton.com
91 Arenson, Gloria, M.S., M.F.T., Five Simple Steps to Emotional Healing, 2001, Fireside, Rockefeller Center, 1230 Avenue of the Americas, New York, NY 10020.

92 Martin, Art, D.D., N.D., M.A., Your Body Is Talking, Are You Listening? 1997. Personal Transformation Press, 8300 Rock Springs Road, Penryn, CA 95663. 916.663.9178; 800.655.3846.
93 Video: Steve B. Reed, Healing an Abandonment Trauma. A REMAP demonstration video. 2003, www.psychotherapy-center.com. 972.997.9955.
94 Video: Jan Yordy, Indigo Child, The Next Step in Human Evolution, www.energyconnectiontherapies.com
95 Video: Art Martin, D.D., N.D., M.A., Changing Paradigms, A TV Interview with Patricia Hill on The Practice of PsychoneuroImmunology.
96Audio CD: Mary T. Sise, CSW-R, TFTdx, Transforming the Trauma of The World Trade Center. 518.785.8576. msise3@aol.com
97a Trivieri, Larry, "Reversing Arthritis with the Jaffe-Mellor Technique," Alternative Medicine Magazine, November 2000: 38.

97b JMT Advance Technique, 928 Penn Ave., Wyomissing, PA 19610. 610.685.1800. jmtseminars@aol.com. www.jmttechnique.com

98 Contact ASHAC@ aol.com for more information, tapes, seminars etc.
99 Schmidt, W. H. Jr., and Leisman G. "Correlation of Applied Kinesiology Muscle Testing Findings with Serum Immunoglobulin Levels for Food allergies," pp. 237-44: "These serum tests confirmed the 19 of the 21 food allergies (90.5%) suspected based on the applied kinesiology screening procedures." International Journal of Neuroscience, December1998: 96 (3-4).
100 Ludtke, R., B. Kunz, N. Seeber, and J. Ring, "Test-Retest-Reliability and Validity of the Kinesiology Muscle Test," pp. 141-5: "The results suggested that the use of kinesiology as a diagnostic tool is not more useful than random guessing." (Test of insect venom allergy.) Complementary Therapeutic Medicine, September 2001: 9 (30).
101 Gerber, Richard, A Practical Guide to Vibrational Medicine: Energy Healing and Spiritual Transformation, 2001, Quill Publishing. Cost: $15.00 (amazon.com).
102 Lonegren, Sig, The Pendulum Kit, 1990, Fireside; Book and Access Edition. Cost: $21.95 (Amazon.com)
103 "Scientific Validation of the Mind/ Body Paradigm and Muscle Testing," Reprint of Research Study "Muscle Test Comparisons of Congruent and Incongruent Self-referential Statements," Our Net Effect Research Foundation, 1991 Village Park Way, Suite 201-A, Encinitas, CA 92024. 760.633.1663.
104 Association for Comprehensive Energy Psychology, P.O. Box 910244, San Diego, CA 92191-0244. 858.748.5963. www.energypsych.org
105 Dishinger, Ronald C. Bad Behavior and Illness Are Caused by Biochemical Imbalances. 270.684.9233. Free Downloadable @ www.biochemimbal-behavior.com
106 Sutherland, Caroline M., The Body "Knows" How to Tune into Your Body and Improve Your Health, 2001, Hay House, Inc., P. O. Box 5100, Carlsbad, CA 92018-5100. 800.654.5126. www.hayhouse.com

107 http://www.labcorp.com/datasets/labcorp/html/chapter/mono/sc030400.htm
108 kcremasco@earthlink.net
109 Dr. Steel, Chatham, Ontario. 519.354.3660.
110 Aller Air, 2373 Michelin, Laval, Quebec, Canada H7L 5B9. 888.852.8247.
111 Epstein, Samuel, M.D., The Politics of Cancer Revisited, 1998, East Ridge Press, USA, Freemont, NY. Cost: $17.00 (plus S&H).
112 Klaire Laboratories, 800.859.8358, www.klaire.com.
113 www.hyperimmuneegg.org/background.htm
114 http://www.mercola.com/2003/may/3/water_safety.htm
115 Passalacqua, G., et al., "Oral and Sublingual Immunotherapy in Paediatric Patients," Curr Opin Allergy Clin Immunol., Apr 2003: 3(2)139-45.
116 Metagenics, www.healthcomm.com
117 MetaMetrix Medical Laboratory, 5000 Peachtree Industrial Boulevard, Suite 100, Norcross, GA 30071. 404.446.5483
118 www.utoronto.ca/forest/termite/termite.htm
119 http://www.herbsofhealth.com/ki_sweet.htm
120 Geier, Mark R., M.D., "Thimerosal in Childhood Vaccines, Neurodevelopment Disorders, and Heart Disease in the United States," Journal of American Physicians and Surgeons, Spring 2003: 8 (1).
121 NuFern Homeopathic Hormone Rejuvenation System, www.wellnesscenter.net

CHAPTER 4

Can Chemicals Affect Behavior, Activity, Learning and Child Development?

We must ask how many attitude, behavior, learning and developmental problems in children and adults can be caused by:

- The polluted air we breathe.
- The contaminated water we drink.[52]
- The pesticide sprayed foods we eat.
- The chemically contaminated places where we live, study, work and play. [1-5, 37]

It has been reported that the thinking ability, behavior, activity and personality of a child seems to be determined by about 50% genetics and the other 50 % by environmental exposures.[26c]

Here are some critical questions that need answers:

- Do chemicals affect certain children and adults so they cannot think clearly or keep up with their peers?

- Do they really affect the physical and mental development of humans, as well as animals?

- Can they cause some youngsters or adults to become inordinately angry, active, withdrawn, upset or violent from ordinary minimal daily life stresses?

- Can poor motor control while driving or engaging in sports, such as golf, cause rages because of chemicals in the air or on the grass?

- Are chemicals one unsuspected reason why children, wives, mothers, husbands and even the elderly are battered?

- Can synthetic feminizing chemicals create hormonal imbalances that lead to unprovoked aggression, depression or even suicide?

- Can these same estrogenic substances affect sex organ development, before and after birth, and affect expressions of sexuality throughout a person's life?

- Can temporary or permanent changes in memory and behavior be caused by exceedingly minute exposures to chemicals for tiny critical periods of time during fetal development?

The answer to all the above questions appears to be a definite "yes," in animals and quite often, also in humans. This chapter will attempt to provide only a small portion of the scientific evidence available that documents and supports this statement.

There is, for example, an unending stream of studies that suggest minute levels of chemicals and trace metals can adversely affect the brains and nervous systems of animals and humans.[1a, 5, 7b, 26a,b, 45] It has been pointed out that some fetuses are sensitive to chemicals that are diluted to one part in a trillion to quadrillion.[7b, 26b, 46-50] Animal and human studies suggest organochlorides, PCBs, dioxin, organophosphates, pyrethroids, solvents (toluene, benzene, xylene, styrene), alcohol, tobacco and fluorides all can have adverse effects on human behavior, learning and development, as well as possibly contributing to other types of illnesses, including cancer.[26b] Toxic reactions or allergic sensitivities to chemical exposures can persist for years or a lifetime, and unfortunately, all too often, no one suspects or recognizes the symptoms might be related to some past innocent-appearing exposure to chemicals or other environmental forms of pollution.[2]

What Has Wildlife Research Shown Us?

In general, researchers have found evidence of altered learning, behavior and sexuality in animals long before they recognized similar signs of reduced intelligence, altered activity and impaired fertility in humans.[1b] For example, the most obvious and reported behavioral sign of neurological damage observed in laboratory rats, mice and monkeys after exposure to PCBs in the womb and early life is hyperactivity.[26d] Might this not provide a possible neglected clue in relation to the many behavioral problems and attention deficit hyperactivity disorder or ADHD epidemic presently evident in millions of today's youngsters? (See companion book, *Can Chemicals Cause Epidemics?*)*

Making a connection or extrapolation from animals to humans is always open to justifiable criticism. However, since such striking parallels exist between the neurological changes noted in animals and what is presently evident in the behavior of children and adults and their ability to learn, possible cause and effect relationships should be examined more closely. At a minimum, the animal data should serve as a compelling impetus for us to be more cautious about chemical exposures until more definitive studies can be conducted.[1c]

In Monkeys

- Exposure to PCBs in the womb and through breast milk can cause monkeys to have deficits in memory and learning, as well as hyperactivity and problems in coordination.[1c, 26d]

---

* *Can Chemicals Cause Epidemics?*, Doris J. Rapp, M.D. ERF, P. O. Box 60, Buffalo, NY 14223-0060, 800.787.8780, www.drrapp.com.

In Rats

- If rats are exposed to PCBs before birth they have visual problems, decreased activity levels and impaired learning.[26d, 27-29]

- Rats exposed to PCBs in the womb show more errors in running a maze and appear to have problems learning to swim.[1c, 28]

- A recent study at Johns Hopkins demonstrated that low doses of chlorpyrifos, (Dursban®), decreased the learning ability of weanling rats. This effect was not related to cholinesterase but to changes in the molecular function of the cells in the immature brain.[3] *(This chemical legally contaminates millions of homes because of present day termite control policies in relation to purchasing new or different houses or buildings. In spite of being banned, Dursban® is still being used at the present time. (See Chapter 10.) This trend continues in spite of the fact that safer better methods have been available for years.)*

- Helen Daly studied the offspring born to mother rats that had eaten pesticide or other chemically contaminated fish.[4a,b] These rats seemed intelligent, healthy and normal sexually, but showed definite changes in behavior and, in particular, hyperactive responses to mildly negative stresses or events. In addition, these offspring also had lower birth weights and smaller heads. This combination tends to be associated with health, behavioral and intellectual deficits.[7a-e, 8]

- Studies of male rats located between two females in the uterus can cause the male rats to become less masculine or more feminine. The eventual expression of sexuality of the unborn rats appears to be inordinately affected by the most minute hormonal exposures prior to birth.[1d, 32a,b]

- Even more disturbing is preliminary evidence that a single low dose chemical exposure at a critical time during gestation can affect not only a mother rat's offspring but possibly her succeeding generations of progeny.[15a,b] These findings appear to be applicable to humans.[5] *(Is it possible that even if we find and eliminate the cause of aggression in today's children, their offspring in future generations might in turn continue to produce aggressive youngsters? We simply do not know.)*

In Mice

- Few would deny that hormones such as testosterone affect both the activity and assertive behavior in male animals. Separate studies by Peterson and by vom Saal, however, indicate female mice also can become more assertive than normal when exposed to more than usual amounts of male sex hormones. This can happen when females are positioned between male siblings while developing in the uterus.[1d]

- Other studies by vom Saal showed pregnant mice exposed to relatively low levels of pesticides, such as DDT and methoxychlor, had excessively aggressive male offspring.[1b,9a]

- Dr. Warren Porter and associates studied mice that were exposed to a combination of pesticides, herbicides and fertilizers at levels found in groundwater.[7a-e] In their thorough evaluation they found:

  a. The mice had changes in their endocrine system affecting the levels of their thyroid and growth hormone. Changes in thyroid function have been linked to increased irritability, inattention and aggression, as well as diminished intellectual ability.[14]

  b. The mice seemed to have exaggerated responses to ordinary minor stresses such as increased irritability from being touched.

c. Their immune function was depressed. This caused their antibody production to decrease making them more prone to infection.

d. Their brains and nervous systems were altered. They had more problems with their ability to learn, agility, coordination and aggression control.[1a,c, 7a-e]

e. These exposed mice also had reduced body weights and disrupted uterine development.

- Mice exposed to PCBs in the womb and early in life commonly showed behavioral abnormalities as adults. The offspring of some mice fed PCBs developed a "spinning syndrome" and constantly circled their cage. Other exposed mice manifested learning deficits.[1c]
- Neonatal mice exposed to organophosphate pesticides can manifest hyperactivity by four months of age.[31]
- In another published study, certain mice were found to lack a gene to make a brain chemical, nitric oxide. They became so aggressive they killed their cage mates. Their actions changed so much that they acted like "rapists."[9a]

If pesticides can cause significant sexual changes in various animals and aquatic life, sometimes in concentrations diluted one to one quadrillion, should we not be concerned about how these same chemicals, often in higher concentrations in our air, water and foods, affect growing infants, children and adults?[46-50]

- Researchers gave laboratory rats and mice water that contained the same levels of chemical contaminants and pollutants found in rural Wisconsin wells. They discovered that these animals showed unpredictable outbursts of aggression.[2, 5]

- These same researchers noted similar effects in rats and mice given free access to water containing mixtures of pesticides commonly found in well water in Dane County. The effects on male rodents were more evident than in females.[2, 5]

In Salmon and Gulls[1e]

- The Great Lakes fish and salmon appear to have developmental, reproductive and endocrine problems such as enlarged thyroids from living in heavily chemically polluted water.[51] If gulls ingest chemically contaminated salmon, they too develop symptoms of thyroid disease. *(We must keep asking, what about the present day thyroid epidemic. Can the thyroids of humans be affected adversly by eating chemically contaminated fish or drinking water contaminated with pesticides?*[14]*)*

In Fish [1f, 47a]

- Adult male guppy fish were exposed to pesticides, such as DDT and vinclozolin, in food and they had shrunken testis, decreased sperm counts and disrupted male courtship behavior.[47a] The biological effects were magnified at lower, rather than higher doses.

- In England, massive numbers of fish were found to be "intersexed", which means they were neither typical male nor female but had both types of sex organs. The cause was thought to be detergents that degraded into estrogen or other feminizing alkyl-phenols or bisphenols released in the water from plastics and pesticides.[1f] One billionth of a gram per liter of an estrogenic chemical can affect fish. *(How much would it take to affect humans, especially pregnant women, infants and children who drink water or eat fish which contains these substances? We simply do not know. We do know that certain feminizing estrogens, such as estradiol, are so potent that they can adversely affect humans when one drop is diluted in a trillion drops of water.*[46-50] *Is it not common sense to want to determine how many of which chemicals and estrogenic drugs are in our drinking water. We need to know the degree to which our polluted water affects infants, children and adult humans sexually as well as how they feel, act, behave and learn.)*

Let's Look in More Depth at Just One Herbicide, Triclopyr

The herbicide Triclopyr is part of the chlorpyrifos group of organophosphates.[16] It has extensively contaminated the soil, ground water and wells in vast areas of the United States.[16] It has been found to be toxic to plants, fish and newborn wildlife.

For example, exposure to this chemical can be associated with the following defects:

- Duck, fish, spider and beetle populations decreased because of reproductive problems.

- Vole populations decreased as much as 80%.

- As many as 20% of ducks had difficulty hatching.

- Rat and baby duck embryos were born deformed or died before birth.

- Rats and mice developed breast cancer and/or adrenal tumors.

- Rats and dogs developed kidney defects.

- Rabbit offspring were stillborn or had skeletal abnormalities.

- Trout had difficulty swimming and rapid respiration.

- Tadpoles lost their protective instinct. They were twitchy and did not move away from danger as normal tadpoles do.

Considering how all these forms of life can be adversely affected, does it not seem sensible that we determine what Triclorpyr and others chemicals, as well as hormones and drugs in our water, air, soil and food, do to humans of all ages?

What Has Human Research Shown Us?

In view of the previous information on animals, we must consider what insight this provides in relation to humans. Our bottom line is what can these same chemical exposures do to the health, behavior, activity, memory or learning ability of children and adults? The following represents some of the impressive but relatively scanty research in humans. It clearly suggests that certain distressing adverse health, learning and sexual effects discussed earlier in animals, are now also becoming evident in humans. In one follow up study it showed that the prolonged adverse effects of pesticide exposures on attention, memory, intelligence and reading comprehension could continue to be evident at least to the age of 11 years.[26d]

Data in Infants, Children and Adults

Some have estimated that at least 5% of babies in the United States are exposed to sufficient contaminants of PCBs or other chemicals in breast milk to cause neurological impairment.[1c] (*To detect breast milk chemicals, call Dr. Rea: 214.373.5161.*) Some babies literally are marinated in a soup of chemicals as they float about in the uterine fluid throughout their entire gestation.[36, 44, 45] In one Australian study it showed that an array of as many as five chemicals were found in the first bowel movements of some unfed newborn infants. Some of these same chemicals also can be found in the breast milk fed to the infants.[11, 7] (*See Chapter 5.*)

Offspring of Pregnant Women Who Eat Great Lakes Fish

It is estimated that there are as many as 2,800 chemicals in the Great Lakes water. PCBs are only one of the suspect chemicals that potentially can cause harmful effects on aquatic life forms.[51]

The Jacobsons studied mothers who ate Lake Michigan fish, polluted mainly with PCBs, two to three times a month for six years prior to their pregnancy.[1a, 5, 33] They found the differences between infants born to fish-eating mothers and non-fish eaters were clearly evident at birth. The babies of fish-eating mothers had smaller heads and weighed less at birth. They tended to be more jerky or twitchy, had poorer balance, weaker reflexes and handled minor stresses poorly. They had problems concentrating and with tests of recognition. The infants with higher levels of PCBs were found to have more learning difficulties as they grew up. When these children were retested at four years of age, those exposed to the highest PCB levels had the lowest verbal and memory test scores.[1a, 5, 33, 34] These findings are similar to the research by Helen Daly showing behavioral and learning changes and poor stress handling in female rats when they were fed salmon contaminated with PCBs or other chemicals as discussed previously.[1a,b,g,j, 4a,b]

Prenatal Exposure to PCBs or Other Chemicals

There is no doubt that PCBs and other chemicals can and do pass through the placenta into the unborn and into breast milk. In fact, toxic chemicals concentrate in a mother's breast milk as a natural way for mothers to lower their own body pesticide levels but unfortunately this is done at the expense of their newborns.

- A study in North Carolina of 866 infants compared their performance level during neurological tests to the amount of PCBs in their mother's milk. The higher the PCB levels in the mother's breast milk, the more these breast fed infants had evidence of a compromised nervous system.[1a] They had weak reflexes at birth and by six to twelve months of age, showed impaired fine and gross motor coordination.[1a, 33, 34]

- A Netherlands study published in 1994 showed a correlation between umbilical cord and maternal PCB/dioxin blood levels and slower reaction times, hyperactivity and problems thinking. The children with the highest PCB levels also had small reductions in their thyroid hormone levels at two weeks and three months of age, which again could contribute to a diminution of their ability to learn in the future.[35]

- A study of Dutch children in 2002 showed that higher prenatal PCB levels influenced childhood behavior. Boys appeared to manifest less masculine play, while the girls developed more masculine activity.

- In contrast to PCBs, higher level of dioxin in the prenatal period appeared to be associated with more feminized play in both the boys and girls as they grew older. These effects suggest that maternal exposure to different chemicals during pregnancy can cause hormonal changes or imbalances of different types in both their male and female offspring. It appears the effects of chemicals can alter the activity and other significant aspects of a child's future behavior.[43]

- Another study began in 1979 when a number of Taiwanese mothers accidentally ingested cooking oil that was contaminated with PCBs.[1a] Between 1985 and 1992, a study was conducted on 128 offspring of these mothers who were exposed to the PCBs when they were in the uterus, as well as later on. These children developed a number of permanent physical and neurological problems. Like the pesticide exposed Lake Apopka alligators, the boys had shorter penises than the unexposed youngsters.[17] These children also had movement, mental and behavioral problems, along with increased activity levels. They appeared to be less bright and their thought processes were slower than normal.[18, 19] The data showed striking similarities in the studies discussed earlier in animals that had a similar type of PCB exposure.

- One particularly outstanding study by Elizabeth Guillette, Ph.D. and her team of scientists compared two groups of Mexican/Indian children whose culture and way of life were basically similar.[20] Half were exposed to pesticide spray 90 times a year and to the daily use of pesticides in their homes. The other half was exposed to pesticides only during the annual DDT spraying for malaria.

  The breast milk of the overly pesticide-exposed mothers, as well as the cord bloods of their newborns, contained five different pesticides in levels above the safe limits suggested by the United Nation Food and Agricultural Agency. When the scientific team evaluated these newborns as children aged four to five years, they found they could not jump up and down very well, draw a stick figure, had poor eye/hand coordination and were less sociable and creative. They also had less stamina, poor short-term memory and more behavioral problems, particularly in the form of irritability and aggression. For example, they were more apt to hit a sibling who passed by or to manifest sudden unprovoked anger when their parents spoke to them.

Unfortunately, measurement of the size of the boy's genitals was not part of the original study design. In view of the numerous wildlife studies that have shown decreased size and abnormal formation of the genitals, as well as changes in adult sexual behavior associated with pesticide exposures, this kind of information might provide valuable insight about human sexual development, preferences and fertility. With proper funding at this time, it might be possible to obtain this type of ongoing, pertinent information from this select, well-studied population.

How Prevalent Are Potentially Harmful Pesticides?

In Chapter 6 of this book there is ample evidence that chemicals are routinely found in the blood, urine and other body secretions of many children and adults. Does this mean these individuals, who appear to be healthy now, will be in jeopardy in the future? We do not know. We do know, however, that you can easily check the chemical levels in your own and your family's blood and urine. (*Accu-Chem: 972.234.5412 and ImmunoScience: 800.950.4686.*) We also know there are ways to eliminate many toxic chemicals stored in our bodies as discussed in Chapter 3 and this should make you less prone to their potential harmful effects in the future.

Can Chemicals Alter Human Intelligence?[45]

Long before concentrations of synthetic chemicals can reach levels to cause physical illness or abnormalities they can impair learning and cause dramatic changes in behavior, such as hyperactivity, as discussed before.[1c] There is little doubt that some animals are less able to learn when they are exposed to chemicals.[45] What about humans? Why have the scores from Scholastic Aptitude Tests fallen since 1973?[1b] Is there a correlation between these test results and increased pesticide use and exposure?

Studies by Elizabeth Guillette et al. and the Jacobsons suggest pesticides do, indeed, directly and indirectly diminish the ability of humans to learn.[5, 20] If the thyroid gland is not constantly up to par while the young is developing in the uterus and throughout the first two months after birth, the brain will not develop normally.[9, 14, 29, 35] There is a similarity in the type of nervous system damage noted in thyroid disorders and those noted after PCB and dioxin exposure. It is not a stretch to assume that these chemicals can decrease a child's ability to learn because of how they affect the thyroid gland.[7d,e, 10a,b, 14] The question is how often and how much is it a factor and how many children are being or have been affected?[35, 51]

The association of nervous system impairment noted in thyroid disorders and following PCB or dioxin exposures suggests that the neurotoxic effects of these chemicals, in particular, impair normal thyroid function.[10a,b, 14, 26, 29, 30, 35] Thyroidal dysfunction and environmental chemicals potentially impact the development of the brain and the ability to learn.[26, 30] Other chemicals also seem to specifically target the thyroid and these similarly can lead to developmental delays and learning difficulties.

In 2002, Dr. Elizabeth Gillette presented research in Japan that indicated the children who were exposed to multiple pesticides had definite problem-solving difficulties and evidence of increased frustration and anxiety when they could not accomplish certain tasks.[53] Specific testing was required to bring these hidden deficits to light.

Unfortunately, on a daily basis, both animals and humans are typically exposed to hundreds of potentially harmful chemicals in our food, water and air. (*Most humans have an average of at least five to seven pesticides in their urine.*)[7] Would it not be of value to monitor both the thyroid function and the pesticide levels in the blood in all learning disabled or aggressive problem children and adults more carefully?[29] It is certainly possible that simple adjustments in their thyroid hormone levels or measures to eliminate some of the chemicals stored in their bodies might help their memories and make the behavior and activity of some more socially acceptable. (*See Chapter 3.)*

If what we desire is truly quality medicine, however, we need always to go one step further. The preferred and best bottom line answer may not be a prescribed thyroid medication, which some might need, but to stop the chemical exposures that are adversely affecting the thyroid. Even if there is proven evidence of thyroid malfunction, we must still ask why the thyroid is a target. What caused the problem leading to this type of illness? If we can eliminate the basic cause, the need for treatment often disappears.

Observations in My Buffalo Practice

In my many years of clinical practice, it was not uncommon for children's grades to improve, sometimes significantly, after an allergy diet, after allergy environmental control measures were adopted in their homes and schools and/or after Provocation/Neutralization Allergy testing and treatment.[25a,b] In a matter of minutes, one drop of ordinary allergy extracts for dust, molds, foods, pollen and chemicals could interfere with a child's physical health, causing hay fever, asthma and itchy skin. In addition, this form of allergy testing would also suddenly change their ability to write, draw, read, think, speak, walk or act appropriately. Treatment with these same extracts, in a different dilution, typically eliminated or neutralized these provoked symptoms in minutes. Thousands of videos of single blinded allergy tests were taken of children and adults during routine office hours for over 25 years that repeatedly documented these changes.[25a,b] Parents often commented on how their child's ability to concentrate improved in hours to days after they began treatment with the substances to which they were sensitive.

In addition to the above-mentioned obvious memory and learning changes, it was also possible to repeatedly document on videos, what was also noted in animal studies. The slightest stress, at times, could suddenly precipitate significant alterations in activity or behavior. This often happened when a child was being tested for some item that caused behavior problems at home or school. Removing a child's shoes or simply saying "no" while testing for a problem allergenic substance or chemical could easily and repeatedly trigger a dramatic, sudden hyperactivity response in a previously quiet youngster. These types of responses would occur in less than 10 minutes after an injection of one drop of an allergy skin test extract, and a drop of a weaker solution of the *same* substance would eliminate a child's heightened activity level or the sudden onset of inappropriate behavior in less than ten minutes.[25a,c]

When samples of common items that contain harmful chemicals (synthetic carpets, mattresses, etc.) were sent for a special bioassay test *(Chapter 3)* it was not unusual for some exposed mice to suddenly be unable to walk, climb or turn over. Others became withdrawn and untouchable. Some developed breathing problems, congestion, body swelling or rashes, aggression and some died. One video documents how these types of changes occurred within three to four hours after some mice merely breathed air blown over a synthetic carpet from a refurbished school.[25b,d] This laboratory has other videos showing these types of dramatic changes can occur in some mice exposed to school air, or other items, sometimes within 15 minutes. (*Anderson Lab: 802.295.7344.*)

Children who received environmental medical treatment generally were better to such a degree that it was clearly evident to parents, teachers and friends, as well as the other patients and parents or physicians who were in the office at the time of testing. Their academic performance, as well as their behavior and activity typically improved. Schools called to find out what drug had been prescribed, but the only change was an allergy diet, an air purifier and/or treatment with the correct dosage of an allergy extract.

Long term follow up of some of the most severely ill children showed that many of these youngsters surprised everyone by completing high school and college. It is highly doubtful this would have been possible without environmental medical treatment. When these children were initially seen, many were discouraged, confused, depressed, fearful and angry because they felt stupid, unwanted and unloved. Like their parents, they did not understand why they did not feel well, had intermittent or constant difficulty learning or acted so inappropriately at times. *(See Chapter 3.)*

Summary

A large number of wildlife research data and laboratory experiments, plus a growing number of human studies, support the probability that major disruptions in human intelligence and behavior can be caused by exposures to chemicals such as pesticides. These exposures can be minute and occur while in the uterus, as well as later on. The chemicals can affect learning, behavior (aggression, fatigue, hyperactivity, etc.), fertility and conceivably even parenting and mating behavior.[1h] The amazing aspect of all this is that there seems to be a lack of belief, appreciation and concern about a possible connection between the observations in animals to what is presently so clearly evident in humans. Obviously there is no one single answer, but pesticides and allergenic exposures certainly can explain *exactly* why many children and adults cannot remember or learn, and why they act, feel and behave as they do. In today's world the massive amount of chemical pollution is one neglected piece of the pie. This aspect appears to be much larger and more significant than most could imagine. One sensible answer appears not to be the need for another mind-altering overpriced drug, but recognition and elimination of the environmental causes of behavior and learning problems.

Chapter 4 References:

1 Colborn, Theo, Dianne Dumanski and John Peterson Myers, Our Stolen Future: Are We Threatening Our Fertility, Intelligence, and Survival? 1996, Penguin Books, Inc., New York, NY. Cost: $15.64.

1a pp. 190-97.
1b pp. 235-239.
1c pp. 186-194.
1d pp. 34.
1e pg. 158.
1f pp. 131-135.
1g Chapter 10.
1h pg. 232.
1j pp. 282-288.

2 Spyker, Joan, "Assessing the Impact of Low Level Chemicals on Development: Behavioral and Latent Effects. Current Status of Behavioral Pharmacology," Federation Proceedings, August 1975:34 (9)1835-1843.

3 Jett, D.A., et al., "Cognitive Function and Cholinergic Neurochemistry in Weanling Rats Exposed to Chlorpyifos," Toxicol. Appli. Pharm, , June 15, 2001:174(2) 89-98. Dept. of Health Science, John Hopkins. djett@ihsph.edw.

4a Daly, H., "Laboratory Rat Experiments Show Consumption of Lake Ontario Salmon Causes Behavioral Changes," J of Great Lakes Research, 1993: 19(4) 784 - 88.

4b Daly, H., "Reward Reductions Found More Aversive by Rats Fed Environmentally Contaminated Salmon," Neurotoxicology and Teratology, 1991:13, 449-53.

5 Jacobson, J., et. al., "Prenatal Exposure to an Environmental Toxin: A Test of Multiple Effects Model," Developmental. Psychology, 1984:20 (4) 523-32.

6 Tilson, H., et al., "Polychlorinated Biphenyls and the Developing Nervous System: Cross Species Comparisons," Neutotoxicology and Teratology, 1990:12, 239-48.

7a Porter, W. P., et al. "Endocrine, Immune and Behavioral Effects of Aldicarb (Carbamate), Atrazine (Triazine) and Nitrate (Fertilizers Mixtures At Groundwater Concentrations," Toxicology and Industrial Health, 1999:15 (1-2) 85, 133-150.

7b Midthun, Teresa, Interview with Dr. Warren Porter, University of Wisconsin Foundation, 1848 University Avenue, Madison, WI. 53706- 1992, from lecture at Santa Barbara, CA to group of environmentalists.
wporter@mhub.zoology.wisc.edu or http://www.wisc.edu/zoology/faculty/fac/Por/Por.html

7c Porter, W. P., et al., "Behavioral and Neurochemical Changes Associated with Chronic Exposure to Low-Level Concentrations of Pesticide Mixtures," Journal of Toxicology and Environmental Health, July 1990: 30 (3) 209-221.

7d Porter, W. P., et al., "Groundwater Pesticides: Interactive Effects of Low Concentrations of Carbamates Aldicarb and Methamyl and the Triazine Metribuzin on Thyroxine and Somatotropin Levels in White Rats," Journal of Toxicology and Environmental Health, September 1993: 40 (1)15-34.

7e Porter, W.P., et al., "Toxicant-Disease-Environment Interactions Associated with Suppression of Immune System, Growth, and Reproduction," Science, June 1, 1984: 224 (4652)1014-1017

8 Fagin, Dan and Marianne Lavelle, Toxic Deception, 1996, Center for Public Integrity. Birch Lane Press Book, pg. 16. Cost: $29.95 (paperback $12.57).

9 Colborn, Theo and Coralie Clement, Advances in Modern Environmental Toxicology, Chemically-Induced Alterations in Sexual and Functional Development: The Wildlife/Human Connection, 1992, Vol. XXI, Princeton Scientific Publishing Co., Inc., P. O. Box 2155, Princeton, NJ 08543. 609.683.4750.

9a Saal, Frederick S. von, et al., Chapters 3 and 10.

9b Chapter 3.

9c Chapter 10.

9d Chapter 13 and 14.

10a Porterfield, S. et al., "Vulnerability to the Developing Brain to Thyroid Abnormalities," Environmental Health Perspectives, l994102 (2)125-30.

10b "Thyroid Hormones and Neurological Development: Update l994," Endocrine Reviews, 1994:3(1) 357-363.

11 Deuble, L., et al., "Environmental Pollutants in Babies First Bowel Movement," April 2000, Dept. of Neonatology, Kirwan Hospital for Women, Townsville, Dept. of Pediatrics, Wayne State University, Michigan.

12 Chensheng, Lu, et al., "Biological Monitoring Survey of Organophosphorus Pesticide Exposure Among Pre-school Children in the Seattle Metropolitan Area," Dept. of Envir. Health, Univ. of Washington, Seattle, WA. Environmental Health Perspectives, March 2001: 109 (3) 1996.

13 Rice, Deborah C., Environmental Health Perspectives, June 2000:108(Supp 3) 405-408.

14 Porterfield, S. P., "Thyroidal Dysfunction and Environmental Chemicals-Potential Impact on Brain Development," Medical College of Georgia, Augusta, GA. sporterf@mail.mcg.edu,

15a Colborn, Theo, Ph.D. and Coralie Clement, Chemically-Induced Alterations in Sexual and Functional Development: The Wildlife/Human Connection, 1992, Volume XXI, pp. 358-9. Part of series, Advances in Modern Environmental Toxicology. Editor: M.A. Mehlman, Ph.D. Princeton Scientific Publication Co., Princeton, NJ.

15b pg. 5.

16 Journal of Pesticide Reform, Winter 2000: 20 (4)12-19.

17 Guillette, L., et al., "Developmental Abnormalities of the Gonad and Abnormal Sex Hormone Concentrations in Juvenile Alligators from Contaminated and Control Lakes in Florida," Environmental Health Perspectives, 1994: 102, 680-688.

18 Yu, M., et al., "Disordered Behavior in the Early-Born Taiwan Yucheng Children," Chemosphere, 1994: 29(9-11) 2413-2422.

19 Rogan, W., et. al, "Congenital Poisoning by PCBs and Their Contaminants in Taiwan," Science 1988: 241, 334-336.

20 Guillette, Elizabeth, et al., "An Anthropological Approach to an Evaluation of Preschool Children Exposed to Pesticides In Mexico," Environmental Health Perspectives, June 1998: 106 (6) 347-353.

21 National Health and Nutrition Examination Survey (NHANES 111, 1988-94).

22a National Resources Defense Council, "Toxic Chemicals and Health; Kids Health. In Depth Report: Trouble on the Farm- Growing up with Pesticides in Agricultural Communities" Chapter 6 "Confirming Exposure: Pesticides in Blood and Urine."

22b nrdc.org/health/kids/farm/chap6.asp no.

23a Hill, et al., "Pesticide Residues in Urine of Adults Living in the United States: Reference Range Concentrations," Environ Research. 1995: 71, 99108.

23b Hill, et al., "Residues of Chlorinated Phenols and Phenoxy Acid Herbicides in the Urine of Arkansas Children," Arch Environ. Contam. Toxicol., 1989: 18, 469-474.

24 Wong, Brad, "Pesticide traces found in kids here," Seattle Times, August 10, 2001.

25 Environmental Medical Research Foundation ERF (Formerly: PARF or Practical Allergy Research Foundation), P. O. Box 60, Buffalo, NY 14223-0060. 800.787.8780

25a Is This Your Child's World? 1996, Cost: $15.00 (plus S&H).

25b Environmentally Sick Schools, 85 minute video. Cost: $25.00 (plus S&H), Spanish video also available.

25c Video: Lanette, Dennis and Billy. Cost: $25.00 (plus S&H).

25d Video: Chemical Reactions in Children and Adults. Cost: $25.00 (plus S&H).

26 Greater Boston Physicians for Social Responsibility, In HARM'S Way: Toxic Threats to Child Development, January 2001. 11 Garden St., Cambridge, MA 02138. 617.497.7440.

26a pg. 54.

26b Chapter 6.

26c pg.49.

26d pp. 75-81.

27 Holene, E., et al., "Behavioral Effects of Pre and Postnatal Exposure to Individual Polychlorinated Biphenyl Congeners in Rats," Environ Toxicol Chem., 1995: 14(6):967-976.

28 Lilienthal, H. and G. Winneke, "Sensitive Periods for Behavioral Toxicity of Polychlorinated Biphenyls: Determination by Cross-Fostering In Rats," Fundament Appl. Toxicol., 1991:17, 368-375.

29 Zoeller, R. T., et al., "Developmental Exposure to Polychlorinated Biphenyls Exerts Thyroid Hormone-Like Effects on the Expression of RC3/Neurogranin and Myelin Basic Protein Messenger Ribonucleic Acids in the Developing Rat Brain," Endocrinal, 2000: 141, 181-189.

30 Porterfield, S., "Thyroidal Dysfunction and Environmental Chemicals-Potential Impact on Brain Development." Env. Health, Pers., June 2000: 108 (Suppl. 3) 433-8.

31 Ahlbo, M.J., A. Fredriksson, and P. Eriksson, "Exposure to an Organophosphate (DFP) During a Defined Period in Neonatal Life Induces Permanent Changes in Brain Muscarinic Receptors and Behavior in Adult Mice," Brain Res, 1995: 677, 13-19.

32a Crime Times, 1996: 2 (1) 4.

32b www.crime-times.org/96a/wd6op5.utm.

33 Rachel's Environment and Health News, #372 "PCBs Diminish Penis Size."

34 Gladen, B.C. and W.J. Rogan, "Effects of Perinatal Polychlorinated Biphenyls and Dichlorodiphenyldichloroethene on Later Development," J Pediatr, 1991: 119, 58-63.

35 Koopman-Esseboom, C., et al., "Effects of Dioxins and Polychlorinated Biphenyls on Thyroid Status of Pregnant Women and Their Infants," Pediatr Res., 36(4) 468-473.

36 Researchers at Cedars-Sinai Medical Centre to Present First Documentation of Man-Made Chemical Contaminants in the Amniotic Fluid of Unborn Babies, http://www.poptel.org.uk/panap/archives/ddtbabe.htm.

37 Garry, V., et al., "Birth Defects, Season of Conception, and Sex of Children Born to Pesticide Applicators Living in the Red River Valley in Minnesota, USA," Environ. Health Persp., 110 (supple.); J. Pesticide Reform, fall 2002: 22 (3) 9, 441-449.

38 Fenski, Richard A., et al., "Children's Exposure to Chlorpyrifos and Parathion in an Agricultural Community in Central Washington State," Environmental Health Perspectives, May 2002:110 (5).

39 Starr, H., et al., "Contribution of Household Dust to the Human Exposure to Pesticides," Pet Monit J., 1974: 8, 209-212.
40 Shealy, D., et al., "Correlation of Environmental Carbaryl Measurements with Serum and Urinary 1-Naphthol Measurements in a Farmer Applicator and His Family," Environ Health Persp., 1997: 105, 510-513.
41 Richter, E., et al., "Sequential Cholinesterase Tests and Symptoms for Monitoring Organophosphate Absorption in Field Workers and Persons Exposed to Pesticide Spray Drift," Tox. Lett., 1986: 33, 25-35.
42 Simcox, N., et al., "Pesticides in Household Dust and Soil: Exposure Pathways for Children of Agricultural Families," Envir. Health Persp., 1995: 103 (13) 1126-1134. Dept. of Env. Health, Univ. of Washington, Seattle, WA 98195.
43 Hestien, J.I., et al., "Effects of Perinatal Exposure to PCBs and Dioxins on Play Behavior in Dutch Children at School Age," Env. Health Perspect 2002:110, A593-A598.
44 Whyatt, R.M. and D.B. Barr, "Measurement of Organophosphate Metabolites in Postpartum Meconium as a Potential Biomarker of Prenatal Exposure: A Validation Study," Environmental Health Perspectives, 2001: 109(4) 417-420.
45 Manuel, John S., "Pondering on Pesticides: Long-Term Low Levels Impair Thinking," Environmental Health Perspectives, August 2001:109 (8).
46 "Why Do You Think They Call Them DIE-oxins?" Teen Source Endometriosis Association Newsletter, spring 2002.
47a "Paracelsus Revisited - Part 2," Rachel's Environment and Health News, October 31, 2002: (755).
47b Environmental Health Perspectives, October 2001:109 (10) 1063-1070.
48. Brucker-Davis, Francoise, et al., "Significant Effects of Mild Endogenous Hormonal Changes in Humans: Considerations for Low-Dose Testing," Environmental Health Perspectives, March 2001:109 (Supplement 1).
49 Padungtod, Chantana, Harvard School of Public Health, J Occup. Environ Med., 2000: 42, 982-992.
50 http://www.ourstolenfuture.org/NewScience/broadtrends.htm
51 Durnil, Gordon, The Making of a Conservative Environmentalist, 1995, Indiana University Press, Indianapolis, IN. Cost: $19.95.
52 The Pure Water Place, inc., 3347 Longview Blvd., Longmont, CO 80504. 888.776.0056. www.purewaterplace.com
53 Guillette, Elizabeth, "Hidden Exposures, Hidden Outcomes," International Symposium of Environmental Risk Assessment, Minamata, Japan, March 2002.

CHAPTER 5

Sex and Chemicals

As impossible as it seems, it is apparent that the many chemicals to which we are all exposed on a daily basis can alter the appearance and type of sex organs in animals and in unborn infants. [1a, 2, 3, 4] These chemicals, also, can diminish the ability of animals and man to reproduce as adults. Even sexual attitudes and preferences appear to be affected, mainly by the many synthetic chemicals that have a definite estrogenic or feminizing effect. Known hormonal disrupting chemicals include 209 PCBs, 75 dioxins and 135 furans, to name only a few. [1, 152] Of the 51 synthetic chemicals that have been identified as hormone disrupters, at least half, including PCBs, are persistent in our soil and water. These may prove to be a terrible legacy for the generations to come.[69, 140]

Can Pesticides Before Birth Affect the Size of the Genitals?[90]

The answer appears to be a definite yes. It is surprising to find how many studies and reports suggest the higher the concentrations of estrogenic-mimicking chemicals in animal or human tissues, the smaller the reproductive organs.[7, 27c, 28] Some of these changes, related to exposure to either low or high concentrations of chemicals while the young is developing in the uterus, can be evident at birth and others at puberty. Some of these effects apparently can last for a lifetime.[1j, 2, 3, 23, 70a-c, 79, 81, 91-98] Many aspects of sexuality are unquestionably determined long before birth. Exposure to the minutest amount of synthetic estrogenic-like pesticides, during very brief but critical periods prior to birth, appear to affect many aspects of a developing offspring, in particular, the reproductive and nervous system. *(See Chapter 4.)*

Natural Estrogen-Mimicking Substances

There are natural estrogenic-mimickers such as soy products called phytoestrogens. These appear to be better tolerated than the many synthetic chemicals found in so many of today's daily contacts. They are readily excreted from the body in one day in contrast to synthetic estrogens which tend to be stored in the body for years. Unfortunately, we simply do not know nearly enough about how either prenatal and postnatal or synthetic versus natural, estrogenic-mimicking chemicals affect animals or humans. Some of what is shared in this chapter certainly shows that this topic warrants immediate and serious consideration. In particular, the frequent use of soy formulas in infancy needs more evaluation. There is some concern because rat studies at the University of Birmingham indicate soy (genistein) damages the reproductive organs of males and the rat's ability to ejaculate. How does this same substance in human baby formulas affect infants?[182]

Without considering the immense, potentially adverse effects of chemically-engineered soy, the above indicates we must be much more cautious about exposures to both common natural estrogens and synthetic phytoestrogens until we have more information.[1i] (*See Chapter 9.*)

---

[*] *Can Chemicals Cause Epidemics?*, Doris J. Rapp, M.D. ERF, P. O. Box 60, Buffalo, NY 14223-0060, 800.787.8780, www.drrapp.com.

More about Synthetic Mimicking Substances[78, 99-111]

Synthetic feminizing chemicals are found in many pesticides, as well as in items containing phthalates or isophenols. Phthalates appear to cause infertility and feminizing effects in some male animals. In human females, there is evidence they cause precocious puberty.[78, 99-111]

Phthalates are found in plastic items such as toys and food wraps, some disposable diapers and fingernail polish. Up to 80% of plastic linings in food cans can release this estrogenic hormonal substance.

The polycarbonate plastics found in baby bottles and water jugs are also suspect. How many plasticizers leave baby bottles and enter the milk formula, especially after microwaving? One preliminary study shows chemicals can leave plastic wrap and enter oil that is microwaved.[144] Even the tiny amounts of chemicals released from plastic test tubes appear to be enough to interfere with some animal research because of their potent hormonal effects. The bottom line, how do these minute amounts of plasticizers affect bottle-fed infants?

Consider for a moment the increasing number of foods and beverages sold in plastic containers. Other stored items, such as cheese, can and do absorb the chemicals from plastic wrapping material. If you microwave the plastic covered foods, the effect is even greater.

We must ask if the chemicals in plastic coated infant mattresses and crib guards are safe.[75] How safe are the hospital plastic bags and tubing used for intravenous fluids? These can be stored for months in hot warehouses before their use in hospitals to administer intravenous fluids and medicines.[75, 134] They are less expensive and bulky than glass, but how safe are they when potentially harmful chemicals leak into the contents?[75a-c]

As indicated above, the many daily exposures to phthalates and other feminizing chemicals, such as certain pesticides, can potentially have extensive sexual effects. (See companion book, *Can Chemicals Cause Epidemics?)*[*]

What is the Evidence of a Need for Concern?

In an organized manner, let us look at the evidence in relation to sexual concerns noted in many forms of wildlife and then look at how the unborn, infants, children and adults appear to be affected. We must ascertain exactly how and in what ways these chemicals can change humans and their offspring.

Studies of the Estrogenic Effects of Chemicals in Animals [2, 3, 5a,b, 6a]

Many scientists are now becoming more vocal about the extent of the hormonal effects of estrogen-mimicking pesticide exposures in animals. In general, these chemicals make the male offspring more effeminate and the female animals more masculine, assertive and aggressive.[76] Due to the lag time between exposure and illness, the full effects of pesticides and other chemicals on today's animals (or children) may not be recognized for many years.

The ultimate effects depend upon the amount, frequency, timing and specific types of chemical exposures. Some relatively new and most disturbing aspects of this problem are illustrated in the following examples:

In Alligators[1c, 5a, 8, 42]

- There was a chemical spill of dicofol, similar to DDT, in Lake Apopka in 1980. A few years later, growing numbers of young male alligators were noted to have deformed penises and abnormal testes. In some, the penises were only one third normal size, and in addition, sperm movements or motility were abnormal. The males had lower testosterone levels than normal, while both the males and females had elevated estrogen levels. The bodies of the male and female alligators contained an excessive amount of a DDT-like substance. Some of the alligators had both male and female sex organs. The females laid abnormal eggs and had difficulty reproducing. During research studies, some alligator eggs were painted with estrogen. This caused the eggs not to hatch and if they did, the offspring were mainly females.

It is known that common pesticides have been reported to cause a feminizing effect in male animals. In addition reports indicate that infertility, significantly smaller male sex organs, hormone changes and testicular cancer can occur. If this is happening in male animals, why are these chemicals continuing to be used in and around children in schools or anywhere else? While we wait for more scientific studies, why can't we use the safer pest control measures that are already known and readily available?[166]

In Mice [9]

- A 1999 study in a selenium polluted area in Kesterson National Wildlife Reserve in Merced County, California showed some significant changes in mice. It was found that 25% to 50% of field, house and deer mice and voles had both male and female reproductive organs. In 1995 only 3% had this problem.[9] Could the selenium, the extensive use of pesticides or other forms of pollution in the soil in this area be related to this change in the mice in this area? What about other areas of the country where selenium is present or pesticides are used heavily? What about the humans who live there? We need more research.

- In one report, mice were given synthetic estrogen. They developed testicular cysts, non-descended testes and abnormal sperm.[165]

- Another study in mice revealed that mice exposed after birth to soy, a known common and supposedly safe plant form of an estrogen-mimicker, developed uterine cancer later in life.[1i] The dosage of the natural plant estrogen in the soy (genistein) was at the same level as found in a soy formula.[14] Are soy fed infants at risk later in life? We simply don't know.

- In one report, Dr. C. Barratt, an authority on reproductive medicine from Birmingham University, claimed mouse sperm is less sensitive to female sex hormones than human sperm. The fundamental question remains: How dangerous are extremely low levels of estrogenic mimicking chemicals in relation to human sperm?[112]

In Rats[2, 10]

- Chemical emissions from diesel fuel were found by Japanese researchers to cause young male and female rats to become masculinized and male sperm counts to drop as much as 33%. The testis, ovaries and thymuses of exposed pregnant rats were altered. These exposures caused progesterone levels in pregnant mother rats to drop, while their testosterone levels rose sharply.[10a, 146]

  Again, we cannot directly extrapolate this information to humans. It is obvious that studies should be conducted to ascertain exactly what does happen to infants, children and adults, and especially pregnant females, when they are exposed to heavy diesel fumes. Possible exposures include expressways near homes, schools, office buildings and factories, or from simply riding in diesel cars or trucks. [2, 10a, 43]

- Three new studies have shown that as little as one dose of dioxin in the form of TCDD in pregnant rats causes the male offspring to have low sperm counts, smaller penises and testicles, low testosterone levels, delayed testicular descent and feminine sexual behavior as adults.[27c] The effects were 100 times greater in unborn rats in comparison to similar exposures when they were sexually mature.

- Tests have shown that even though certain toxic chemicals can eliminate 99% of a rat's sperm, they can still reproduce. *(Humans, by comparison, are inefficient breeders and require much more than 1% sperm for successful fertilization.)*[1f]

- In other studies, the sperm of rats, mice and rabbits were 80% to 85% normal. In sharp contrast, other studies suggest that humans sperm are only 15% normal [70a-c]

- A single dose of dioxin, a chlorinated chemical that is not a hormone mimicker, administered during pregnancy can permanently reduce the sperm counts in rats by about 60%.[48] Low doses of either dioxin or PCBs have been reported to cause significant changes in sperm counts. *(See Chapters 4, 6, 7, 8.)*

- In one study, estrogenic chemical exposures caused changes in the mammary and pituitary glands, as well as in the brain structure of rats.[1b]

- Hexachlorobenzene, an insecticide and fungicide, is toxic to the ovaries of rats.[74, 113]

- It takes only 1/8 the dose of the chemical DBCP (dibromochloropropane) to cause infertility in a pubescent rat compared to a mature adult rat. *(This same chemical is reported to cause infertility in exposed adult male factory workers.)*[70a-c]

- In cellular research, a common pesticide, methoxychlor, has been shown to lower male testosterone in rats and decrease their fertility.[63]

- A estrogen-mimicking chemical, bisphenol A, causes early puberty in female rats and reduces fertility in rats.[5a,b, 78] In males it appears to cause enlargement in the male rat prostate glands.[78] We do not know if this chemical might be related to prostate cancer in humans.[5a,b]

- A chemical called nonyl phenyl ethoxylate can mimic estrogens and can cause inflamed vaginas, endometriosis and a decrease the sperm counts by as much as 10% to 20% in rats.[89a-d]

- It has been reported that malathion can cause breast cancer, testicular atrophy and stillborns in rats.[135, 157]

- In one report, when pregnant rats were fed malathion, their weanling rats were twice as susceptible to the effects of malathion as adults. *(See Chapter 8.)*[114]

In Fish[1e, 3b, 11]

- In one study, up to 100% of male fish living in fresh water in five of seven European countries had become feminized.[11] Affected fish had both male and female sexual organs. This was thought to possibly be due to the fact that the fish lived in water that contained female-mimicking chemicals downstream from the sewage waste or effluent that contaminated the water. *(See Chapter 6.)* The breakdown products of industrial detergents, alkyl phenols, phthalates and other so-called "inert" ingredients in pesticides also were suspect causes of these changes in the fish. If chemicals in concentrations of one to a billion, trillion or quadrillion can have effects on animals, what do these same or higher concentrations of exposure do to us?[48, 79, 80]

- About half the fish in Britain's lowland waters have sexual abnormalities. The male fish have testicles that contain eggs or other evidence of being hermaphrodites. About 33% of Britain's drinking water is taken from below the discharge area containing sewage. Their government and water agencies say no hormone-disrupting chemicals have been detected in their water supply. When German scientists, however, used more sophisticated and sensitive testing methods to test the water, they found 40% of it had tiny amounts of feminizing hormonal substances.[48] Little is known about the effects of these hormones on the offspring of pregnant women.

- In one study, male guppies exposed to certain pesticides in their food had shrunken testes, lower sperm counts and severe disruptions in their male courtship behavior. The effects were evident at low levels of exposure.[81] The biological effects were surprisingly magnified at lower rather than higher doses

- The Great Lakes region contains fish with high PCB and DDT levels due to contamination of the water. Some of the terns and gulls that eat these fish become hermaphrodites, having both male and female sex organs. Their male offspring are feminized. *(The Great Lakes contains 20% of all the fresh water on earth and it is a vast and badly polluted ecosystem.)* [23]

- Nonyl phenyl ethoxylates in plastics are reported to mimic estrogens causing decreased fertility and sperm counts in fish.[89a-d]

In Salmon[1c, 1e, 17, 42, 65]

- The salmon in Lake Erie presently show evidence of early puberty and a loss of their secondary sexual characteristics. They have markedly enlarged thyroids, as do the gulls that eat them. There are so many chemicals in the Great Lakes it is difficult to pinpoint the specific culprits, but estrogenic effects of certain pesticides are once again a prime suspect.[23, 42]

- In the pesticide-contaminated Columbia River, 84% of the Chinook salmon offspring appear to be females.[1c, 7, 65]

In Guinea Pigs[42]

- In 1985, the EPA found that when female guinea pigs were

exposed to a common fungicide, they adopted masculine behaviors, including mounting other females when they were in estrus or heat.

In Panthers[1c, 19]

- In 1989, Florida panthers were discovered to have so many serious health problems that they could not reproduce. Their sperm were abnormally shaped and lower than normal in amount. Up to 67% had atrophied testicles and many were sterile. They had weakened immune systems, excessive infections and malfunctioning thyroids. Some males were found to have very high levels of estrogen and low levels of testosterone. Their fat contained DDE, DDT, PCBs and mercury. The changes are so extensive there is concern that this animal is about to become extinct.

In Monkeys

- A study on monkeys found that dioxin exposures in concentrations of five parts per trillion could cause endometriosis and immune system defects. This is about as much as a teaspoon of this chemical in an Olympic-sized swimming pool.[80]

In Dogs[27d,e,i, 153]

- Reports claim that Vietnam scout dogs used to detect landmines in the Agent Orange sprayed soil were approximately twice as likely to develop atrophy, cancer or degeneration of their testicles, as well as lowered sperm counts than non-exposed dogs.[27d]

- Malathion and the antibiotics in the tetracycline category also are reported to cause testicular atrophy and decreased sperm quality in dogs and humans.[271] *(See Chapter 8.)*

In Rabbits

- The plasticizer, nonyl phenol ethoxylate, can cause inflamed vaginas in rabbits and appears to be able to alter their secondary sex characteristics and behavior.[89a]

In Gulls [3e, 27a,b, 42, 59, 60]

- In the Great Lakes the male offspring from eggs of gulls that were exposed to DDT had deformed genitals and were feminized. The female offspring had genital malformation, growth retardation and deformities. The chick mortality was higher than normal.[3e]

- In another report the male gulls had female ovaries which were thought to be due to high DDT exposures when the gull eggs were developing.[59]

- Studies by Dr. Michael Fry at the University of California on Santa Barbara Island showed that female to female pairing or "lesbian" gulls became more apparent as the male gulls, with smaller than normal genitals, showed progressively less interest in the females.[42, 60]

In Bald Eagles and Birds[1c, 18]

- The higher the levels of DDE and PCBs in their bodies, the less capable the bald eagles are of breeding successfully. Other birds appear to be similarly affected.

In Frogs[1b, 12]

- Although many factors were considered in relation to the innumerable deformities found in frogs in Vermont and Michigan in the 1990s, pesticides remain a prime suspect. Some of the frogs lacked legs, eyes, spines and intestines.

Others had deformed bladders and sexual abnormalities including smaller than normal sex organs. The chemicals atrazine, diazanon, methoprenediuron, dithane and temephos have all been linked to these types of disturbing changes.[12] Atrazine is the most widely used herbicide in the United States. *(See Chapters 5, 6, 8.)* It has been associated with sexual abnormalities, including demasculization of male frogs in concentrations of 0.1 parts per billion which is 1/30th the amount that is allowed in your drinking water by the EPA.[48, 79]

In Turtles

- When turtle eggs are painted during experimental research with PCBs, the male hatchlings become females, complete with ovaries.

In Polar Bears[1c, 1d, 7, 13, 14]

- In Norway, some female bears have stunted male penises and damaged immune systems when they swim in water contaminated with PCBs (polychlorinated biphenyls) and other chemicals.[7, 14]

In Beluga Whales[1c, 15, 16]

- These whales in the St. Lawrence River have been studied extensively. Those living in contaminated water were found to have a number of sexual and other serious medical problems. DDT, PCBs and mercury were found in their body fat. Some were hermaphrodites with both testis and ovaries. Some had stomach ulcers, cysts on their thyroids, bladder cancer and evidence of excessive infection. They were less able to reproduce. It was discovered that the affected whales had ingested chemically-contaminated fish. The fish, living in the same chemically polluted water, also have the same types of medical illnesses, as is increasingly evident in the whales and even in humans who drink the same water.

In Seals[1c 20]

- The decrease in the ability of the seals to reproduce has been correlated to the level of PCBs in the contaminated water. In addition, these female seals are reported to have more tumors and uterine abnormalities.

In Otters[1c, 21]

- The testes of the otters in the Columbia River in Portland, Oregon are much smaller than normal. The penises can be a third normal size. The most affected otters have the highest levels of PCBs, heptachlor, mirex and dioxin-like chemicals in their tissues.[1c, 7]

In Deer

- A number of studies report that as many as 67% of deer have abnormal genital development. Their offspring tend to be skewed towards a preponderance of males. The possible suspect cause is again exposure to some feminizing endocrine disrupting pesticide or chemical.[82]

In Sheep[150]

- One report found malathion exposure in pregnant ewes appeared to be related to aborted fetuses, stillbirths and low birth weight offspring.[115] *(This is one of the chemicals repeatedly sprayed in NYC to help control mosquitos and the West Nile virus.) (See Chapter 8.)*

- Many animals eat plants that make or contain estrogens. Estrogen-rich clover is reported to cause increased miscarriages and infertility in sheep.[150]

In Pigs

- Moldy, estrogen-rich corn causes uterine overgrowth in pigs. It can feminize males, stop ovulation and produce infertility.[150]

Summary of Effects of Feminizing Chemicals on Animals[150]

It appears that low levels of estrogenic-mimicking chemicals before birth can certainly affect the fertility, genital type, size, development, sperm count, testosterone levels and sexual appearance and behavior in many forms of wildlife. There is also evidence that the higher the levels of chemicals in the environment and body tissues, the more certain types of changes will become evident in animals. Humans are breathing the same polluted air and drinking the same chemicals in their own water supply. We have no idea about the degree to which all of the above applies to humans, but in view of the seriousness of the changes, we surely need to find out. The following observations and studies in humans indicate definite reasons for immediate concern.

Studies of the Estrogenic Effects of Chemicals in Humans[70a-c]

Sexual Concerns in the Unborn[86b, 177]

We do know an unborn human is particularly vulnerable during certain brief, critical periods of intrauterine development, especially at about 20 days and again at about seven weeks after conception. This can occur before most females know for certain they are pregnant. Researchers believe the male urinary and genital systems are particularly vulnerable to damage in the womb shortly before and after birth.[1a, 2, 45] Brief exposure to feminizing chemical hormones during these small windows of time can cause some most surprising and dramatic lifetime changes in the unborn or newborn of many forms of wildlife, including humans.[1a, 2, 3] Similar to animals, some of these effects may not become apparent until puberty or adulthood.[45] Again, it is apparent that prenatal exposure of animals to feminizing pesticides or chemicals (dioxin or PCBs) appears to cause more feminine activity in male offspring and more masculine activity in females.[77] There are even a few reports suggesting that exposure in one generation can affect future generations.[35, 168-171]

> **What we are doing to our unborn and infants is so sobering that I personally believe we are unknowingly guilty of monumental infant and child abuse.**

Consider the following:

- The fluid in which an unborn baby floats and is totally immersed, inside and outside, for nine months can contain one to several pesticides. One study showed one third of the unborn babies floated in intrauterine fluid that contained DDT, lindane and PCBs. DDT can interfere with the reproductive system's biochemical pathways. PCBs have been linked to birth defects and problems with the thyroid and learning disabilities. Both DDT and PCBs can damage nervous and immune systems.[53a-c, 72a,b]

- In another study in June 1999, researchers confirmed the presence of DDE (a breakdown product of DDT) and PCBs in 30% of the uterine fluid of pregnant American and Canadian mothers.[72a]

- One chemical called DBP or dibutyl phthalate is reported to cause severe birth defects in animals and sexual problems in human males. This chemical is used by females in shampoos, cosmetics, sunscreens, hair preparations, antiperspirants and especially in nail polish.[48] Many young married women paint nails in beauty parlors and, along with any others who have hair appointments, breathe many toxic fumes for hours. Most beauty salons have little to no protection in the form of ventilation or air purification systems.[48] We must wonder what effect this can have on the unborn of young women who are exposed.

Sexual Concerns In Infants

- The infant's first bowel movement, prior to any oral feeding, has been reported to contain the same chemicals or pesticides found in the uterine fluid, including several of those banned in the 1970s.[55]

- A mother's breast milk typically contains these same chemicals.[54, 143, 151]

- Some disposable diapers contain chemicals such as plastics in the form of bisphenols, nonyl phenols and sodium polyacrylate. Nonyl phenols are a family of chemicals that are known to affect sexual development, secondary sexual characteristics and reproduction. These are known to feminize males and reduce fertility in laboratory animals.[84, 89a-d] In addition some diapers also contain another chemical, polypropylene, to keep the urine from touching the baby's skin. *(Polypropylene is also used as a plastic in food containers so they are safe in dish washers and as a fiber to make indoor/outdoor carpets. Tushies make disposable diapers that contain no plastics, gels, chlorine, dioxin or polyacrylates. They use polyethylene which is not a plasticizer in their diapers.[84, 89a-d])*

- Professor Wolfgang Sippell at the University of Kiel, Germany has found that exposure to plastic in disposable diapers can significantly raise the temperature of the scrotal area for prolonged periods of time. He theorizes this might be one factor related to the decrease in male fertility in the past 25 years. Cotton diapers do not have this effect.[85a,b, 134]

(When I was in practice in Buffalo in the 1980s and 1990s, some mothers had the "impression" that their son's genitals seemed to shrink when they wore disposable diapers in contrast to their more normal appearance when cotton diapers were used. This anecdotal "impression" proves nothing until it is documented scientifically, but maybe the testis contracted in synthetic diapers to protect that area. It might provide valuable insight to conduct a study comparing adult sexuality of men who wore disposable diapers during infancy versus those who wore cotton diapers during their first few years of life.)

- Some infant baby foods contain pesticides.[73a-b] Natural varieties are available. (*See Pregnancy and Fertility sector later in this chapter.*)

Sexual Concerns in Children

- A 30% to 40% increase in abnormal placement of the opening of the penis or hypospadias, non-descended testicles *(located in the abdomen rather than the scrotum)* and bisexuality or feminization of males has occurred in the past 30 to 40 years.[5ab] These types of changes are evident in European countries, as well as in the United States.[67]

- In Denmark, it has been reported that approximately 5% of boys have testicles that are not descended into the scrotum. Nearly 1% have some abnormality in the formation of the penis. In addition, over 40% have subnormal sperm counts when they grow up.[48]

- A study published in 2000 revealed a strong association between non-descended testicles in boys and the presence of two organochloride chemicals (like DDT) stored in their fat tissues.[1j]

- Groups of boys exposed in the uterus to PCBs or dioxin were reported to have smaller penises than normal.[23, 27a, 48, 116]

- In another report from Yucheng, Formosa, pregnant women who were accidentally exposed to PCBs and furans had offspring that had smaller than normal penises and increased behavioral problems.[23, 25a-b,27a ,b, 28, 116, 117*]

- The sons of Michigan women whose breast milk contained the flame-retardant chemicals (TRIS or PBB) had a higher incidence of testicular abnormalities and smaller penises than normal.[23]

- Between 1948 and 1971, many pregnant women who took DES (diethylstilbestrol) to prevent spontaneous abortions gave birth to girls who had genital abnormalities and boys who had abnormally small penises.[1a] (*Dioxin has had a similar estrogen-like effect on the males born to exposed pregnant rats.*)

- Some research indicates that if pregnant women are exposed to PCBs, their sons can have a diminished penis size, and children of both sexes can have an array of other genital, hormonal, and immune system abnormalities, as well as cancer.[1, 118]

If these sorts of problems are evident in the unborn, infants and children, what can happen when these youngsters grow up? Hormone-disrupting chemicals have been found in human blood, urine, feces, breast, fat, semen, ovarian tissue and oviducts.[56, 147] *(See Chapter 6.)* Keep asking yourself if you should be concerned not only about what these chemicals can do to children, but what are they doing to you and possibly to future generations.

A Possible Source for Reliable Answers Regarding Children

An outstanding study by Dr. Elizabeth Gillette observed two select groups of children. One was exposed and the other essentially not exposed to pesticides over a number of years.[119a,b]

The degree to which these children might have been adversely affected sexually by pesticide exposures as they matured unfortunately was not part of this original study. Unfortunately, this type of research requires funding that is not typically available from regular sources. With additional funding, a continuation of this study might provide immense valuable and reliable insight because these well-studied children are now approaching pubescence.[119a,b] *(See Chapters 3, 4.)*

Sexual Concerns in Human Females

Infant Deaths

- In 1988, 600,000 women experienced a miscarriage or fetal death, but the cause was not always clear. In 1999, seven of every 1000 American babies did not live. This is more than twice the mortality found in Hong Kong. The infant mortality rate in the United States is ranked 28th when compared to most other countries. Why?

- Pesticides are suspected as a possible cause of the Washington Shoalwater Bay Indian tribe's 50% rate of stillbirths and miscarriages. In one report in 1998, eight of nine pregnancies terminated in the loss of the infant.[136]

- One study indicated that if women are exposed to pesticides for one month, during the first three months of their pregnancy, they have a 70% increased risk of having a stillborn baby. Similar findings were noted if they were exposed to home insecticides used to control ants or roaches early in their pregnancy.[88b]

- Some women who have elevated levels of pentachlorophenol (from wood preservatives, leather upholstery and carpets) or lindane (from lice treatment preparations) in their blood are

---

* *Can Chemicals Cause Epidemics?*, Doris J. Rapp, M.D. ERF, P. O. Box 60, Buffalo, NY 14223-0060, 800.787.8780, www.drrapp.com.

more apt to have habitual abortion, unexplained infertility, menstrual disorders and premature menopause.[120, 127]

Breast Milk

Breast milk appears to store toxic substances.[147, 27b] Females tend to concentrate chemicals in their breast milk. This appears to possibly be one of nature's ways to help females excrete excessive amounts of chemicals from their bodies.

- In 1976, 25% of the human breast milk was contaminated with chemicals.[162]

- In 1998, Japan's breastfed babies ingested six times the daily tolerated amount of dioxins. Dr. H. Miyata at Setsunan University is reported to have advised mothers to stop breast-feeding at three months of age. It was even reported that Japan suggested that contaminated breast milk be treated as a toxic waste.[163]

Breast Fat

- Women who have DDE (a breakdown product of DDT) in their breast fat appear to have a four times greater risk of developing breast cancer than women whose fat is free of chemicals.[122]

Breast Cancer Studies[156a-d]

Breast cancer is another full-blown epidemic as discussed in more detail in the companion book, Can Chemicals Cause Epidemics?* The incidence has doubled in the past fifty years. One woman is diagnosed with this illness every three minutes and one dies from this disease every 12 minutes.[149] Breast cancer was uncommon early in 1900 but it affected one in 20 by 1960. It has increased by 1% each year since World War II.[123] Statistics now indicate that as many as one in two or three women will develop breast cancer in her lifetime.[83]

A family history of genetically prone breast cancer explains only 10% of this problem. Radiation before puberty is said to account for another 50%. There is evidence suggesting the remaining 40% can be linked to estrogen-mimicking pesticides, such as dieldrin.[36-38]

Possible Chemical Causes of Breast Cancer[156a-d]

- Breast cancer is supposedly five times more common in women who have the organochloride, DDT, in some form in their blood or stored in their breast fat. It is reported to be seven times more common if the fungicide, HCB (hexachlorobenzene), is in that tissue. The scientists are correct, that this does not conclusively prove a cause and effect relationship but it does suggest there is a connection.[178] Read about some other evidence, however, and see what you think.

- In one study, breast cancer was associated with elevated blood levels of DDE, but not PCBs, implicating organochloride chemicals.[15]

- Industrial chemicals have been connected to the increased incidence of breast cancer in both females and males.[27b]

- Breast cancer was reported in Germany to be elevated two fold in women who worked in factories exposing them to dioxin.[143]

- Women living near organochloride chemical plants in Minnesota were found to have significantly higher levels of breast cancer.[90, 143, 172a, b]

- The incidence of breast cancer in Long Island, NY is 27% higher than in the rest of the country. One suspect factor is the pesticides used to grow potatoes in that area. Another is the organochloride chemical plants in that area.[143]

- Professional chemists, hair dressers and those who use hair dyes are also at a greater risk of developing breast cancer.[143,164]

- Our bottom line is not so much proving to scientists that a cause and effect relationship exists, but what can we do now to eliminate the cause of this terrible illness. Well, surprisingly, the proof that it can be done is exemplified in one outstanding but rarely quoted Israeli study. It provides evidence that it is definitely possible to diminish breast cancer by decreasing pesticide exposure.[37] Israel had the same high incidence of breast cancer affecting older and younger women as 28 other countries prior to 1976. Some astute women convinced their negative legislative authorities to limit the use of a few chemicals that they believed might be causing the problem. Between 1976 and 1985, while other countries had a 20% rise in breast cancer, in Israel, it fell by 8%! In the youngest age group the drop was 34%, as opposed to the expected rise of 20%.[37, 143] The three organochlorides that were banned were alpha-benzene hexachloride (BHC), lindane (gamma benzene hexachloride) and DDT. These were heavily used in cowsheds in Israel and contaminated their milk and milk products. This Israel study confirmed the animal experiments done in the 1960s that suggested that organochlorides were associated with breast cancer in rats.

For over 30 years it has been known that organochlorides concentrate in animal and human fat tissue.[143] DDT, HCB, dioxin and atrazine all contain chlorine. Organochlorides are also found in herbicides, detergents, spermicidal foam, polychlorinatedbiphenols (PCBs), paper, polyvinylchlorides (PVCs), lubricants and plastics. Every woman should be made more aware of the importance of strict avoidance of these types of products so they can try to reduce their chances of developing this horrible illness.[151] We must influence our legislators to listen and act, as the women did in Israel. Maybe we can decrease breast cancer in the United States.

Endometriosis

- In 1934, only 21 cases of endometriosis existed in the entire world but now this illness, which causes infertility, affects as many as five million women in the United States alone.[122]

- High levels of PCBs have been found in the blood of German women who have endometriosis.[116]

- Female monkeys exposed to high doses of dioxin were found to develop endometriosis.[116, 118, 179a,b]

Again we have more questions than answers. We need to know exactly how low dose, short-term exposures of dioxin affect humans? How are so many women exposed to dioxin and why does the genital tract seem to be so vulnerable? Maybe it is related to the dioxin that is supposedly used to bleach some tampons and sanitary products to make them white. Again, in this regard, the answers are unclear because the literature provides conflicting information.[158, 159, 160*] *(See Chapter 6.)*

Sexuality of Female Offspring

- One study indicated that a female needs only one exposure to a pesticide at a critical stage during her pregnancy to adversely affect the sexuality of her offspring.[121]

- Other investigations in humans suggest that anxieties, phobias and other behavioral changes, in addition to many reproductive and sexual problems, are possible after exposure of female offspring to estrogen-like substances. *(See Chapter 4.)*

- Extremely weak amounts of estrogen can cause surprisingly dramatic changes and totally different responses than those noted from higher concentrations in both animals and man.[150]

- Androgens or male hormone exposures also play a role but these appear to be less well studied than the effects of estrogens.

Sexual Concerns In Human Males

1h,6b,27f,29-31,47,48, 57, 61, 64, 68, 70a-c

Sperm Counts and Infertility

- The numbers vary, but there is absolutely no doubt that the sperm counts have dropped precipitously in the last 60 years. In many industrialized countries the sperm count has dropped by 50%, both in quantity and quality, in the past 50 years. Some reports say the drop in the sperm count has been decreasing as much as 2% per year for the past 20 years.[48]

- Although data is sparse in the Third World and Africa, subnormal sperm counts appear to be a worldwide problem.[48]

- The average male sperm count decreased from about 120 million per milliliter (M/ml) in 1938 to 20 to 80 M/ml or less by 1991.[48]

- In one report, the sperm count of 30-year-old males in 1975 was 102 million/ml.[140] In another report in 1992, the sperm count of 30-year-old males was said to be only 51 million/ml. If this trend continues, by 2005 the count is estimated to be 32 million. This is only 25% as high as the sperm count was in males born in 1925.

- There is genuine concern that males will be sterile in 65 to 80 years unless this trend is stopped.[48, 64]

- In one report, there was a three-fold increase in infertility in men whose sperm counts are below 20 million/milliliter. This means their fertility is severely jeopardized and conceiving a child will be most difficult when the sperm count reaches this level. When counts reach five million per milliliter or fewer, men are considered to be sterile.[48]

- It is presently thought that about 85% to 90% of the human male population would not be eligible as sperm donors because their counts are too low. This is in contrast to hamsters in whom only 15% of their sperm counts are dangerously low.[48] In addition, the average man has only 1/3rd as many sperm as a hamster.[33, 42, 48]

- Scientists worldwide are now aware there is not only a decrease in the quantity of sperm, but also in the quality. It is estimated that about 85% of sperm produced by healthy humans can be DNA-damaged.[33]

- About 50 different pesticides have been linked to reproductive problems.[140]

- Male sperm can be genetically altered for 90 days from one pesticide exposure.[27b]

- Chinese workers in an organophosphate pesticide factory had less active and decreased sperm. A later study showed these men also had decreased testosterone.[128]

- In 1,000 Chinese men, one report claimed only 20% had a sperm count in the range that was considered to be highly fertile.[48]

- Men who work as printers, painters, builders, beauticians, decorators and anesthesiologists are at risk because of their occupational exposure to organic solvents such as glycol ethers, toluene, xylene, and benzene. A decrease in sperm counts has been correlated with the degree of solvent exposure and similar findings have been noted in animals.[47, 129]

- A small study has shown that men's aftershave, shampoos, cologne and hair products cause breakdown products of phthalates (DBP) to be found in their urine and semen.[33, 147] These substances are suspect causes of decreased sperm production and birth defects in animals and man.[13, 130, 147, 164] Immense loopholes in laws allow unlimited amounts of known toxic substances to continue to be included in many cosmetic products used on a daily basis.[48, 137]

- One study showed that farmers exposed to the herbicide 2,4-D had sperm that were less active, less able to swim, more deformed and fewer in number than non-exposed farmers.[27d,i, 47]

- Another study showed 2,4-D, in the most minute concentrations can pass into a female during intercourse and go directly into the fertilized egg.[125,147] This means from the moment of fertilization, it is possible for a chemical that can damage the brain, nervous, immune, endocrine and reproductive systems to be present. Should we be worried?

How low will the human sperm count have to drop before we become concerned enough to do something about it? [1h, 6b, 29-31, 47, 48, 57, 61, 64, 68, 70a-c]

Why Are Sperm Counts Dropping?

Chemicals are again major suspect causes of the decline of sperm in both quantity and quality.[1h] Some of this drop has been attributed to marijuana, cocaine, alcohol and sexually transmitted diseases, but many forms of wildlife are manifesting similar problems reproducing.[150] They don't drink alcohol, use narcotic drugs or smoke. The sexual problems in men do not appear to be confined to any particular country. The major causes appear to be pesticides, herbicides and fungicides in the water, air and food. Specific major offenders include dioxin, PCBs, solvents such as benzene, xylene, toluene, trichloroethylene (cleaning solution, spot removers), ethylene glycol (in paints, printer's ink and paint thinners), vinyl chloride (plastic, PVC pipes), acetone (nail polish), phenol (common disinfectant cleaning products), phthalates (plastics), heavy metals, personal body care products (colognes, cosmetics, fingernail polish) and electromagnetic radiation.[48, 137] Other suspects include medications taken for birth control, other hormones and a wide variety of pills found in our sewage and regular drinking water.

Infertility and Sterility

- In the United States, one report stated infertility increased over 4% in the past forty years.[48]

- In China, one report states fertility problems affect 15% of married couples, 5% being due to male inadequacy.[48] Might this be related to the report indicating only eight of 46 major Chinese cities meet their own government's air and water pollution standards?

- It has been claimed that exposure of adult men to pesticides may alter not only their own fertility but the health of their newborn infants.[118]

- In June 1992, at a congressional hearing, the Assistant United States Surgeon General announced a study by NIOSH (National Institute for Occupational Safety and Health) found abnormally low levels of testosterone in the blood of the male workers exposed to high levels of dioxin.

- The pesticide DBCP (dibromochloropropane - a fumigant that kills worms) is said to have been conclusively proven to cause reproductive problems, not only in animals, but it is known to cause infertility in human males.[150]

- An expert panel found credible evidence that bisphenol A and the insecticide methoxyclor can cause reproductive damage at very low levels of exposure that are well below the so called "no effect" levels.[48]

- In one report infertility had risen from 0.5% to 25% in one cross-section study of college males.[27b, 116]

- In another report in April 2001, the infertility rate in Chinese university students was reported to be as high as 85%.[48]

- Infertility, sexual dysfunction and impotence was stated to affect 20% to 30% of Chinese males in one study.[48]

Male Sex Organs and Cancer[5a, 34, 48]

We do not know to what degree chemicals contribute to the marked increase in testicular and prostate cancer, but we do know: [5a, 34, 48]

- Cancer of the prostate has doubled in the past 50 years.[23]

- Testicular cancer now affects approximately 1% of men, mainly in young men under 30 years.[48]

- Testicular cancer has risen 66%, or tripled, in the past 50 years.[122]

- In England and Wales, testicular cancer increased 80% between the 1970s and the 1990s. Chemicals again are suspect.[48]

- In Denmark, they have noted a 300% to 400% increase in testicular cancer compared to fifty years ago.[5a]

- In the June 1992 Congressional meeting, Dr. Fingerhut reported that if workers were exposed to dioxin for at least a year, as long as 20 years ago, they developed 46% more cancer than the average U.S. male. An earlier report had suggested dioxin was only a weak human cancer-causing agent.[27h, 143]

- Increasing reports suggest that non-descended testicles and malformed or tiny penises are increasing in a number of countries.[48]

Sexual Problems in Male Veterans

- Many Gulf War veterans were exposed to a plethora of harmful chemicals.[126,154] The Gulf War Syndrome is complex because they were exposed to germs as well as chemicals in their clothing, in the air, inoculations of vaccines and hydrocarbons from space heaters in their sleeping areas. Many soldiers had symptoms of sensitivities to multiple chemicals and definite evidence of impaired neurological, musculoskeletal, respiratory, reproductive and immune function.[154] Common complaints included nausea, chronic fatigue, joint pains and body aches. These types of symptoms suggested that sensitivities to chemicals could be part of their problem. Preliminary information indicates that some of these individuals have been helped by environmental medical care. (*AAEM: 316.684.5500, Dr. William Rea 214.368.4132.)*

- Vietnam veterans showed a 2.5% increase in testicular cancer, compared with men who were not in Vietnam.[27d] A number of chemical exposures, including malathion, dioxin, 2,4- D and "inert" substances are thought to be at fault.[27g,i, 153, 180, 181] (*See Chapter 8.*)

- Twenty-some years after the war, some of Vietnamese soldiers continue to have dioxin (TCDD or tetrachlorodibenzo -p-dioxin) from Agent Orange in their semen.[118, 124, 148] Could this form of pollution be related to the findings of a questionnaire study of hundreds of U.S. veterans that indicated that their children had more evidence of impaired immune systems, severe and chronic infections, allergies, chemical sensitivities, asthma, learning and attention disorders, unusual mood swings, food reactions, cysts and cancer than normal?[118, 148]

- Could Agent Orange's dioxin be a factor in relation to the report that Vietnam veterans are reported to have 50% to 70% more birth-defective children than normal?[124, 174] The dioxin exposed Vietnamese have noted similar abnormalities in their offspring.[180, 181] Even more upsetting is the observation that the third generation of Viet Nam children now have evidence of possible dioxin-related birth defects.[180, 181] The water, soil and food in Viet Nam will be contaminated for many years.

- The offspring of American veterans and the Vietnamese exposed to chemicals appear to be inordinately sick with multiple medical complaints.[148, 154, 174] Their symptoms suggest possible food allergies and chemical sensitivities, as is typical of those who suffer from environmental illness. Some of these children appear to be classically allergic, but because the army surprisingly does not evaluate for allergies until a child is five years old, no official data is forthcoming. It is not unusual for allergies to begin early in infancy.[132b,c]

- Some veterans' wives are reported to complain of vaginal burning after intercourse and difficulties conceiving babies.[147, 161] Is it possible that the soldier's contaminated semen has chemically sensitized their wives? We don't know but that is possible.

- Maybe a damaged male-mediated genetic factor is also related to the inordinate number of congenital anomalies that are evident in some of the veteran's infants.

- The government has the capability to do SPECT brain imaging which can show characteristic changes after toxic chemical exposures.[139] If it is possible that veterans have evidence of abnormal brain function, why are they not being given this test?

We must ask: Are defective sperm one more missed reason for the increased infertility in the adult population? Can abnormal sperm be related in some way to the epidemic increases in birth defects, developmental delays and learning problems in children?[48] *

New Sexual Concerns

- It appears estrogenic-mimicking pesticides are one suspect cause of a marked increase in transexualism, or the feeling of being one sex but stuck in the body of the opposite sex.[59] Male to female transsexuals increased from one in 45,000 in 1980, to one in 18,000 by 1986, to one in 11,900 by 2001. These changes are possibly attributed to hormonal exposures, especially endocrine-disrupting chemicals such as pesticides and plastics.[59]

- If adult males are given estrogen, their gonads become smaller than normal and their testes shrink. It is also well-known that if either testosterone or progesterone is given to a pregnant woman, genital abnormalities such as pseudohermaphrodite changes can occur in their female offspring.

- In a study of eight to 10 year olds it was reported that the girls who were exposed to pesticides had less mammary tissue than normal, even though their breasts were well defined.[119b]

The best answer for the epidemic of sexual problems affecting humans is not psychotherapy, which is also needed, but prevention and avoidance. It is imperative to recognize and eliminate the cause, whenever possible. Until we know more, we should start by reducing chemical exposures of all types, as much as we can.

It appears that prenatal exposure to synthetic and natural estrogenic hormone disrupting chemicals are unquestionably capable of jeopardizing not only the survival of animal populations, but also the human race.[1h,k,150] The public urgently needs to know to what degree estrogenic mimicking and other pesticides influence our well-being. Could these be related to the upsurge of inappropriate behavior and activity, memory problems, muscle weakness and twitching, rages, violence and sexual problems in today's children and adults? The answer appears to be a definite yes.

The scope of adverse affects will not be easy to ascertain because the bottom line for too many is money and deception, not the health and future of our children, our human race and our planet. A recent report from Texas A and M contends that hormone-mimicking chemicals are not the cause of much that has been stated in this chapter.[173] Until we know more, you can decide for yourself if all the above reports in animals and man, from all over the world, are not at least enough to make you aware that you should become more cautious until we have more information.

It appears that miniscule exposures to feminizing hormone-like substances during brief critical windows or periods of time can cause significant changes in the sex organs of a developing fetus. Delayed effects can include changes in sexual attitudes and preferences. These changes might not become apparent until sexual activity begins in adolescence.

We Must Learn from Past Mistakes

Three reports of accidental exposures in humans in the past have clearly shown how harmful estrogenic-like chemicals can be when no one seems to be listening.

1.
The TRIS Flame Retardant Tragedies [22a, 23]

The tragedy of what happened to the sons of Michigan women whose breast milk was accidentally contaminated with an industrial flame retardant 2, 3-dibromopropylphosphate or TRIS is well-documented. The male offspring had a higher incidence of testicular abnormalities and smaller penises than normal.[23] In addition, TRIS exposure was associated with an increase in cancer and genetic defects.[22a, 24]

2.
More on Fire Retardants[141]

What about the effects of the fire retardant called polybrominated biphenyl or PBB on human female offspring and on cows? In a 1973 report in Michigan, this chemical was accidentally mixed in some animal feed.[141] This feed caused the cows to produce less milk and to have stillborn or deformed calves. The daughters of the exposed pregnant women, who drank milk from these animals that had been fed this contaminated feed, had early menses and puberty. The higher the PBB blood levels in the mothers, the more their daughters were affected. It is possible the offspring had a combined exposure from this chemical while in the uterus, as well as more PBB when they were breast fed.[109, 142]

3.
The DES (diethylstilbestrol) Tragedy[1a,g, 117]

About 60 years ago, the hormone estrogen in the form of DES, was frequently prescribed by physicians to prevent miscarriages. Few suspected that it might significantly affect the unborn offspring at birth, and certainly no one expected it might influence a child's future sexuality in adolescence and throughout adulthood.

At birth, and as some DES-exposed female offspring grew older, they were found to have a variety of serious congenital anomalies and deformities of their reproductive system.[27f] As adults, some had miscarriages, stillbirths, evidence of decreased fertility and some developed cancer of the vagina. In addition, about 24% of exposed female offspring reported bisexuality, homosexuality and/or depression by adulthood.[1a]

Some of the DES-exposed male offspring had non-descended and underdeveloped testicles at birth, stunted penises and, as adults, they were found to have abnormal sperm.[1a] DES did not appear to influence their adult male sexual orientation or preferences.[1g,e]

Warnings Regarding DES from Animals

The effects noted from this DES exposure parallels that which had been seen in wildlife and laboratory animals exposed to estrogenic-mimicking pesticides in the past.[1a,g, 22]

One major disappointment in relation to this drug is that scientists, physicians and politicians ignored clear-cut evidence that DES might prove to be a serious problem. No one spoke out.

- Research in 1939 with rat pups, many years before the human DES fiasco, indicated this hormone could cause severe reproductive tract abnormalities. DES was found to affect both female and male rat offspring [138, 167a,b]

- In the 1940s, pellets of DES were placed under the skin to fatten chickens and suppress the male hormone. It accomplished both purposes. The heads and intestines of these chickens were then used for mink food.[22d] The mink farmers reported what happened at the Congressional hearings in 1951. After mink were fed chicken parts containing DES as food, they noted these mink had hair loss and problems reproducing.[22b] *(Could hormones injected into our meat sources be one reason for the present increased hair loss, especially in human adult females?)*

- Studies in the 1940s in rats, mice and mink showed that DES in the feed to animals caused changes in the genitals of the newborns that survived. Hormonal chemicals in animals have also been shown to stimulate breast development and malignancies.[22d]

- The amazing fact is that DES continues to be allowed to be injected into food supplying animals at the present time. For this reason, organic meat is preferred. *(Why is hormone contamination of our meat allowed?*[143] *This suggests that we should possibly eat only organic meat, less fat and certainly less liver, because this is where hormone-affecting chemicals tend to be stored.*)

In many forms of wildlife, exposure to either too much estrogen or androgens at critical times in the development of females appears to cause aggression or increased masculine and less feminine behavior. [1g, 22b, 25] These types of changes in animals are similar to what is presently being seen in humans. Toxic pollutants can cause these types of complaints, especially if they contain estrogenic-like hormones.[155]

The TRIS and DES examples clearly show how more understanding and appreciation of what happens in animal studies could have prevented lifetimes of heartache and tragedy for many humans. Because no definitive action was taken, many women and their offspring were needlessly exposed and hurt for long over 20 years. Once again humans suffer when we ignore the obvious warning signals from the animal kingdom.[1]

Unfortunately There Is a New Potential Opportunity to Learn [26, 66]

Much will be eventually learned from the repeated and prolonged multiple chemical exposures of millions of children and adults in the New York City area, along the Eastern seaboard and in many other cities in the United States in an effort to control mosquitos. (*Unfortunately, I personally believe it will not be long before we have more than an inkling of the scope of the tragic adverse health effects caused by the purposeful and repeated spraying of toxic aerial pesticides.*) We know relatively little about the effects of malathion on the reproductive system, but there are studies that indicate sexual or birth defects have been noted in a variety of animals, for example, in turtles, fish, hens and frog/tadpoles.[66, 135, 148] Sexual dysfunction was said to be one of the medical complaints of the spray applicators who were so heavily exposed.[71] (*See Chapter 8.*)

One reassuring study, however, claims to have followed many pregnancies after malathion spraying in California. They found *no* association with malathion and miscarriages, stillbirths, spontaneous abortions, abnormal fetal development or genital defects.[66] More confirmatory and long term impartial studies, however, are needed to reassure the public and scientists that there are no sexual harmful effects, such as infertility or increased birth defects from malathion or other pesticide spraying

Other Sexual Concerns

Pregnancy and Fertility

Many couples who want to reproduce are totally unaware of the possible harmful hormonal effects of many common daily chemical exposures. If they use more caution and have more awareness, their unborn children will have a better chance of being normal.[86a,b]

- Infertility is a major concern at the present time. It rose from 14.4% to 18.5% in 1995.[48] As many as 5% of couples cannot conceive unless artificial reproductive techniques are used.[48]

- There are measures that both the males and females can take prior to considering conception that should significantly increase their chances of producing a healthy, normal baby.[86a,b] Massive education programs are needed to help teach couples how to prepare their bodies so they are more able to conceive healthier infants.[86a,b]

- They must thoroughly understand that very brief minuscule exposures to estrogenic-mimicking pesticides or other chemicals, early in a pregnancy, can possibly cause significant changes in their offspring's sexual and nervous system development in the uterus and their baby's future ability to learn.[49]

- In addition, women must know that chemicals in the air, water, foods, beverages, tobacco and alcohol can pollute their unborn infant, as well as their breast milk. No formula can compare with human breast milk but pesticided breast milk is not what nature had in mind. *(To check breast milk for chemicals contact Dr. William Rea: 214.368.4132 or Accu-Chem: 972.234.5412.)* If pregnant women stringently avoid chemicals, their breast milk should not only be safer, but much more nutritious.[86a,b]

- Many chemicals have been linked to miscarriages, stillbirths, birth anomalies or congenital defects. Couples must be warned not to live near rural areas at the time when pesticides are heavily applied or near sludge waste sites or dumpsites containing buried toxins such as Love Canal. These types of areas have been associated with numerous serious infant, child and adult health and emotional problems.[50-52, 70a-c] *(If you are pregnant, ask your health department how far away you are from sprayed or buried toxic chemicals.)*

- People who live within 2600 feet of agricultural areas can have a six to seven fold increase in brain tumors.[87]

- In another study, fetal death was more likely if pregnant women lived in areas where commercial pesticide sprays had been applied within a nine square mile radius of their homes.[88a]

- Briefly breathing pesticides sprayed inside or outside your home to control insects or weeds or breathing fumes from a diesel-fueled trucks or nearby expressways can be potentially harmful to an unborn baby.[10a,b, 14]

- How often does a mother realize that breathing chemicals associated with the preparation of a newborn's nursery can be fraught with possible danger for her unborn child? The wallboard, paint, synthetic carpeting, carpet pad or glue, lighting, mattress, bedding, clothing, disposable diapers and plastic toys, all can expose a pregnant woman to chemicals that potentially might be harmful to a fetus or infant.[131a,b, 132a,b, 133]

- Something as commonplace as washing a dog with a flea solution or using a flea collar when pregnant can increase the propensity for that unborn child to develop cancer in the form of leukemia or brain tumors before the age of six years.[32, 39a,b] (*See Chapter 2.*)

Applications for Teenagers

There is no question that children are admittedly more sensitive to pesticides and chemicals than adults. There is also no doubt that sexually developing adolescents think and worry about their sexuality more than most adults. Many are concerned about the size and appearance of their breasts or penises, as well as their sexual preferences, and they desperately want to be considered sexually attractive. The girls need to know that the foods they crave before their menses are the ones, which might affect their weight, moods and behavior. They must be aware that unavoidable hormonal exposures before birth not only affect sexuality, but also might be related to the increasing evidence of aggression, depression and inexplicable drastic mood changes noted in so many of today's youngsters.[132d,e,155] It does not seem a stretch to realize that some estrogenic-like chemicals affect the emotions, attitude, learning and behavior of pubescent and pre-menstrual females and adolescent males. And finally, is chemical pollution just one more unsuspected and under-investigated factor playing a role in our inability to find the cause of certain teenage and adult physical illnesses, memory problems, panic or rage disorders, violent actions, depression or suicide?[132d,f] We have many medications to mask symptoms but at some point the real challenge must be faced. Why is all this happening? We must take the time to find and eliminate the possible causes of medical complaints.

Perplexing Basic Questions to Ask Our Legislators[176a-c]

If our government unquestionably knows specific toxic substances cause birth deformities, nerve cell damage, serious illness, cancer, behavioral problems, sexual aberrations and even death, consider the following:

- Why do they allow continued and expanded pollution? (*See Chapter 6.*) They quickly informed the public about defective tires but allow toxic chemicals to continue to be used for years after they know their frightening dangers.

- Why would they continue to permit proven, known extremely harmful, toxic substances to be discharged into our water, air and soil?

- Why do so many toxic chemicals continue to be allowed (or even legislated to be used) in our buildings, on our food supply and in our cosmetics and perfumes? [137]

- Why would the legislators permit the continued or indefinite use of proven banned poisons under certain circumstances after it has been determined that they are so toxic or poisonous that they must be banned? When there is a compromise between the health of the public and big business or the economy, the health issues seem to consistently lose.

- Why would they allow known banned solvents for example to be labeled deceptively as "inert" on Material Safety Data Sheets?

- Why would legislators allow known toxic chemicals to be sold to third world countries?

- Is it possible that the EPA allows misdirected or concealed research, poor test designs and even collusion of their own employees with chemical corporations? If they find this type of problem exists, why do they not take appropriate action? Can problems related to funding pressures, selective apparent bribery, withholding of material facts and altered, false, incomplete, inaccurate or no records really exist? Why is it possible for products, shown to be unsafe after investigation, to be released for use by trusting Americans?[175a,b]

- Why are some FDA and other public officials in protective agencies given lucrative incomes and positions in chemical corporations? Could these be given in return for political and other favors related to approval of products that are unquestionably unsafe for the American public? *(See Chapter 7.)*

Perplexing Basic Questions We Need to Ask Ourselves:

- Why is the public not more concerned? Why are we not all violently objecting to what is happening?

- How many sterile couples, miscarriages or deformed or developmentally delayed or autistic babies will it take to make the public object?

- How much breast, prostate and testicular cancer has to occur before we stop emphasizing treatment and start to think more about recognizing and eliminating the cause?

Adults must try to understand more about why so many sexually-related issues are prevalent in today's world. Smaller genitals and cancer of the breasts, testicles and prostates appear to be only part of the many possible serious effects estrogen-mimicking pesticides can have on humans. We surely need more understanding and funded unbiased research in this area, and we need it now.[119a,b]

Observations from My Clinical Practice

In the 1980s and 1990s, a few mothers in my pediatric allergy practice began to complain that their son's penises seemed to be too small. I had to admit that they did seem smaller than I had seen in my previous 30 years in practice. I had no idea at that time why this was happening.

In the past few years, I have shared some of the information in this chapter at medical conferences and doctors have approached me after my talks to comment that some of their patient's penises are enlarging only 1/2 inch when they have erections. Another anecdotal observation occurred after a recent television program in Mexico concerning impotence. There was a surprising response, not from older listeners, but from younger men. They were upset and wanted help because they knew they had erectile dysfunction. The "need for Viagra" epidemic is certainly not just affecting the middle aged and older men. In doctor's offices or on television, many common sexual problems are discussed more openly and candidly than ever before. However, many young and older men continue to be reluctant to tell anyone about their personal sexual concerns. It is obvious we need large-scale, properly conducted studies to find out exactly how prevalent certain sexual health problems are in our society. We are drinking the same water, breathing the same polluted air and eating some of the same pesticided foods, as some forms of aquatic and animal wildlife. The concentrations of certain estrogenic-like chemicals are reported to be higher in human bodies than the levels found in those animals that have manifested serious sexual and other significant abnormalities.[1a] How much longer can we afford to wait before we try to find out why? Those who want to check their blood or urine levels of estrogenic-mimicking chemicals should ask their physician to contact Accu-Chem: 972.234.5412 or ImmunoScience Labs: 800.950.4686. (*For nearest environmental medical physician call 316.684.5500.)*[46]

The Glimmer of Good News

If you make the changes discussed in Chapter 3, you definitely can delay, minimize or avert the trends discussed in this chapter and throughout this book in yourself and in your family. For obvious reasons, sperm banks and cloning are not the best or only answers to resolve our many present-day infertility and sexual problems. We simply must find and eliminate the causes of the many sexually-related changes that are so increasingly apparent in today's world.

Summary

As skeptics read this, they will correctly point out that the amount of solid scientific evidence in humans about feminizing pesticides is insufficient. What happens to animals certainly cannot always be applied directly to humans. But in both animals and humans, similar noteworthy and frightening scientific studies and observations already exist to show relationships between synthetic feminizing hormone pesticides or other chemical disrupters and sexual changes. These publications are mounting at a steady and alarming rate. These are the facts:

Male fish, birds and mammals are being de-masculinized and feminized; female fish, birds and mammals are being masculinized and de-feminized. In addition, their immune systems, brains and nervous systems are being compromised. The sexuality of animals and man is being affected in many previously unrecognized ways by the plethora of chemicals to which we are exposed on a daily basis in our food, water, air, homes, schools and workplaces. The animal studies indicate that the genitals and behavior patterns that differentiate males from females can be altered by exceedingly minute chemical exposures while the unborn are developing in the uterus. This observation cannot be glibly discounted. Should we not be concerned about what might be happening to unborn human infants in the uterus when our exposure to dioxin, for example, is so prevalent and unavoidable? Should we not immediately take some sensible precautionary measures and demand more impartial scientific research in this area?

Until we know more, precaution should be the rule. Rachael Carson, in no uncertain terms, warned us in the 1960s in her book Silent Spring, as did Theo Colborn in the more recent environmental update, Our Stolen Future.[1] Both books provide ample, substantive, frightening and alarming evidence of how rampant the problems briefly discussed in this chapter have become.[1, 7, 40] The environmental issues are many times worse now than 40 or even 10 years ago. Is funding for research and education in this area not as important as a new football stadium or travel into outer space? What we are talking about is indeed a matter of life or death. It is that important. We are talking about the future of our children, ourselves and all forms of life on our planet. We are all truly one. This is not just a catchy phrase. Polluted air and water know no borders.

CHAPTER 5 REFERENCES:

1 Colborn, Theo, et al., Our Stolen Future: Are We Threatening Our Fertility, Intelligence, and Survival? A Scientific Detective Story, 1996, Penguin Books USA, Inc., 375 Hudson Street, New York, NY 10014 USA.

1a pp. 253-5.

1b Chapter 10 and pp. 161-164.

1c pp. 145-159.

1d Chapter 6.

1e pp. 192-195.

1f pg.111and Chapter 7.

1g pp. 56-66.

1h pp. 173-6.

1i www.ourstolenfuture.org

1jhttp://www.ourstolenfuture.org/NewScience/reproduction/cryptorchidism/2000hosieetal.htm

1k pg. 170.

2 Jett, D. A. et al, "Cognitive Function and Cholinergic Neurochemistry in Weanling Rats exposed to Chlorpyifos," Toxicol. Appli. Pharm., 6/15, 2001:174 (2) 89-98. djett@ihsph.edu Dept. of Health Science, Johns Hopkins.

3 Colborn, Theo, Ph.D. and Coralie Clement, eds., Chemically-Induced Alterations in Sexual and Functional Development: The Wildlife/Human Connection, Vol. XXI, Advances in Modern Environmental Toxicology, 1992. Series Editor: M.A. Mehlman, Ph.D., 1992, Princeton Scientific Publication Co.

3a pp. 358-9.

3b pg. 282.

3c pp. 195-202.

3d Chapter 2.

3e Chapter 8.

3f Chapter 7.

3g Chapter 14 and 15.

4 www.nfm-online.com.

5a Skakkebaek, Dr. Niels, "Sexual Abnormalities: Assault on the Male," 1993, Horizon video BBC.

5b Video: Front L-ine, "Fooling With Nature," 1998.

6a Porter, M.D., et al., "Endocrine, Immune, and Behavioral affects of Aldicarb (carbamate), Atrazine (triazine), and Nitrate (fertilizer) Mixtures at Concentrations," Toxicology and Industrial Health, 1999:15 (1-2) 85, 133-150.

6b Midthun, Teresa, Dr. Porter's Washington Toxics Coalition Interview in Santa Barbara to Environmentalists, 1992, U. of Wisconsin Foundation, 1848 University Av., Madison, WI 53706. 206.632.8661

7 Ross, Gerald, M.D., "President's message," Environmental Physician, Summer 1996: 30 (2). 7701 East Kellogg, Suite 625, Wichita, KS 67207. 316.684.5500.
8 Guillette, L. et al., "Developmental Abnormalities of the Gonad and Abnormal Sex Hormone Concentrations in Juvenile Alligators from Contaminated and Control Lakes in Florida," Environmental Health Perspectives, 1994: 102, 680-688.
9 Earth Island Journal, "Mickey/Minnie," Fall 1999:14 (3), Gary Santolo of the Sacramento, California consulting firm of C2HMHill, headed the Kesterson field study.
10a "Diesel Gases Masculinize Fetal Rodents," Science News, January 20, 2001:159, 39.
10b "Unthinkable Risk: How Children Are Exposed and Harmed When Pesticides Are Used at School," April 2000, Northwest Coalition for Alternatives to Pesticides, P.O. Box 1393, Eugene, OR 97440-1393. 541.344.5044, www.pesticide.org
11 BBC News on Line's Helen Briggs, September 6, 2000: GMT 17:11. UK and British Festival of Science in London, Prof. Alan Pickering presentation.
12 Pfeiffer, Okyan, "The Fate of Frogs: A Closer Look at Frog Deformities," 802.223.5221. www.vpirg.org.
13 Norheim, G., et al., "Some Heavy Metals, Essential Elements, and Chlorinated Hydrocarbons in Polar Bear[s] (Ursus maritimus) at Svalbard," Environmental Pollution, 1992: 77(1) 5157.
14 Science Magazine, September 11, 2000. www.envirolink.org/environed.
15 Be'land, P., et al., "Tumors in St. Lawrence Beluga Whales (Delphinapterus leucas)," Veterinary Pathology 1994: 31, 444-49.
16 DeGuise, S., et al., "Possible Mechanisms of Action of Environmental Contaminants on St. Lawrence Beluga Whales (Delphinapterus leucas)," Environmental Health Perspectives Supplements 1995: 103 (4) 73-77.
17 Daly, H., "Laboratory Rat Experiments Show Consumption of Lake Ontario Salmon Causes Behavioral Changes: Support for Wildlife and Human Research Results," Journal of Great Lakes Research, 1993: 19(4) 784-88.
18 Giesy, J., et al., "Deformities in Birds of the Great Lakes Region: Assigning Causality," Environmental Science and Technology, 1994: 28(3) 128-35.
19 Facemire, C., et al., "Reproductive Impairment in the Florida Panther: Nature or Nurture?" Environmental Health Perspectives Supplements, 1995: 103(4) 79-86.
20 Reijnders, P., et al., "Reproductive Failure in Common Seals Feeding on Fish from Polluted Coastal Waters," Nature 1986 (324) 456-57.
21 Foley, R., et al., "Organochlorine and Mercury Residues in Wild Mink and Otter: Comparison with Fish," Environmental Toxicology and Chemistry 1988: 7, 363-74.

22 Sherman, Janette M., Chemical Exposure and Disease: Diagnostic and Investigative Techniques, Princeton Scientific Publishing Co., Inc. P.O. Box 2155, Princeton, NJ 08543. 609.683.4750. Fax: 609.683.0838.

22a pg. 94.

22b pp. 176-7.

22c Chapter 2.

22d pp. 122-123.

23 Durnil, Gordon, The Making of a Conservative Environmentalist, 1995, Indiana University Press, Bloomington, Indianapolis, IN. Pp. 85-86.

24 "IRAC Monographs on the Evaluation of the Carcinogenic Risk of Chemicals to Humans: Some Halogenated Hydrocarbons," International Agency for Research on Cancer, Lyon, France, 1979: 20, pp. 575-85.

25a Crime Times, "Is Estrogen a Culprit in Teen Aggression?" 1998:4 (1) 6.

25b http://www.crime-times.org/authors.htm. The Wacker Foundation, Dept.132-1106, N. Gilbert Road, Mesa, AZ 85203.

26 "Legal Ramifications of WNV Mosquito Control," http://www.meepi.org/wnv/overkill.htm, pg. 26.

27 Rachel's Environment and Health News, P.O. Box 5036, Annapolis. MD 21402-7036. 410.463.1584. Fax: 410.263.4894. www.rachel.org

27a #372. "PCB's Diminish Penis Size," January 13, 1994.

27b #438. "Warning on Male Reproductive Health," April 20, 1995.

27c #290. Birnbaum, Linda, "Young Male Rats Are Demasculinized and Feminized by Low Doses of Dioxin," June 6, 1992.

27d #250. "Pet Dogs Get Cancer from Weed Killers," September 4, 1991.

27e #726. Science, "Precaution and Pesticides," June 7, 2001.

27f #432 "Two More Studies Show Human Sperm Loss," March 9, 1995.

27g #463 "Dioxin and Health," October 12, 1995.

27h #249 "Dioxin Dangers - What's Going On," September 4, 1992.

27i #436, "The Dogs of War," April 6, 1995.

28 Dold, Catherine, "Hormone Hell," Discover, September 1996, pp. 52-59.

29 Skakkebaek, Dr. Niels, et al., British Medical Journal, September 12, 1992:305 (6854) 609-13.

30 Auger, J., et al., "Decline in Semen Quality among Fertile Men in Paris During the Past 20 Years," New England Journal of Medicine 1995: 332 (5) 281-85.

31 Sharpe, R. and N. Skakkebaek, "Are Oestrogens Involved in Falling Sperm Counts and Disorders of the Male Reproductive Tract?" British Medical Journal "The Lancet," 1993: 341, 1392-95.

32 David Steinman and R. Michael Wisner, Living Healthy In A Toxic World. 1996, The Berkley Publishing Group, 200 Madison Ave., New York, NY 10016. Cost: $12.95 (plus S&H).

33 Murray, Rich, Alkalize For Health: montrealgazette.com: Aitken:
33b Earth Crash Earth Spirit, June 22, 2001: "Scientists suspect pesticides, heavy metals, electromagnetic radiation in dramatic decline in human sperm quality – up to 85% of sperm produced by healthy men now DNA-damaged, causing male infertility and possibly, birth defects, brain cancer, leukemia, other cancers in children." See: http://eces.org/health/ malerepreductiveproblems.shtmt
33d http://www.alkalizeforhealth.net/Lspermdamage.htm.
34 Frederick vom Saal, F., et al., "Prostate Hyperplasia and Increased Androgen Receptors in Adulthood Induced by Fetal Exposure to Estradiol in Mice," Abstract for the Fall Meeting of the Society for Basic Urologic Research, Stanford University, 1994.
35 Technical Report, "Beyond Pesticides," NCAP, August-September 2001: 19 (88). 202.543.5450.
36 Cohen, Ronnie, "Cancer Watch," Pacific Sun, October 4, 2000.
37 Westin, J. B. and E. Richter, "The Israel Breast Cancer Anomaly," Annals of New York Academy of Sciences, 1990 (609) 269-279.
38 Pujol, P., et al., "Rising Levels of Estrogen Receptor in Breast Cancer over 2 Decades," Cancer, 1994: 74(5):1601-1605.
39a Davis, J. R., et al., "Family Pesticide Use and Childhood Brain Cancer," Archives of Environmental Contamination and Toxicology, 1993: 24, 87-92.
39b Ames, R. G., et al., "Health Symptoms and Occupational Exposure to Flea Control Products among California Pet Handlers," Journal of the American Industrial Hygiene Association, 1989: 50(9) 466-472.
40 Carson, Rachel, Silent Spring,1962, Houghton Mifflin Company, Boston MA.
41 Crime Times, "Aggression Research: of Mice, and (Maybe) Men," 1996: 2 (1) 4.
42 Luoma, J.R., "Havoc in the Hormones," Audubon, July/August 1995. www.magazine.audubon.org.
43 www.safe2use.com/ca-ipm/00-03-21c.html.
44 Colborn, T. and C. Clement, eds., "Toxicity of Polychlorinated Dibenzo-p-Dioxins, Dibenzofurans, and Biphenyls During Early Development in Fish," in Chemically Induced Alterations in Sexual and Functional Development: The Wildlife-Human Connection, pp. 195-202. 1992, Princeton Scientific Publishing.
45 "Significant Effects of Mild Endogenous Hormonal Changes in Humans: Considerations for Low-Dose Testing," Environmental Health Perspectives, March 2001: 109 (Supp. 1).
46 American Academy of Environmental Medicine (AAEM),7701 E. Kellogg, Suite 625, Wichita, KS 67207. 316.685.5500.
47 Skakkebaek, N., British Medical Journal, December 8, 2001 (323) 1317-18.

48 "Male Infertility and Other Reproductive Problems in Men," Environmental Health, March 17, 2002. http://eces.org/ec/health/malereproductiveproblems.shtml.
49 New York Coalition for Alternatives to Pesticides, Winter 1991-92: 3 (1) 8.
50a www.mercola.com/2001/feb/28/pesticides_miscarriage.htm
50b www.mercola.com/1997/jul/13/stillbirths.htm.
51 Occ. and Env. Med., 1997:54, 511-518.
52 Epidemiology, March 2001: 22, 148-56.
53a"Endocrine Disrupting Chemicals: Effects on Human Reproductive Health," Early Pregnancy: Biology and Medicine, April 2001: V (2) 80-112.
53b www.orionsociety.org/pages/om/01-4om/d/steingraber.html.
53c http://www.psr.org/endofs.htm
54 Kimbrough, R.D., "Human Health Effects of Polychlorinated Biphenyls (PCBs) and Polybrominated Biphenyls (PCBs)," An Rev Pharmacol Toxicol., 1987: 27, 87.
55 "Environmental Pollution in Meconium in Townsville, Australia, Study of babies first bowel movement," Pesticides and You, Spring 2000: 20 (1) 8. 202.543.5450, www.watoxics.org.
56 Colborn, Theo, Ph.D. and Coralie Clement, Environmental Estrogens: Health Implications for Humans and Wildlife.
57 Paulozzi, L., et al., "Hypospadias Trends in Surveillance Systems," Pediatrics, 1997: 100 (5).
58 Deutsch, Nancy, "Pesticides May Impair Male Fertility," Biology of Reproduction 2000: (62) 51-58.
59 Johnson, Christine, "Endocrine Disrupting Chemicals and Transexualism," www.transadvocate.org/news/htm.
60a Raloff, Janet, "The Gender Benders: Are Environmental 'Hormones' Emasculating Wildlife?" http://www.sciencenews.org/sn_edpik/ls_7.htm.
60b Raloff, J., "Perination Dioxin Feminizes Male Rats," Science News, May 30, 1992: 14, 359.
61 Krimsky, Sheldon, "Hormonal Chaos: The Scientific and Social Origins of the Environmental Endocrine Hypothesis," Johns Hopkins University Press, $34.97.
62 "Declines in Sperm Counts: Largest Analysis Ever Confirms Earlier Findings", Northwest Coalition for Alternatives to Pesticides, NCAP, Fall 2000: 20 (3) 7.
63 Akingbemi, B.T., et al., "A Metabolite of Methoxychlor,2,2-bis(p-hydroxyphenyl)-1,1,1-Trichloroethane, Reduces Testosterone Biosynthesis in Rat Leydig Cells Through Suppression of Steady-State Messenger Ribonucleic Acid Levels of the Cholesterol Side-Chain Cleavage Enzyme," Biology of Reproduction 2000: 62, 571-578.

64 "World Decline in Sperm Count," Scottsdale Ear, Nose and Throat Allergy/Environmental Health Center, February 15, 1998: 3 (Issue No. 5). 7301 E. 2nd St., Suite 106, Scottsdale, AZ.
65 Nagler, James J., et al., "High Incidence of a Male-Specific Genetic Marker in "Phenotypic Female Chinook Salmon from the Columbia River," Environmental Health Pers., January 2001: 109 (1).
66 www.chem-tox.com/malathion/research/index.htm.
67 Paulozzi, et al., "Hypospadias Trends in Surveillance Systems," L. Pediatrics, 1997: 1 (5).
68 Deutsch, Nancy, "Pesticides May Impair Male Fertility," Biology of Reproduction, 2000: 62, 51-58.
69 Ohanjanyan, Olga, "Persistent Organic Pollutants and Reproductive Health." CSD NGO Women's Caucus women-csd@egroups.com. www.egroups.com/group/women-csd/info.html.
70a Paigen, Beverly, Ph.D., "Children and Toxic Chemicals," J of Pest Reform, Summer 1986.
70b Paigen, Beverly, Ph.D., "Health Hazards at Love Canal." Testimony Presented to the House Sub-committee on Oversight & Investigations. March 21, 1979. Roswell Park Memorial Institute.
70c Regenstein, Lewis and Paul G. Irwin, Cleaning Up America the Poisoned: How to Survive Our Polluted Society, 1993, Acropolis Books, Inc., pp. 138-9. (Book is currently out of print.)
71 Garry, V., et al., "Birth Defects, Season of Conception, and Sex of Children Born to Pesticide Applicators Living in the Red River Valley in Minnesota," USA, Environ. Health Persp., J. Pesticide Reform, fall 2002,: 22 (3)10 (supple.) 9, 441-449.
72a Researchers at Cedars-Sinai Medical Centre, "First Documentation of Man-Made Chemical Contaminants in the Amniotic Fluid of Unborn Babies," http://www.poptel.org.uk/panap/archives/ddtbabe.htm.
72b http://benson.niehs.nih.gov/sbrp/newsfeatures/News2000/success.html
73a "The Food Quality Protection Act (FQP) Background: A Visit to the EPA's Office of Pesticide Programs." www.epa.gov/opppsps1/fopa/backgrnd.htm
73b www.parentcenter.com/refcap/health/food/29644.html.
74 Foster, W. G. et al., "Ovarian Toxicity of Hexachlorobenzene (HCB) in the Superovulated Female Rat," J. Biochem. Toxicol, 1992: 7, 1-4,.
75a. "Contents of Common Plastic Packaging Items," Mothers and Others for a Livable Planet. 888 ECO- INFO.
75b "Hormone Mimics Hit Home: Tests of Plastic Wraps and Baby Foods," http://www.consumerreports.org/main/detailv2.jsp?CONTENT%3C%3Ecnt_18999&F
75c Diane Welland, "Should You Ban Plastic Products from Your Kitchen?" Environmental Nutrition, June 2000.

76 Environmental Health Perspectives, 110:A593-A598 September 2002.
77 PCB, "Dioxin Exposure Linked to Altered Play Behavior," Crime Times, 2002: 8 (4) 1.
78 www.mercola.com/2001/may/19/canned_foods.htm.
79 Nature, October 31, 2002.
80 "Why Do You Think They Call Them DIE-oxins?" Endometriosis Association Newsletter, Spring 2002. 414.355.2200.
81 Environmental Health Perspectives, October 2000:109 (10)1063-1070.
82 Hoy, J., et al., "Genital Abnormalities in White-Tailed Deer in Western Montana: Pesticide Exposure a Possible Cause," J of Env. Biol, 2002: 23(2) 189-197.
83 Epstein, Samuel, M.D., The Politics of Cancer Revisited, East Ridge Press, USA, Freemont, NY 1998. $17.00 (plus S&H).
84 www.tushies.com
85a Sippell, W., et al., Archives of Diseases of Children, September 2000.
85b "Use of Disposable Diapers May Lead to Low Sperm Count," British Medical Journal, http://www.bmj.com
86a Buttram, Harold E., M.D., Woodlands Healing Research, 5724 Clymer Rd., Quakertown, PA 18951-3266. 215.536.1890.
86b Caton, Helen, et al., The Fertility Plan: A Holistic Program for Conceiving a Healthy Baby, 2000, Fireside Books, Rockefeller Center, 1230 Avenue of the Americas, NY, NY 10020. Cost: $15.00 (plus S&H).
87 USA Today, June 29, 2001.
88a Bell, E.M., et al., "A Case Control Study of Pesticides and Fetal Death Due to Congenital Anomalies," Epidemiology, 2001: 22, 148-156.
88b "Pesticides Linked to Still Births," Occup.and Env. Medicine, 1997: 54:511-518.
89a Cox, Caroline, "Nonyl Phenol and Related Compounds," J of Pesticide Reform, Spring 1996:16 (1) 15-20.
89b White, R., et al., "Environmentally Persistent Alkylphenolic Compounds are Estrogenic," Endocrinal., 135(1) 175-182.
89c Soto, A.M., "p-Nonyl phenol: an estrogenic xenobiotic released from 'modified' polystyrene," Environmental Health Perspectives, 92: 167-173.
89d Naylor, C. G., et al., "Alkylphenol ethoxylates in the environment," J. American Oil Chem Soc., 1992: 69(7) 695-703.
90 In Harm's Way: "Toxic Threats to Child Development," Report by Greater Boston Physicians for Social Responsibility, January 2001.
91 Hamm, Keith, "What's in the Mix," Santa Barbara, Independent, April 15, 1999: pg. 21. Interview with Dr. Warren Porter.
http://www.independent.com/007/001/003.html

92 Park, D., et al., "Endosulfan Exposure Disrupts Pheromonal Systems in the Red-Spotted Newt: A Mechanism for Subtle Effects of Environmental Chemicals," Env. Health, Persp. 109: 669-683.
93 Hayes, T. B., et al., "Hermaphroditic Demasculinized Frogs after Exposure to Atrazine at Low Ecologically Relevant Doses," PBNAS, 2002:99 5476-5480.
94 www.SaveOurEnvironment.org Action Center
95 Spyker, Joan, "Assessing the Impact of Low-Level Chemicals on Development: Behavioral and Latent Effects." Current Status of Behavioral Pharmacology, Federation Proceedings August 1975: 34, (9)1835.
96 Cavieres, M., et. al., "Developmental Toxicity of a Commercial Herbicide Mixture in Mice: I. Effects on Embryo Implantation and Litter Size," Environmental Health Perspectives, November 2002: 110 (11).
97 Ashford, N. and C. Miller, Chemical Exposures: Low Levels and High Stakes, 1998, Van Nostrand Reinhold, NY. $52.50.
98 Williams, Rose Marie, "Dioxin, The Universal Toxin," Part 1. Townsend Letter, April 2001, pp. 158-60.
99 Rachel's Environment and Health Biweekly, "Here We Go Again," September 14, 2000 (708).
100 Biology of the Neonate, November 2000: 78, 269-276.
101 Reproductive Toxicology, November 1, 2000: 14, 513-532.
102 http://www.ithyroid.com/phthalates.htm.
103 Environmental Working Group, EWG Science Policy, http://www.ewg.org.
104 News on Earth, October 2000, 101 W 23rd St., PMB 2245, N.Y., NY 10011.
105 Herman-Giddens, et al., "Secondary Sexual Characteristics and Menses in Young Girls Seen in Office Practice," Pediatrics, April 1997: 99 (4) 505-512.
106 Raloff, Janet, "Girls May Face Risks from Phthalates," Science News, September 9, 2000: 158 (11).
107 ephnet1.niehs.nih.gov/docs/2000/108p895-900colon/colon-full.html.
108 Welland, Diane M.S., "Should You Ban Plastic Products for Your Kitchen," Env. Nutrition, June 2000.
109 Colon, I. et al., "Identification of Phthalate Esters in the Serum of Young Puerto Rican Girls with Premature Breast Development," Env. Health Persp., September 2000: 108 (9).
110 Sharpe, R. M., "Hormones and Testis Development and the Possible Adverse Effects of Environmental Chemicals," Toxicol Lett., 2001: 120 221-242 [Medline].
111 Holmes, P., Harrison PTC. "Environmental and Dietary Endocrine Disruptors and Women's Health," J Brit Menopause Soc., 2001: 7, 53-59F.
112 Associated Press, "Study Shows Chemicals Affect Sperm," July 3, 2002.
113 Agency for Toxic Substances and Disease Registry, "Hexachlorobenzene," September 2002. http://www.atsdr.cdc.gov/tfacts90.html

114 EXONET Pesticide Information Profile, "Malathion Revised," June 1996.
115 Brenner, Loretta, "Malathion," J. of Pest. Reform, Winter 1992:12 (4) 29-37.
116 Davis, "Fathers and Fetuses"; "Estrogen in the Environment."
117 Regenstein, Lewis G., Cleaning Up America the Poisoned, 1993, Acropolis Books, Washington, DC.
118 Holloway, Marguerite, "Dioxin Indictment," Scientific American, January 1994, pg. 25.
119a Guillette, Elizabeth, et al., "An Anthropological Approach to an Evaluation of Preschool Children Exposed to Pesticides in Mexico," Environmental Health Perspectives, June 1998: 106 (6) 347-353.
119b Guillette, Elizabeth, "New Ways to Investigate Contamination and Health," International Symposium on Environmental Endocrine Disrupters, November 2002, Hiroshima, Japan.
120 Gerhard, Ingrid, "Prolonged Exposure to Wood Preservatives Induces Endocrine and Immunologic Disorders in Women," American Journal of Obstetrics and Gynecology, August 1991: 165 (2) 487-88.
121 Moses, Marion, M.D., "Designer Poisons," 1995. Pesticide Education Center, P.O. Box 420870, San Francisco, CA 94142-0870. 415.391.8511. Cost $19.95.
122 Lawson, Lynn, Staying Well in a Toxic World, 1993. Noble Press, Chicago.
123 FAIM, Innovation, No. 1, 1995.
124 Clapp, R. W., et al., "Human Health Effects Associated with Exposure to Herbicides and/or Their Associated Contaminants—Chlorinated Dioxins," Agent Orange and the Vietnam Veteran, April, 1990. www.birthdefects.org/information/env_immteral.htm
125 The Delicate Balance, 1991: IV (3-4)18. 609.429.5358.
126 G. Ziem, "Multiple Chemical Sensitivity: Treatment and Follow-up with Avoidance and Control of Chemical Exposures," Toxicology and Industrial Health, 1992: 8 (4) 73-86.
127 Personal communication.
128 Padungtod, Chantana, Harvard School of Public Health, J Occup Environ Med., 2000: 42, 982-992.
129 Health News September 22, 2001. www.intelihealth.com/IH/ihtIH/EMIHC000/333/333/333738.html
130 www.the-scientist.com/yr2003/jan/research_030127.html
131 Jacqueline Krohn, M.D., 1991, Hartley & Marks, Inc., Box 147, Roberts, WA 98281.
131a The Whole Way to Allergy Relief and Prevention, 1991. Cost: $24.95.
131b Natural Detoxification: A Practical Encyclopedia: The Complete Guide To Clearing Your Body of Toxins, 2000. Cost: $24.95.

132 Environmental Medical Research Foundation ERF (Formerly: PARF or Practical Allergy Research Foundation), P. O. Box 60, Buffalo, NY 14223-0060. 800.78.78.78.0 www.drrapp.com

132a Is This Your Child's World? Cost: $15.00 (plus S&H).

132b Is This Your Child? 1991. Cost: $12.00 (plus S&H).

132c "Infant Allergic Reactions." Cost $15.00 (plus S&H)

132d Video, Chemical Reactions in Children and Adults_$25.00.

132e Video, Mold Reactions in Children and Adults. Cost: $25.00.

132f Video: Environmentally Sick Schools, 90 min. Cost: $25.00 (plus S&H).

133 Sherry Rogers, M.D., Wellness Against All Odds, 1994, Prestige Press, P.O. Box 3068, 3500 Brewerton Rd., Syracuse, NY 13220. 800.846.6687; 315.468.4417. Fax: 315.468.8119. Cost: $17.95 (plus S&H). www.prestigepublishing.com

134 Schmitt, Laura, "Crazy for Cloth, The Benefits of Cotton Diapers," Mothering Magazine, January-February 2003, pp. 37-46.

135 Cabello, G., et al., "A Rat Mammary Tumor Model Induced by the O Phosphorous Pesticides Parathion and Malathion," Env. Health Persp., 5-01:109, 471-9.

136 "Pesticides Suspected as Washington Shoalwater Tribe Suffers 50% Rate of Stillbirths, Miscarriages," Earth Crash, March 4, 2001. http://eces.org/articles/static/9836856009742.shtml

137 Erickson, Kim and Samuel Epstein, Drop-Dead Gorgeous: Protecting Yourself from the Hidden Dangers of Cosmetics, March 2002. McGraw-Hill Companies. Cost: $16.95.

138 Sharpe, Richard, et al., "Gestational and Lactational Exposure of Rats to Xenoestrogens Results in Reduced Testicular Size and Sperm Production," Environmental Health Perspectives, December 1995: 103 (12) 1136-1143.

139 Simon, T. R., et al., "Abnormalities in Scintigraphic Examinations of the Brains of Desert Storm Desert Shield Veterans," presented at the twelfth annual international symposium on Man and His Environment in Health and Disease, Dallas, TX, 1994.

140 J of Pesticide Reform, 16 (2):2-7 or www.pesticide.org

141 www.niehs.nih.gov/oc/news/PBBlate.htm

142 Epidemiology November 2000:11 (6).

143 Spangler, Luita D., "Xenoestrogens and Breast Cancer: Nowhere to Run."

144 Lehourites, Chris, The Associated Press, CNews, "Girl Finds Cancer-Causing Particles from Plastic Wrap Seeping Into Food," April 28, 2000. http://www.canoe.ca/CNEWSScience0004/28_phenom.html.

145 NIEHS Press Release, "Increased Uterine Cancer Seen in Mice Injected with Genistein, a Soy Estrogen, as Newborns," May 31, 2001. http://www.niehs.nih.gov/oc/news/genist.htm.

146 Kilburn, Kaye H., M.D., Chemical Brain Injury, pp. 296-305, 1998, International Thomson Publishing Company, Van Nostrand Reinhold, 115 Fifth Avenue, New York, NY 10003.
147 CBC News, "Common Pesticide Ending up in Semen of Farmers," May 27, 2002. www.cbc.ca/stories/2002/05/27/consumers/weedkiller
148 Mekdeci, Betty, Association of Birth Defect Children, Warren Statement for Committee on Veterans Affairs, 5400 Diplomat Circle Suite 270, Orlando, FL, 32810.
149 Williams, Megan, "Breast Cancer and the Environment The Chlorine Connection," http://www.voiceofwomen.com/articles/breastcancer.html
150 Lyons, Ron, "Estrogens and Estrogenic Exposure," Spring 1994. http://casswww.ucsd.edu/personal/ron/CVNC/estrogens/estrogen_paper.html
151 Wolff, Mary S., et al., "Blood Levels of Organochlorine Residues and Risk of Breast Cancer," J of National Cancer Institute. April 21, 1993: 85, 648-52.
152 Ohanjanyan, Olga, Health and Environment officer, WECF, "Persistent Organic Pollutants and Reproductive Health, 'Hormone Disrupters,'" September 5, 1999. http://www.earthsummit2002.org/wcaucus/Caucus%20Position%20Papers/agriculture/pest.
153 Hayes, Howard, et al., "Case Control Study of Canine Malignant Lymphoma: Positive Association with Dog Owner's Use of 2,4 Dichlorophenoxyacetic Acid Herbicides," J. of Nat. Cancer Insti., September 4, 1991: 83 (17).
154 Duehring, Cindy, "Recommendations for Gulf War Syndrome Conference and Research," Our Toxic Times, September 1993: 9 (9)1-7.
155 Montague, Peter, "Toxics and Violent Crime," Rachel's Environment and Health News, June 19, 1997, P.O. Box 5036, Annapolis. MD 21402-7036. 410.463.1584. Fax: 410.263.4894. www.rachel.org.
156a Anditti, Rita and Tatiana Schreiber, "Breast Cancer: The Environmental Connection," Sojourner, December 1992, 13-15.

> **156b** Epstein, Samuel S., "Environmental and Occupational Pollutants are Avoidable Causes of Breast Cancer," International Journal of Health Services, 1994: 24, 145-150.
> **156c** Greene, Gayle and Vicki Ratner, "A Toxic Link to Breast Cancer?" The Nation, June 20, 1994: 866-869.
> **156d** Raloff, Janet, "EcoCancers," Science News, July 3, 1993: 10-13; Joe Thornton, "Chlorine, Human Health and the Environment: The Breast Cancer Warning," Washington: Greenpeace, 1993.

157 Weisenburger, D.D., et al., "A Case Control Study of Non-Hodgkin's Lymphoma and Agricultural Factors in Eastern Nebraska", American Journal Epidemiology, 1988, 128: 901.
158 "Tampons and Asbestos, Dioxin, and Toxic Shock Syndrome," USFDA, July 23, 1999. www.fda.gov/cdrh/oed/tamponsabs.html

159 "Dioxin is a Burning Health Issue: Incinerators Get Blamed as Public's Pollution Fears Grow," Center for Health, Environment and Justice, June 2, 1998, P. O. Box 6806, Falls Church, VA 22040, 703.237.2249.cchw@essential.org
160 Scialli, A.R., "Tampons, Dioxins, and Endometriosis," Reprod. Toxicol., May/June 2001: 15 (3): 231-8. Review PMID: 11390166 (PubMed- Indexed for MEDLINE).
161 Bernstein, J., et al., "Antibody Responses in Civilian Couples with Seminal Plasma Protein Hypersensitivity and Gulf War Couples with Burning Semen Syndrome," J. Allergy Clin Immunol., 1999: 103(1) S226.
162 Massachusetts Precautionary Principle Partners. 800.649.6222
163 "For Japanese, Dioxin is a Burning Health Issue: Incinerators get blamed as Public's Pollution Fears Grow," June 2, 1998, Center for Health, Environment and Justice, P. O. Box 6806, Falls Church, VA 22040. 703.237.2249. cchw@essential.org
164 Zahm, S. H., "Use of Hair Coloring Products and the Risks of Lymphoma, Multiple Myeloma and Chronic Lymphocytic Leukemia," Am. J. Public Health 1992: 82, 990-997.
165 McLachlan, J., et al., "Reproductive Tract Lesions in Male Mice Exposed Prenatally to Diethylstilbestrol," Science 190:99.
166 Get Set, The Bug Stops Here, downloadable free book. Get Set, Inc., www.getipm.com 800.221.6188.
167a Greene, R., et al., "Experimental Intersexuality: The Paradoxical Effects of Estrogens on the Sexual Development of the Female Rat," Anatomical Record 1939: 74(4) 429-38.

167b. Greene, et al., "Experimental Intersexuality: Modification of Sexual Development of the White Rat with a Synthetic Estrogen," Proceedings of the Society for Experimental Biology and Medicine 1939: 41, 169-70.

168 Daly, H., "Laboratory Rat Experiments Show Consumption of Lake Ontario Salmon Causes Behavioral Changes," J of Great Lakes Research, 1993: 19(4) 784-88.
169 Daly, H., "Reward Reductions Found More Aversive by Rats Fed Environmentally Contaminated Salmon," Neurotoxicology and Teratology, 1991: 13, 449-53.
170 Brenner, Loretta, "Malathion," J. of Pest. Reform, Winter 1992:12 (4) 29-37.
171 "Next Generation Effect," see "Malathion," Health Library Index, pg. 6, "Health Prof. for Malathion in 2nd generation," November 4, 1961, Nature.
172a National Resources Defense Council, "Toxic Chemicals and Health: Kids Health," In Depth Report: Trouble on the Farm- Growing up with Pesticides in Agricultural Communities, Chapter 6 "Confirming Exposure: Pesticides in Blood and Urine,"

172b www.nrdc.org/health/kids/farm/chap6.asp

173 Safe, Stephen and Kavin Ramamoorthy, "Disruptive Behavior: Endocrine Disrupters, Sperm Counts and Breast Cancer," 1998, Forum for Applied Research and Public Policy.
174 Razak, Dzulkifli Abdul, "Poison Control: Agent Orange – A Deadly Legacy Continues to Devastate." www.prn.usm.my/bulletin/nst/2000/nst19.html
175a Martini, Betty, "Former FDA Investigator Exposes Aspartame as Deadly Neurotoxin that Never Should Have Been Approved," April 22, 2003. http://www.rense.com/general37/ddly.htm

175b http://www.dorway.com (Experts on Aspartame, government records, UPI and CDC investigations, books by physicians, protest of National Soft Drink Assn. Class Action, support groups, etc.)

176a Heavens, Alan J., "EPA Bans Residential Use of Lumber Treated with Pesticide CCA after 2003," November 3, 2002, The Philadelphia Inquirer.

176b Hurst, Pamela S. Hadad, "New Research Indicates Toxic Playgrounds in Capital Region," July 2002, New York Coalition for Alternatives to Pesticides. 518.426.8246. http://www.crisny.org/not-for-profit/nycap/nycap.htm

176c Feldman, Jay, "Beyond Pesticides Asks EPA Administrator Whitman to Immediately Suspend Registration of Wood Preservatives; Calls on Governors to Initiate Phase-out," National Coalition Against the Misuse of Pesticides. 202.543.5450. www.beyondpesticides.org

177 Brucker-Davis, Francoise, et al., "Significant Effects of Mild Endogenous Hormonal Changes in Humans: Considerations for Low-Dose Testing," Environmental Health Perspectives, March 2001:109 (Supplement 1).
178 Occupational and Environmental Medicine, May 2003.
179a Reir, Sherry, et al., "Endometriosis in Rhesus monkeys following chronic exposure to 2 3 7 8 Tetrachlorodibenzo-p-dioxin," Fundamental and Applied Toxicology, l993: 21 443.

179b Reir, Sherry, et al., "Serum Levels of TCDD and Dioxin-like Chemicals in Rhesus Monkeys Chronically Exposed to Dioxin: Correlation of Increased Serum PCB 151 Levels with Endometriosis," Reprinted from Toxicological Sciences, 2001: 59 (1) 147-159.

180 Scott-Clark, Cathy and Adrian Levy, "Spectre Orange – Nearly 30 Years after the Vietnam War, a Chemical Weapon Used by US Troops is Still Exacting a Hideous Toll on Each New Generation," Guardian Unlimited © Guardian Newspapers Limited 2003, March 2003.
181 Pesticide Action Network Updates Service, "More Were Exposed to Agent Orange," April 25, 2003. www.www.panna.org
182 Kirk, Chris, University of Birmingham, BBC News World Edition, February 2003. http://news.bbc.co.uk/2/hi/health/2753675.stm

CHAPTER 6

Just How Contaminated Are We?

(There is repetition for emphasis in this Chapter)

How Contaminated Are We?[1, 53, 57, 107]

The potential scope of health problems from chemical exposures can be immense as demonstrated earlier. In Chapter 1, the symptoms and common causes of sensitivities to numerous chemicals were discussed. Chapter 4 contained information about the relation of pesticide exposures to behavioral or learning changes in both animals and man.[22] There is an unending stream of studies that show that high, as well as miniscule levels of chemicals and trace metals can adversely affect the immune, nervous (brain), endocrine and reproductive systems of animals and humans.[2a-d, 6b, 14, 16, 18b, 48a,b, 64b, 85a, 88b,c, 102a, 121, 144-5, 154, 170-2]

Most distressing is the research that indicates exposure in the uterus to extremely tiny levels of certain toxic chemicals can apparently cause significant damage from birth through adulthood in relation to both the development and sexuality of any exposed offspring.[6b, 14, 18b, 19, 88b,c, 121, 144, 145] Some of these effects are even passed on to the next or future generations.[156, 183a-d]

In this chapter we continue with more insights concerning other unsettling aspects of this problem. Numerous studies will be presented that show how chemicals routinely can be found in human urine, blood, feces, fat, breast milk and semen. (*See*

*Chapter 5**) This should not be too surprising because chemicals, such as pesticides, have been shown to contaminate our water, air, soil, foods and homes, as well as other unsuspected aspects of our lives.

Let us look at just two examples of why we must become more concerned.

1. There are at least 20 studies published in peer-reviewed journals showing a relationship between pesticide exposure and the increased risk of cancer in children in the form of brain tumors, leukemia and lymphomas.[5, 87a, 116, 153, 154, 156] The incidence of this illness in young children has now become a frightening epidemic.

2. As discussed in Chapter 5 and the companion book entitled Can Chemicals Cause Epidemics?* the potential immediate and long term sexual effects in unborn infants and mature adults can be equally distressing.* [85a,b, 144] What will it take to get the attention of parents whose children are presently well?

How Many Humans Are Sensitive to Chemicals?[1, 6a,b, 51a,b]

- A 1996 study suggested that 4% to 7% of the United States population becomes ill each day from chemicals.[1a] This means at least 11 million people are affected, some very seriously.[48, 85a] Typical low estimates of sensitivities to multiple chemicals suggest that 10% to 16% of the public have "unusual" sensitivities to common everyday chemicals, while the high estimates in randomly selected adults suggests as many as 30% might be "especially" sensitive to chemicals.[2a] Physicians who are familiar in diagnosing environmentally-related medical problems from chemicals would estimate this percentage to be considerably higher

* *Can Chemicals Cause Epidemics?*, Doris J. Rapp, M.D. ERF, P. O. Box 60, Buffalo, NY 14223-0060, 800.787.8780, www.drrapp.com.

than 30%.[72] The vast majority who have this problem, are totally unaware of it, but only until they learn more about the possible effects of chemical pollution.

Among the ill Gulf War veterans who were known to be heavily exposed to chemicals such as Agent Orange (dioxin), about 86% complained of chemical sensitivities.[2a] In contrast, only 30% of non-chemically exposed veterans thought they had this problem. Similar to adults with numerous chemical sensitivities, Gulf War veterans frequently complained about memory loss, anxiety, nausea, fatigue, balance problems, chronic muscle and joint pains, sexual dysfunction and burning painful skin spots. In addition, the wives of exposed veterans were more apt to have miscarriages and infants with birth defects.[98a,b] Chemical exposures certainly can be one major possible cause of all these symptoms.[2a-c, 129, 156]

Other Pertinent Chemical Exposure Information[4a, 15, 176a,b]

The EPA has data that 1.2 billion pounds of chemicals harmful to children were released into the air and water nationwide in 1998. According to a federal estimate in 1989, these emissions account for only about 5% of the total release of chemicals, which is thought to be about 24 billion pounds annually.[4a, 15, 176a,b]

- We have inadequate medical information concerning over 78% of the 2,863 major chemicals produced in the United States, including the most commonly used pesticides.[2a-d, 3]

- Nearly every one of the 21,000 known pesticides contain "registered" toxins (or known poison). In spite of this they do not have to be specified but are lumped into a deceptive so called "inert" category that does not have to be revealed on the Material Safety Data (MSD) information sheets.[5] *(See Chapters 1, 7, 8, 9.)*

- It is estimated that adults can have as many as 500 different chemicals stored in their bodies.[2a-d, 3]

- The National Academy of Sciences estimates that 360,000 children have developmental and neurological disabilities due to toxic exposures.[17]

- The EPA considers 90% of all fungicides, 60% of all herbicides and 30% of all insecticides to be potential causes of cancer.[20c, 50]

- The National Cancer Institute in 1973 found a connection between pesticide exposures and a 50% increase in lymphomas in Americans.[89]

- In 2003, the Environmental Working Group extensively checked nine adults and found their bodies contained a total of 167 different chemicals. Their urine or blood had an average of 91 different industrial compounds or pollutants.[131]

- It is known that 33% of pesticides are suspect or proven causes of cancer, another 30% are known or suspect causes of reproductive problems and about 25% are known or suspect causes of genetic damage.[87a]

Surprisingly, in spite of all of the above, there is no pesticide toxicity data in 40% of pesticides in relation to cancer, in 36% in relation to reproductive effects and in 35% in relation to genetic effects.[87a]

- In California, five of the top nine pesticides used on cotton are known to cause cancer. Pesticides can be absorbed into the body from cotton fabrics.[20a] This is one reason why new clothing should be washed before wearing and why organically grown cotton is so desirable. Some hospitals use cotton bedding permeated with pesticides in an effort to control germs so the bodies of the sick are further polluted with toxins. It has been reported that the chemical companies are even attempting to encourage the public to purchase bedding that is impregnated with toxic germ-controlling chemicals which can be absorbed into the body.

- In 1991, they found dogs appear to double their chances of developing lymphomas when exposed to crabgrass killing herbicides containing 2,4-D.[49a-c]

We must continually keep asking how much do chemicals contribute to the epidemics of illness such as cancer that are so prevalent at the present time.* What more can we do as individuals to prevent this from happening?

Studies of Chemicals in Human Urine, Blood, Bowel Movements, Fat, Breast Milk and Semen[6, 176a,b]

Pesticides residues can be detected in the tissues of every human because of their worldwide distribution and their chemical properties.[142] The vital question that you must ask yourself is: How many chemicals are in your own or your loved one's urine, blood, bowel movements, fat, breast milk, ovaries or semen? Measuring the levels of chemicals in these body fluids and tissues can sometimes reveal the specific cause of common, as well as some perplexing or elusive forms of illness. (*Accu-Chem: 972.234-5412, ImmunoScience, Inc.: 800.950-4686,*) Can these stored chemicals cause you to have serious medical problems now or in the future? The answer to both questions is yes. If the levels are too high, there are definitely measures you can take now to increase your chances of remaining well. (*See Chapter 3.*)

Incidence and Studies of Chemicals in Urine[8, 11a, 93a]

- The urine of the average American contains five to seven pesticides.[6a,b, 7]

- One study of 900 adults in a National Health and Nutrition Examination Survey found 98% had a breakdown form of a carcinogenic pesticide, dichlorobenzene, in their urine.[74] This chemical is found in mothballs and toilet deodorizers. About 82% had urine containing breakdown products of chlorpyrifos, an organophosphate pesticide like Dursban®.[74] In addition 41% had evidence of parathion (in herbicides) and 64% had pentachlorophenol, (in wood preservatives).[4a-c, 8, 9, 61] *(See Table 6A)* This suggests that low and high level exposures obviously contaminate a significant number of adults.[2a-d, 6b, 14, 16, 18b, 48a,b, 64b, 85a, 88b,c, 93a, 102a, 121, 144-5, 154, 170-2]

- The urines of 197 children in an Arkansas community had detectable residues of pentachlorophenol at levels as high as 240 ppb. In addition, a metabolite of p-dichlorobenzene was also detected in 97% of the children. In addition, the herbicide 2,4-D was found in the urine of 20% of the children, even though it is extremely short lived in the body. This implies that one in five children had been exposed to this pesticide shortly before their urine was collected for analysis.[73a,b]

- Another study found 92% of 89 school children had traces of chlorpyrifos (Dursban®) in their urine.[8, 11a,b, 59, 61, 91, 93a-c]

- One study in Arizona found 100% of 40 children had detectable levels of chlorpyrifos (Dursban®) in their urine.[109c]

- Similarly a 1998 study of 110 children aged two to five years in Seattle showed that 99% had one breakdown product from organophosphate pesticides in their urine and 70% to 75% had two. The long-term health effects of such exposures are not known but they should be.[12, 164]

- The urine and blood of farm children under six years of age in the fruit growing area of Washington State were examined and 66% had four times more DMTP (dimethylthiophosphate) than non-farm children. The concentration was four times higher in those who lived near the orchards when compared to a control group of children who lived further away.[12] DMTP was also detected in about 40% of nearby non-farm children and this was thought to be from dietary sources, pesticide drift or contaminated soil and dust in this agricultural region.[93a,b]

- In another study scientists examined the urine of farm children exposed to organophosphate pesticides.[73a,b, 165] They found that half the children had dieldrin or pesticides in their blood above the levels considered safe by our government. This was found even though years before, in 1987, dieldrin had been banned as hazardous. In addition, many had chlordane in their blood even though this was banned in about 1988. Their food similarly contained elevated levels of these same pesticides. This means we have probably contaminated our farm soil and this could have serious long-term implications in relation to the health of children and adults. Banning helps but repeated evidence shows it certainly is not providing adequate protection.

We need studies of more farm and nearby non-farm children to be conducted in the future to determine if the levels of these chemicals in their body fluids correlate with the onset of any specific adverse physical, behavioral, learning or sexual problems as they grow older.[73a,b, 165, 166]

Should our little children be exposed to these or other potentially dangerous chemicals? Should we not be more fully aware so we can protect them against the long-term health risks of such contacts?

Incidence and Studies for Chemicals in Blood[93a,b]

- A Center for Disease Control study showed 99.5% of over 5,000 people had a breakdown product of DDE in their blood, even though it was banned over 30 years ago.[51a,b]

- Dursban® is found in the blood of 82% Americans. (National Resources Defense Council). [4b,c, 8, 9, 48, 74, 85a] This chemical was finally temporarily and partially banned in 2002.[60]

- There is evidence that hand-spraying of the herbicide carbaryl not only triples the farmer's blood levels of this chemical, but their spouses and children double their urine excretion of this chemical.[165, 167] This suggests that farm family members are possibly contaminated not only when they are outside but also from the inside because of open windows and doors.[176a,b] *(See Chapter 1 for more details on carbaryl.)*

- Residents near organophosphate sprayed fields have evidence of changes in their blood, as well as symptoms that required visits to an infirmary. Their medical complaints include respiratory symptoms, headaches and eye irritation.[167, 168] How many people, however, would consider that sudden irritability, aggression, rage, muscle aches or an inability to remember might be related to such exposures? Many might have symptoms that few, including those in the health profession, would recognize as possibly due to chemicals. *(See Chapter 2.)*

- In one study, half the children had pesticide levels in their blood above those considered safe by our government. Most uses of the pesticide dieldrin were cancelled by the government in 1974 yet in spite of that, in 1998, it was found in five out of six farm families.[93a,b] Their food similarly contained elevated levels of pesticides, probably because of prolonged soil contamination. Chlordane, banned in foods in 1978 and for termites in 1988, also was found in their blood.[22, 93a]

- Levels of pesticides in the blood of children and adults in a Colorado study correlated with levels found in house dust showing that chemicals from outside air and soil can contaminate the inside of homes. Some of this is due to pesticides used in home construction, tracked in from the outside and those purposely used within and around homes and buildings for insect and weed control.[68, 163, 176a,b]

Incidence and Studies of Chemicals in Bowel Movements

- In an Australian study in 25 newborn infants, the first bowel movement contained, on the average, three pesticides.[10a,b] They found the following:
  78% had lindane.
  59% contained chlorpyrifos or Dursban®.
  52% contained DDT.
  43% had pentachlorophenol.
  34 % had malathion.
  27% had PCBs.

These were found in spite of the fact that Australia outlawed DDT in 1981, lindane in 1985 and chlordane in 1995.[10a,b] It is obvious that the present methods of banning a product do not ensure that human contact with these forms of chemical poison pollution will not continue.

Studies of Chemicals in Fat[48, 85a-c, 95, 120]

Our bodies have become polluted with more chemicals than we can effectively eliminate. When the human body is so overloaded with chemicals that they cannot be excreted, they tend to be stored in the fatty areas of your body. Your fat, in particular, as well as other body areas can literally become your own personal toxic dumpsites. (*See Chapter 3 discussion of practical ways to help you excrete chemicals using detoxification methods to resolve this type of problem.*)

The human body routinely tries to excrete harmful chemicals though the lungs, intestines, urine, skin and even breast milk.[85a,c] *(As noted before, the concentration of pesticides in breast milk is higher than that found in the mother's body be-*

cause her body is trying to protect her, at her infant's expense.) There is even some evidence that ear wax, eye mucus, and skin sebaceous gland secretions increase when chemicals need to be eliminated from the body.

- In one medical report researchers showed that 155 patients with elevated levels of pesticides experienced gradually decreasing levels in their fat, along with diminution of their symptoms, after detoxification treatment.[94] *(See Chapter 3.)* This is one sensible and practical way to help eliminate illness.

- The fat samples from 100% of Americans in some studies have shown styrene (styrofoam), dioxins and the solvent xylene.[13b, 14, 27a]

- In 1982, in one study, the EPA found five environmental chemical toxins in 100% of fat samples.[51a,b, 95] There were nine toxic chemicals in over 90% and 20 in 76%. The major chemicals included styrene, benzene, phenol, xylene, dioxins, furan, PCBs and DDE. Chemicals known to damage the nervous system were found in 83%.

- A Texas study of the fat of older people showed 100% had dieldrin, oxychlordane, heptachlor and para-BHC.[51]

- A study in four-year-olds showed over 70% had DDT, over 50% had PCBs and over 21% had PBBs. Nursing was thought to be the primary source of these exposures.[51, 96]

The good news is that with avoidance of chemicals and detoxification procedures, it is possible to decrease the amount of chemicals stored in your fat. The bad news is that these stored chemicals are probably factors related to many of the epidemic illnesses present in today's world? *

---

* *Can Chemicals Cause Epidemics?*, Doris J. Rapp, M.D. ERF, P. O. Box 60, Buffalo, NY 14223-0060, 800.787.8780, www.drrapp.com.

Studies in Breast Milk[54]

(Some of the following was discussed in Chapter 5.)

For more studies and discussion of chemicals found in breast milk and amniotic or uterine fluid during fetal development, see Chapter 5, in which the serious ramifications of toxic chemicals in relation to sexuality are discussed.

The tragedy of what happened to the sons of Michigan women whose breast milk was accidentally contaminated with an industrial flame retardant (TRIS) is well documented. The male offspring had a higher incidence of testicular abnormalities and smaller penises than normal.[23] In addition, TRIS exposure was associated with a definite increase in cancer and genetic defects.[22a, 24] (*It is known that at least 50 million children were also exposed to TRIS in their nightwear and millions more were knowingly contaminated with this chemical in clothing that was exported overseas.*)[184]

As said before, the 1973 report in Michigan implicated another fire retardant, PBB or polybrominated biphenyl This was accidentally mixed in some animal feed and it created a number of health problems. The cows that ate the feed had stillborn calves with deformities. The daughters of the exposed pregnant women, who drank the milk from the animals that ate the contaminated feed, had early menses and pubescence. It was found that the female offspring whose mothers had the highest PBB blood levels and who were also breast-fed had the earliest menses. Again, some males had a higher incidence of testicular abnormalities and smaller penises than normal.[18a] It was thought the most severely affected children had a combined exposure to the chemical before birth while in the uterus and again, after birth from the breast milk.[109, 142]

Studies on Uterine Fluid in the Unborn[86b]

We do know the unborn human is particularly vulnerable during certain brief critical periods of intrauterine development, especially at about 20 days and again at about seven weeks after conception. This can occur before most females know for certain they are pregnant. Researchers believe the male urinary and genital systems are particularly vulnerable to damage in the womb shortly before and after birth.[1a, 2, 45] Brief exposure to feminizing chemical hormones during these small windows of time can cause some most surprising and dramatic lifetime changes in the unborn or newborn of many forms of wildlife, including humans.[1a, 2, 3] Similar to animals, some of these effects may not become apparent until puberty or adulthood.[45] Again, similar to studies in animals, feminizing pesticides (prenatal PCB) are associated with more feminine activity in males and more masculine activity in females.[77] There are even a few reports suggesting that exposure to certain chemicals in one generation can affect future generations.[35, 183a-d, 188]

- The fluid in which an unborn baby floats and is totally immersed, inside and outside, for nine months can contain one to several pesticides. One study showed one third of the unborn babies floated in intrauterine fluid that contained DDT, lindane and PCBs. DDT can interfere with the reproductive system's biochemical pathways. PCBs have been linked to birth defects and problems with the thyroid, learning and changes in both the nervous and immune systems.[53a-c, 72a,b]

- In another recent study in June 1999, researchers confirmed the presence of DDE (a breakdown product of DDT) and PCBs in 30% of the uterine fluid of pregnant American and Canadian mothers.[72a]

Studies for Chemicals in Semen and Sperm [5b,c, 97, 103b, 177, 178]

Some of the information about semen and sperm is discussed in Chapter 5 in more detail. Some studies and reports indicate:

- Semen, as well as breast milk, appear to store toxic substances and serve as a means of excretion for chemicals.[177b]

- Twenty-some years after the war, some of Vietnamese soldiers continue to have dioxin (TCDD or tetrachlorodibenzo -p-dioxin) from Agent Orange in their semen.[97, 156, 179, 180]

- A health study in Canada found the herbicide 2,4-D used on lawns and golf courses is transmitted not only into the human urine but also into the sperm. This chemical can therefore have direct access into the female egg and affect the developing fetus from the moment of fertilization.[103a]

- In Argentina, the levels of 2,4-D in semen were 300 times higher in exposed men and these men also had damaged sperm cells.[97, 103a,b]

- High levels of four toxic chemicals, including TCDD (dioxin), were found in the seminal fluid of 132 males at Florida State University.[24, 90]

- A study was conducted on 32 Chinese men working in a pesticide factory who had been exposed to organophosphates, such as the herbicide, parathion. These workers showed excessive sperm abnormalities and decreased testosterone.[181]

- Farmers and pesticide sprayers similarly have been reported to have impaired sperm.[102a,b]

The basic challenge again is to determine if large or miniscule amounts of pesticides or chemicals can be harmful or dangerous to adults or unborn infants. (*See Chapter 1.)* Could the over 50 pesticides that have been linked to serious reproductive problems in males be related to adult infertility and infant developmental problems?[50, 85c, 156] Should everyone not be immensely concerned?[5c, 86, 87a,b, 88a, 103a,b]

Chemicals in Our Environment[4a, 15, 22, 136, 139, 140, 147, 176a,b]

You have just read the evidence that many chemicals can be found in our body and body fluids. These chemicals come from contacts inside our homes, schools and workplaces, the outside air, our water and our foods. There are studies that certainly suggest infinitesimal amounts of chemicals in the range of five parts per billion or even one part per quadrillion can damage the fetus of animals and possibly humans.[2a-d, 6a,b, 14, 16, 18a,b, 48a,b, 64b, 85a, 88b,c, 102a, 121, 144-5, 154, 170-2] Our water alone certainly contains levels which are slightly or, at times, markedly above these concentrations. We have no idea what these exposures are doing to humans.

Again consider this in relation to our daily environmental exposures. Only 3% to 10% of the 85,000, chemicals to which we potentially can be exposed on a daily or infrequent basis, have been evaluated for safety by the EPA. Less than a handful of these chemicals have been thoroughly studied for their short or long term effects in relation to behavior, learning, reproduction or immunity. They have not been investigated for their effects on the thyroid, pancreas or other endocrine organs.[3] They have not been checked specifically for safety in the most vulnerable, namely infants, children, pregnant women or the elderly.[54, 101] Should we not be especially concerned about the extensive contamination of our world with organophosphate and organochloride chemicals that have been shown repeatedly to be hazardous to the brain and nervous, reproductive and immune systems of both animals and humans?[22]

It has been stated that we need pesticides to increase crop yields but Sweden, Norway, Denmark, the Netherlands, Canada and Indonesia have reduced pesticide use by more than 50% *without reduction of crop yields or cosmetic standards.* Maybe, we should learn from them.[114a-c] Maybe we can save more than money.

Table 6A
Locations of Common Indoor Chemicals

Room deodorizers and mothballs
Paradichlorobenzene
2,4-D Weed killers
Dichlorophenoxyacidic acid
Dry cleaning fluid, odors or contacts
Tri, tetra or per-chloroethylene
Wood preservatives used on patios and outside furniture, toys etc
Pentachlorophenol
Paint
Xylene (a solvent)
Gasoline
Benzene
Carpets, plywood, chipboard, room dividers, laminated beams, polyurethane, polyester, synthetic fabrics, tobacco smoke
Formaldehyde
Gas, oil, kerosene, propane or coal heating systems
Polycyclic hydrocarbons
Styrofoam cups, plates and bowls, meat wrapping materials
Styrene
Plastic, foam rubber, pipes, insulation, synthetic carpets, food in tin cans, baby bottles
Phthalates. Furans, polyvinyl chloride

Table 6B
Common Indoor Chemical Exposures

Aerosol sprays
Arts and Crafts
Bleach
Carpet, carpet adhesive
Cleansing materials
Crayons
Deodorizers
Detergents/Disinfectants
Dry-cleaned clothes
Floor polish or wax
Gas appliances
Glue, rubber cement
Insecticides
Mothballs, moth crystals
Newsprint
Oven cleaners
Paint, paint remover
Permanent markers/pens
Personal cosmetics
Pesticides
Plastic
Plywood, fiberboard
Polyurethane, varnish
Pot cleaners
Radon
Scouring powders
Tobacco Smoke
Turpentine

Chemicals in Our Indoor Air [4a, 15, 51a,b, 53, 98a,b, 100, 125, 134-6, 139, 140, 142, 147, 176a,b]

It is now an accepted fact that the indoor air can be up to 10 times more polluted than the outside air.[134-6] We construct with and continually bring substances into buildings that contain toxic chemicals. *(See Tables 6A and 6B.)* Due to the oil shortage in the early 1970s, buildings were made tighter in construction to make them more "energy efficient". This means the heat or cold stays inside, along with all the chemicals, because they cannot escape to the outside. In addition, it is also not unusual to find that some ventilation ducts in buildings (including schools) were sealed in the 1970s and never reopened or cleaned. This combination has contributed greatly to a newly recognized common illness, the Sick Building Syndrome.

Sick Building Syndrome

The common symptoms of this illness include some combination of the following: recurrent or daily headaches, extreme fatigue, eye and nose irritation, metallic taste in mouth, numbness and burning in skin, rashes, problems breathing normally, an irregular heartbeat, dizziness, disorientation, muscle and joint weakness, difficulty thinking clearly or remembering, mood changes, problems walking or talking, agitation and loss of control of emotions. These symptoms may not be recognized by those who are not familiar with unusual forms of allergy or sensitivities to multiple chemicals. Many do not know these symptoms can be caused by things found inside homes, schools and workplaces.

As you read further in this chapter, consider if some unexplained health problems in yourself or family might be due to some form of indoor or outdoor chemical air pollution.[51]

(*Some common chemicals causing sick buildings and people are listed on Table 6A and 6B.*)

Indoor Air Concerns

- Solvents such as benzene, xylene, toluene and styrene (styrofoam) can lower testosterone and sperm levels, contribute to abortions, birth defects, asthma, nose congestion and adversely affect the blood and heart. [98a,b] These chemicals are in many products but are erroneously not specified and listed only as "inert" on the Material Safety Data Sheets. These solvents can be found in the blood and urine in many Americans. *(Accu-Chem: 972.234.5412 and ImmunoScience: 800.950.4686.)*

- Studies have indicated that dichlorobenzene (moth balls, deodorants), was found in the urine of 96% of children in Arkansas and in 98% of 1,000 adults across the United States.[73d]

- Formaldehyde exposures in carpets and construction materials are often unrecognized causes of asthma, hay fever and recurrent infections such as flu, plus many of the other less suspected symptoms associated with environmental illness as discussed in Chapter 2. [62, 85a, 87, 173a,b, 174a]

- Leukemia is several times more likely in children if pesticides are used in and around a home.[87a]

- Some 30 million homes were treated with chlordane prior to 1988, when it was finally banned. There is a 75% chance you continue to breathe this chemical if your home was constructed prior to 1988. In a small percentage of homes, the level, though low, continues to be dangerous. This chemical can persist for 35 years after application.[98a] Chlordane appears to be able to cause many common types of illnesses including learning, emotional and mood problems. Even seizures have been reported. If the cause is not recognized, the necessary steps will not be taken to eliminate this potentially toxic substance. This means many will remain ill indefinitely and require daily medications that only temporarily relieves symptoms because no one examined their blood, urine or fat, or attempted to find the cause.[22]

- The EPA put new synthetic carpets in their Washington DC office in the 1980s. Over 70 employees had to be evacuated because of illness and some continue to be ill and unable to work. The obvious clues were that the employees became ill shortly after the carpet was installed, their symptoms recurred every time they were inside the building and they were better whenever they were elsewhere.[99a,b,100] Does this happen to you when you go to work?

- One non-occupational chemical exposure study showed that the air in the households studied contained five to 20 different pesticides.[91]This does not include the other chemicals in the air.

- The level of pesticides in the air is nearly four times greater at five to 10 inches above the floor, than it is at 24 inches. This puts toddlers and pets at excessive risk.[91] *(Yes, pets are also having more cancer and thyroid disease than ever before.)*[187]

- A study at Rutgers University in New Jersey found the amount of pesticides on toys and on surfaces in a room in which a pesticide had been applied could expose a three to six year old child to a level of pesticides 69 times higher than that level considered safe. If certain toys were exposed to pesticided air and then placed in the mouth, the level was reported as 211 times higher.[23]

Table 6C
Common Outdoor Chemical Exposures

Asphalt
Chemical spills
Clothing exhaust vent odors
Factory odors (paper mills etc.)
Fireplace smoke from artificial chemical logs
Highway exhaust diesel, bus, auto fumes
Outdoor grill smoke and odors
Paints, sealants
Pesticides, herbicides, insecticides – (some aerial)
Refinery odors
Roofing materials, tars and insulation

- Chemicals released from hot Teflon™ pots, microwaved foods and aerosols containing disinfectants, deodorizers, oven cleaners, carpet cleaners, foods and cooking odors, hair or ironing sprays etc. all can contribute to indoor air and body pollution.[185a-d, 186]

- Studies indicate that children and pregnant women are particularly sensitive to chemicals.[101] For this reason, schools are of special concern.

- In California, it was determined that 87% of school districts used highly toxic pesticides.[42] This means 1.5 million children were exposed in schools where it was possible:

    70% used suspect cancer causing chemicals.
    54% used substances that hurt the nervous system.
    52% used chemicals that cause birth defects and prevent normal physical and mental development.[93a,b]
    50% used chemicals that disrupt hormones.[42]

- In Maryland, 17 out of 24 school districts used some highly toxic pesticides.[25a,b] Of these:

88% used pesticides suspect of causing cancer or reproductive problems.
41% contained toxins thought to damage the nervous system.[25a,b]

- A 1994 report estimated that 32% of the surveyed school districts had regular pesticide applications even though no pests had been observed. [157]

What do the chemicals used inside (and outside) your homes, schools or work areas do to you, your children or your grandchildren? When safer and less expensive pest control measures, such as Integrated Pest Management, have been known for years, why are they not being used? [67a,b]

Chemicals in Outside Air [70, 84, 134-6, 139, 140, 147, 176a,b]

There is no doubt that many people are sick all the time because of exposures in the outdoor air. Some of the common causes of these illnesses are listed in Table 6C.

- The EPA admits that breathing outdoor toxic chemicals can expose Americans to a lifetime cancer risk that is 10 times greater than the level considered acceptable by the EPA.[134-6] For 20 million people, this risk is 100 times above the acceptable standard.[110] It is known that the levels of toxic chemical exposures indoors are five to ten times greater.
- Federal monitoring of widespread air pollution studies have shown that the insecticides Diazinon and DDT (banned over 30 years ago) were present in 90% of air samples. In addition, toxic chlorpyrifos (Dursban®) was in 70%, and the weed killers, 2,4-D were found in almost 60%, and Triflualin in almost 50% of the studied air samples.[104]
- In one study, it was found that the death rate in six United States cities was highest in those that had the most air pol-

lution. The most neurological and developmental toxins are found in the air and water in states where there are large petrochemical industries. Texas and Louisiana have the highest levels of petrochemical emissions.[15]

- Factory emissions of harmful chemicals, such as dioxin from power plants, printing shops and industries producing paper, metal and plastics contaminate the air we breathe. (See Chapters 4, 5.) Some pollute the air with a form of dioxin called 2,3,7,8 TCDD that is said to be 470,000 times more potent than DDT.[16]

- Toxic outside air includes a risk from diesel fumes reported by a California air quality study to be another major outside air pollutant causing cancer.[110] Being in buildings located near expressways increases this potential danger.

- The EPA studied 36 most common lawn pesticides[5d, 7, 105]
  24 have never been fully tested by the EPA.
  13 are known to cause cancer.
  21 can damage the nervous system.
  15 can hurt the liver and kidney.

- Maybe it is significant that the most common lawn chemical, 2,4 -D (dichlorphenoxyaceticacid) found in most "weed and feed" preparations is known to cause serious illness. It has been called a plant cancer chemical, but what about humans? Earlier studies gave conflicting information but later reports again suggest the 27 million pounds of this chemical are used each year and it appears to contribute to the development of lymphomas in crop workers and lawn service applicators.[106, 117a-c] *(See Chapters 7, 8.)* In fact, birth defects occur at twice the normal rate in pesticide applicators.[98a,b,106] In addition, non-Hodgkin's lymphoma has increased 75% among farmers in the past 20 years. These increases, in part, are attributed to 2,4 -D. Although the manufacturers of herbicides claimed for years that their products were not harmful, this claim was reported to be false, using the manufacturer's own data.[175]

In spite of all the above information, in 1997 the EPA stopped short of ranking 2,4-D as a possible cause of cancer. It is due for re-registration in the next year or so. We must ask why the jury for our government and federal protection agencies is still out. Can we, as individuals, afford to take a chance and wait any longer to avoid this chemical? In the meantime, personally begin to protect yourself until final decisions are made. In general, it is a good rule to try to avoid any suspect chemicals when serious questions keep recurring about their safety.

- Golf course superintendents' association members who died between 1970 and 1992 had 1.75 times more colon cancer, twice the national rate of brain cancer and non-Hodgkin's lymphoma and three times more prostate cancer.[61, 69] Maybe more chemical studies on avid golfers would provide additional insight.[69]

- Another study compared pilots who applied pesticides to flight instructors. Those who actually sprayed aerial pesticides developed impaired coordination. Some also had a loss of balance leading to increased accidents, leukemia and pancreatic cancer. The brains, muscles and immune systems were affected.[70]

- The chemical routinely used on some domestic and international airlines includes permethrin which disrupts the endocrine system and may be a carcinogen The pyrethroids are suspect endocrine disrupters (thyroid, pancreas, etc). No federal laws require that airline passengers be informed before this is done.[182]

- Other research showed that people living within 2600 feet of agricultural areas had a 6.7 fold increase in brain tumors (astrocytomas). How far away from sprayed chemicals are you? Remember, studies indicate that only 0.1 % of a pesticide reaches a target pest while 99.9 % of a pesticide reaches your outside air, water and soil.[114a-c]

- A landmark decision was passed by the Canadian Supreme Court in June 2001.[115] This decision enabled Canadian municipalities to decide about banning lawn chemicals in their particular provinces. Quebec now restricts the use of pesticides, for example, in public parks and buildings. When will our government act similarly? In the past our EPA usually required at least ten years to accumulate enough evidence to "begin" to ban a toxic substance. Then it routinely takes a few too many more years before it is more fully banned.

Pesticides Found in Farmers and Their Children[73a,b, 92, 93a,b, 111, 176a,b]

It might help if we look at the findings of some studies about farmers who routinely use pesticides, fungicides and herbicides.

- The EPA estimated that 300,000 farm workers have injuries and illnesses caused by pesticides each year.[7] They typically allow their children to help so they are similarly exposed.

- The National Cancer Institute has repeatedly found the farmers have higher than average risks for several types of cancer affecting the blood (leukemia), brain and stomach.[7] In general, they had a six times greater risk than non-farmers in developing cancer. Organic farming eliminated that risk.[20a]

- Diazanon is another common organophosphate insecticide that is reported to be related to non-Hodgkin's lymphomas in farmers, as well as damage to the nervous system and increased brain cancer in children. It is used in homes, on lawns and in gardens. Its use was restricted in December 2000.[116]

- Studies of farmers in the United States and elsewhere indicate they suffer from more depression or suicide than expected.[4a, 43, 44] Is it possible that the immense need for antidepressant drugs by so many in the United States also might be related to our massive exposure to toxic chemicals?[13a,b, 155, 158, 159]

- Children born to farmers who use fumigants and Roundup® (glyphosate) or pesticide applicators were found to have more birth defects, especially if they were conceived in the spring and their offspring were also three times more likely to have some form of the attention deficit disorder (ADD). In addition, reports suggest they have a preponderance of female offspring.[106a,b]

Chemicals in Our Water and Soil[4a,c, 7, 20a,b, 21a,b, 48, 53, 84, 104, 137, 176a,c]

A chemical in the air eventually comes down onto the ground and along with what is put directly onto the soil, eventually finds its way into the ground water. Ultimately, in a most dilute form, it can come out your kitchen faucet. (*Although these chemicals are obviously present in extremely low concentrations, evidence throughout this book indicates the most minute levels can cause major illness in wildlife and sensitive humans.*) [6b, 14, 18b, 19, 88b,c, 121, 144, 145]

Also consider this:

- In 1984, about 50% of the drinking water was found to come from the groundwater.[152]

- The EPA estimates that 74 pesticides, including a number known to cause cancer, presently contaminate the ground water in 38 states.[20b]

- A United States Geological Survey in 1997 showed that Dursban® was found in 25% of the ground or surface water in the United States and in Georgia, Alabama and Florida, the level was reported to be as high as 65%.[4c, 61] This chemical is exceedingly toxic and the EPA finally decided to ban it in 2000. A year and a half later, in December, 2001, they announced that they would "begin to" ban or limit the use of this toxic chemical in certain places. *(See Chapter 10.)* Why a delay of a year and a half?

- Our country's water supply and soil are in serious jeopardy. In 1997 about 270 million pounds of toxic pollution was released into the U.S. waterways.[137] In one report about 30% of the industrial, municipal and federal facilities were in serious violation of the Clean Water Act during a 15 month period.[137, 149a-c] To make it even worse, the water quality was recently weakened again by the Bush Administration when certain legislators slipped a provision into the Homeland Security bill to allow chemicals to pollute our water in emergency situations.[160] *(See Chapter 7.)* Once it is in the water, it cannot easily be removed.

- In addition, more contamination is added to our water by manufacturers who buy cheap toxic waste from industrial facilities to use as fertilizer. This toxic fertilizer can contain a total of 22 trace metals including arsenic, mercury, lead and cadmium, as well as toxic chemicals, such as dioxin.[137] *(See Chapter 7.)*

This unlabeled waste "fertilizer" can be sold for use in homes and gardens so children at play can be directly exposed. When used on agriculture, the components in the fertilizer can enter the ground water, the food grown on the polluted ground, and the bodies of humans who touch it. We must ask why toxic fertilizer is exempted from hazardous waste treatment, storage, and disposal tracking.[137, 140, 141] The fertilizer industry claims the EPA said this waste does not generally pose a threat to human health or the environment. Does the EPA agree?

In relation to our water supply and our health, consider the following:[141]

- The drinking water of 15 to 23 million Americans is contaminated with pesticides according to the EPA.[7, 20b] Extensive herbicide use accounts for much of this pollution.

- A United States Geological Survey found at least one pesticide in 100% of all major river water samples. In addition 90% of urban, 92% of agricultural streams, 50% of urban wells and almost 60% of agricultural wells contain at least one pesticide.[104, 146]

- About 40% of the nation's waterways are considered to be too polluted for safe fishing or swimming.[137]

- Ten million people are exposed to five herbicides in their water at levels that exceed the EPA's negligible cancer risk standards.[21a-c]

- In one study, tap water in 28 out of 29 cities contained herbicides known to cause cancer in wildlife and possibly in humans, as well as other serious health effects.[21a-c]

- Nearly 900,000 pounds of toluene, a reproductive system toxin, were released into U.S. waterways in 1992. This is an increase of 60% over the year before.[137]

- It was reported that more than 2.5 million pounds of carcinogens such as vinyl chloride and benzene were released into our waterways in just one year in 1992.[137]

- Studies of water from municipal wastewater treatment plants can contain from 16 to 38 chemicals, including four suspect estrogenic or feminizing hormone mimickers that can interfere, in particular, with male sexuality.

- About 90% of municipal water treatment facilities lack the equipment to remove toxic chemicals (or the common drugs) found in the drinking water. In fact, they add more chemicals to the water.[21a, 150] Much of the water we drink is not filtered adequately because of cost.[118] We can afford sports stadiums but not good water? Maybe we need to rearrange our priorities. In many cities it is no longer desirable or possible to drink urban tap water because of the taste and the chemicals it contains.[151]

- Our nation's waterways are also contaminated with beauty aids, various cleaning products, food and body products such as perfume, contraceptives, nicotine and caffeine. In addition, the water can contain the residues of innumerable drugs used to treat infection (antibiotics), diabetes, heart disease, elevated blood pressure, depression, high cholesterol, insect bites (DEET) and pain (acetoaminophenol). The presence of the above medications and other items indicates human urine and feces contamination is unquestionably present in our drinking water.[75-77]

The Pollution Problems in the Great Lakes[18a]

This problem is well summarized by Gordon Durnil in his book, The Making of a Conservative Environmentalist. As Chairman of the International Joint Commission, he worked with Canada to oversee the quality of the environment in the Great Lakes area. He was part of a select team which thoroughly studied many aspects of the water and air in that region.

After a most extensive investigation and a thorough analysis, his committee made a number of recommendations. They agreed there was compelling evidence that the toxic environmental chemical exposures very likely were damaging North American children, causing inattention, hyperactivity, decreased IQ's, aggression, anxieties, hostility, behavioral abnormalities and possible excessive anger leading to juvenile violence. They suggested these exposures might also be factors related to the increase of disobedience of today's school children, along with the apparent significant decrease in academic performance. They found extensive evidence of immune system damage along with an associated decreased ability to fight infection and an increase in cancer, thyroid disease and physical deformities in aquatic forms of wildlife. The Commission suggested that toxic pollution of our water and air might be one more logical explanation for the increase in the number of birth defects in newborns.[62]

This panel also concluded there was evidence in both wildlife and humans that prenatal exposure to toxic estrogenic-mimicking pesticides can predetermine certain aspects of adult fertility, as well as sexual organ size, formation, sexual preferences and behavior. No one can argue that hormones strongly influence how we act, behave, feel and learn. This committee found suggestive evidence indicating humans were following trends observed in fish and gulls in the Great Lakes. The levels of the same chemicals found in physically sick and sexually deformed Great Lakes fish and wildlife are similar to or lower than the levels found in humans.[18b] Might this suggest we are simply oblivious to the extent of our potential jeopardy or do we simply have a higher tolerance to chemicals than wildlife before more flagrant illness is noted? No one truly knows how extensive the role of multiple chemical pollutant exposures is in relation to many of our present-day human illnesses. It certainly appears possible that chemicals in our water can be one more missing factor related to the obvious increase in aggression and violence presently seen in some children and adults. It is imperative that we learn more about these possible relationships.

The final recommendations of the committee working with Mr. Durnil were most disconcerting.[18c] They concluded that some serious health problems face the 40 million or so people living around the Great Lakes as a result of the persistent discharge of toxic substances into the waters of the Great Lakes Basin. The problems are not national, but global. The database in the Great Lakes evaluation provides more than enough information to indicate future generations are at risk. In his book, Mr. Durnil states that if policy makers in the United States and Canada "even slightly suspected" that their children and grandchildren might develop learning problems, a weakened immune system and reproductive problems such as lowered sperm counts from the water they drink, they would never allow what is happening. He assumes the American public simply does not fully understand the seriousness of what has occurred and are unaware of the overwhelming evidence indicating we must be concerned and take action soon.

Chemicals In and On Our Foods [20c, 26, 27a-d, 28, 30a,b, 124, 127, 128, 138, 142, 143, 176a,b]

- In the past, "safe" levels of chemicals on or in foods were determined only for adult healthy males, not children. The 1996 Food Quality Protection Act, however, specifies that more protection of infants and children against pesticides and other toxins was necessary. Recently the EPA also concluded that organophosphate pesticides have common harmful effects and exposures to combinations of chemicals should be considered when determining what is "safe" for a child. The EPA requires organophosphate pesticide protection for infants and children and decisions are supposed to err on the side of child safety. In this regard, an extra 10-fold margin of safety was supposed to be applied to ensure safe tolerance levels for children, especially if there was an absence of total scientific certainty. However to date, the EPA has devised and implemented an official policy that appears to disregard this safety factor.[138] Until this is applied, it is estimated that 3.6 million children under the age of five years will be exposed to levels in excess to what is considered safe. Should we not be concerned?[27a-c]

In spite of banning several organochloride pesticides in the 1970s, these pesticides (DDT and dieldrin) along with others, continue to show up in many of the foods that children and adults eat. In part, this is because these chemicals were stockpiled by the farmers and because crops are grown in tainted pesticide-contaminated soil.[34]

Atrazine is the most frequently used herbicide in our country and it is used primarily on corn, sorghum, sugar cane and pineapple.[88a,b, 147] It can remain in the soil for several years. It is often used along with paraquat, another most dangerous chemical. It continues to be sold over the counter in many states, but it is banned in France and other European countries. The following information has been reported about atrazine:

- It contributes to the contamination of 60% to 80% of our ground water, streams, rivers and wells, especially in the Midwestern United States. Almost every water sample in the Corn Belt and 90% of samples from the Pacific Northwest river basin are contaminated with this herbicide. More than a million children and adults are drinking water that exceeds the EPA's standard for this very toxic chemical.

Studies in rats:

- Atrazine is known to cause breast cancer in rats.[87a,b, 88a,b, 147]

Studies in frogs:

- If frogs are exposed to 1/30th the standard amount of atrazine considered by the EPA to be safe, they have severe sexual deformities.[88c] It also causes male and female sex organs to form in the same frog.[86, 88b]

- This chemical feminizes male frogs in concentrations of 0.1 part per billion![88b] Concentrations of 25 ppb cause the levels of testosterone in young male frogs to decrease by 90%.[88b] *(The EPA allowed standard for atrazine is an average of 3 ppb in our water but samples can reach 25 ppb during the spring when herbicides are applied to crops.)*

Studies in humans show:

- Atrazine exposed humans appear to have higher rates of breast, prostate and blood cancer.[88a]
- Workers in factories manufacturing atrazine appear to develop cancer of the prostate at an alarmingly high rate.[87b, 88a,]

We must ask: what can this chemical do, not only to us but to our children?

Do You Know What You and Your Family Are Eating? [21c, 42, 54, 80-83, 176a,b]

General Concerns:

- It is acknowledged that more than 5,000 chemicals and preservatives are put into our food products.[28]
- In 1980, the FDA found 38% of all food samples contained pesticide residues.[45]
- In 1998, the USDA found pesticides in about 55% of nearly 7000 fruits and vegetables; 29% had multiple residues.
- Only about 40% of the possible 496 pesticide residues identified on foods are detected by the current methods used by the FDA. This means 60% are missed![46]
- It is estimated that Americans can eat as many as 20 or more pesticide-like chemicals in their meals every day.[20a-c]
- Of the 25 most commonly used agricultural pesticides:
  - 18 can damage the skin, eyes and lungs.
  - 17 cause genetic damage or birth defects.
  - 12 cause cancer.[5a,c]
  - 10 cause reproductive problems.
  - 6 disrupt normal hormone function.
  - 5 are toxic to the nervous system.[7]

- Even though DDT was banned in 1972, in one FDA Total Diet Survey from 1982 to 1986, it was found in 100% of the samples of some foods (raisins, spinach, beef and beans) and in 87% to 93% of other foods (bologna, hot-dogs, chicken, turkey, lamb, sausage, ice cream sandwiches, butter and cheese).[112]

- In 1992, the EPA indicated Americans were exposed to 300 to 600 times the "acceptable" level of the toxic chemical dioxin every day in food and water. Major food sources of contamination with dioxin include chicken, egg, red meat, fish and dairy products.[16] The FDA has volumes of research showing this chemical can be harmful to humans and wildlife at exceedingly low levels.[16, 31]

- Dursban®, reported for years to cause birth defects and cancer in animals or humans, was found in 22 foods tested by the USDA (the United States Department of Agriculture).[59, 62, 64a,b, 65, 131] No wonder it was found in the urine of over 90% of Minnesota school children.[8, 11a, 47, 48, 93a] The EPA only "began" to ban this chemical in 2001. *(See Chapters 7, 10.)*

- When the immune system is adversely affected by chemicals, it can make someone more prone to develop allergies, such as asthma. For example in 2001, it was estimated that one in 17 children had food allergies. This represents a marked increase.[79] There also has been a definite rise in asthma in the past few years and again, in part, this could be due to herbicides used on the soil and then found in our foods and water. The immune or protection system of humans is further jeopardized by the many pesticides routinely used inside and outside buildings.

- Unfortunately the contamination of our foods is much more than residues of pesticides sprayed on the surface of foods. These chemicals can permeate the inside of fruits and vegetables. Washing and peeling fruit helps but certainly does not completely eliminate the potential problem of numerous chemical exposures. Much of our produce also contains bleach, fumigant residues, artificial colors and flavorings, sulfur, artificial sweeteners, ethylene gas, phenols, wax, desiccating agents such as glycol and innumerable additives.[107, 133, 134, 135]

Special Concerns in Infants and Children[53, 82, 83, 124]

- Pound for pound, babies consume two to four times more fruits and vegetables than adults so they are exposed to a higher proportion of possible chemical contaminants at a time when they are most vulnerable.

- In a study from 1994 to 1996, the government found that 25% of children's most frequently eaten foods contained detectable pesticides known to probably or definitely cause cancer in animals or humans and 34% contained substances known to damage the brain and nervous system.[20a-c, 33, 98a,b]

- Twenty million children under five years of age eat an average of eight pesticides a day.[148]

- One million under the age of five years ingest an unsafe dose of organophosphate insecticides. This includes 77,000 infants, six to 12 months of age, who eat unsafe baby foods.[7, 20, 21b,c, 28, 42]

- Many American two year olds consume organophosphates in amounts 10 times above the levels considered to be safe by the EPA.[7, 20, 28]

- Every day nine of 10 children aged six months to five years are exposed to combinations of 13 different nerve-damaging insecticides in the food they eat, even after washing and processing the food.[112a,b]

- In addition, children live closer to the floor where toxic contaminants are in higher concentrations.[42, 48]

The bottom line is that the foods children eat can expose them to too many potentially harmful chemicals. Even when the levels of allowed toxins in produce are within legal limits, these can be excessive in children.[113]

Reports About Pesticides in Your Foods[30b]

Claims about Vegetables

- Highly pesticided vegetables are reported to include winter squash and green beans. Domestic grown broccoli appears to be safer than the foreign variety.[27d, 36] Some broccoli samples, however, were found to contain 10 different chemicals in or on them.[27a-d, 29]

- It is possible for a single sample of spinach to contain as many as 14 different pesticides.[20c]

- High levels of chlordane have been found in potatoes, carrots, beets, lettuce, dandelion and zucchini.[37] This could be caused by growing them on previously contaminated soil or the use of chlordane that was stockpiled years ago.

- Some winter squash, green beans, spinach, celery and lettuce were found to contain more than the daily safe limit of pesticides for children in one serving.[34]

- Some USDA tests have shown that vegetables, such as squash and cucumbers, can contain high levels of cancer-causing pesticides that were banned years ago.[126]

- The USDA found as many as 108 different kinds of pesticides on 22 fruits and vegetables.[131-4]

- A fungicide, Triphenytin, is used to control beetles on potatoes, pecans and sugar beets. In laboratory studies, it has been reported that is it so extremely toxic that one hour's exposure can cause irreversible damage to the human immune system's "killer" cells. We need to study the agricultural workers, who are exposed to this product, as well as their families.[109a-c] Are they in special jeopardy and are they in need of urgent help? Then we need to ask, what happens to us when we eat foods contaminated with this specific chemical?

Claims about Fruits

- Fruits considered to be relatively high in toxic pesticide residues include peaches, apples, pears, cantaloupe and grapes (except those from Mexico).[27d]

- Recent studies indicate 25% of peaches, 13% of apples, 7.5% of pears and 5% of grapes can expose children to unsafe levels of organophosphate pesticides.[20c, 21a-c, 42]

- The Environmental Working Group (EWG) concluded in 1998, that one million children under five years of age consume foods that contain unsafe levels of organophosphates, including apples, pears and grapes.[23, 38]

- Reports in 2002 indicate that Dursban® was found in star fruit. *(This is the pesticide linked to brain defects in young rats.)*[123a,b]

- The average 25 pound one year old can eat certain fruits such as two grapes or three bites of some apples, pears or peaches and that amount will exceed the EPA safe adult exposure level to organophosphate pesticide.[21b,c, 42]

- The Government urges children to eat more fresh fruit and vegetables but reports indicate pesticide residues in fresh fruit were found on:

  56% in grapes
  47% in nectarines
  32% in peaches [123a,b]

- Canned fruits and fruit juices are less toxic but these can contain phthalates that leak from the metal cans. [27a-d] This chemical can cause precocious puberty in girls.[49c] *(See Chapters 3, 4, 6.)*

- A hormone disrupting pesticide, iprodione, was found in 29% of nectarines and also on kiwi fruit and mangos.[123a,b]

Claims about Bananas[107]

- Bananas can be contaminated with benomy, which has been linked to birth defects and chlorpyrifos (Dursban®), a known nervous system toxin.[62, 113]

- Bananas are often fumigated with ethylene gas to ripen them artificially. These can cause some chemically sensitive individuals to become ill. Gassed bananas tend to have white seeds and large black streaks on the skin while naturally ripened bananas have black seeds and small speckled black areas.[107]

Claims about Apples

- One grocery store apple had been reported to contain as many as 10 different types of pesticides.[30] The USDA found as many as 37 different chemicals on apples.[27a,c] A full page ad in the New York Times by the Environmental Working Group listed pesticides in and on apples, and stated that a child eating an apple a day could be exposed to a total of 30 pesticides in one year.[21a-c, 27a] Apples and apple products account for over half of the unsafe organophosphate exposures in children less than six years of age.[21a-c, 27a, 30b]

- It is possible for a two year old child to have ingested more than the lifetime tolerated amount of pesticides by eating only half of a non-organic pesticided apple.[27a]

- The residue methyl parathion was as much as 10 times higher on some apples than the level the government considers to be safe until it was banned for use on apples (and peaches) in 1999.[30b]

Claims about Peaches [30a,b, 41, 42, 142]

- According to the USDA, peaches contain more residues than any other domestic or imported fruits or vegetables.[30a,b, 41, 42, 142] In another report, however, strawberries have been reported to be the most pesticided of all fruits.[38]

- Twenty five to 40% of peaches contain a level of pesticides that exceeds the EPA safe pesticide limit for one day. This can be true for a single United States grown unpeeled and unwashed peach.[27a,c, 113, 153] For a 25 pound child this can mean about three bites of a highly pesticided peach can be too much.[41, 42, 142]

- One report estimated one in four peaches (and one in eight apples) have levels of organophosphate pesticides that are unsafe for children.[42] This figure should be less now that methyl parathion is no longer used on peaches.

- A recent study of peaches shows that 21% contain the organophosphate, fenitronthion.[124]

Claims about Cereals or Grains

- In one British study, 28% of breakfast cereals and 71% of cereal bars contained pesticide residues.[123]

- USDA found 80% of grains tested in the U.S. were contaminated with pesticides.[80, 132]

- One particular substance, a residue of Dursban®, is used extensively on foods and in the storage bins of grain.[48]

Claims about Meats and Fish[153]

- Fatty foods contain more chemicals, especially dioxin.

- Red meats, fish and dairy account for 95% of this dioxin exposure. Many Americans have dioxin levels hundreds of times above the "acceptable" cancer risk level set by the EPA.

- Many forms of fish contain pesticides or other chemicals due to water pollution.[18a, 158]

Foods Reported to be Low in Pesticides

- Foods that tend to be low in pesticide residues include bananas, broccoli, canned peaches, canned and frozen peas and corn, orange, pineapple and grape juices.[36]

Domestic versus Imported Foods

- In general, domestic food products appear to have more pesticides than foreign produce.[34]

- The FDA published a report in 1991 stating they found no residues in 64% of domestic food samples and 69% of imported samples. Their conclusion is reported to conflict with their own data and that of others.[35]

- Some studies by the USDA's Pesticide Data Program from 1994 to 1998 indicate that apples from New Zealand, grapes from Chile, tomatoes from Mexico and domestic soybeans have the highest chlorpyrifos (Dursban®) residue levels. Dow Chemical Company, which manufactures Dursban®, states that they have 3,600 scientific studies to prove Dursban® is harmless, if used as directed.[27c, 61] We must respectfully ask more about how the studies were conducted, how were the patients selected and how long was the follow up. Were the conclusions scrutinized by any impartial scientists?

- Butter was tested from 23 countries. Czech butter was the highest in PCBs and India had 1000 times more lindane (hexachlorocyclohexane) than Australia's butter.[119]

- Even chocolate can be a problem. In the United Kingdom about 75% of supermarket chocolate is contaminated with lindane. This chemical is banned in most of Europe and California, but it is used in places such as Africa and universal world trade enables it to make its way to the United States market.[108, 119]

Pesticides in Foods Eaten by Pregnant Women and Infants

Women can easily inadvertently ingest damaging pollutants when pregnant.[30a,b, 39] These can pass easily into the unborn baby. After birth it takes from about two to six hours for foods eaten by a mother to reach her breast milk.[161a-c]

- One diet study revealed DDT in 136 foods eaten by pregnant women, dieldrin in 100 and heptachlor and hexachlorobenzene in 31. Unfortunately, dioxin was not evaluated in this study even though it is the most toxic of all the persistent organic pollutants. It commonly contaminates many milk and dairy products.[40a,b] *(See Chapter 9.)*

- Every day 77,000 infants are fed commercial foods (apples, pears and peaches) which can contain an unsafe levels of pesticides.[122]

- The infant foods that most frequently have elevated levels of pesticides are pears, peaches and apple juice.[42]

- One USDA report indicates that 16 pesticides were found on eight samples of processed baby food.[133]

- A 1995 survey of 76 jars of brand name baby foods found them to contain 16 different pesticides.[30a,b] Safer brands of baby food are sold in some regular and health food stores. These include Earth's Best, Organic Baby and Healthy Times.

Summary[67a,b]

This chapter discusses the degree to which humans are presently contaminated with toxic chemicals. If you have been ill for years and no one knows why, this chapter might help you recall when and how some toxic harmful exposure occurred in your life. With this type of knowledge you can certainly find answers that others have missed and be more able to protect yourself in the future.

You have been and are being exposed to many chemicals in the air inside and outside your homes and in your water and foods. There is abundant evidence of this because of the many chemicals routinely found in the urine, blood, fat, bowel movements, breast milk and semen of Americans when they were studied.[48]

In spite of all the evidence of possible danger, there is much you can do that is practical to help protect your own nest and family. This is possible to a significant degree but only after you are more aware of how, where, why and when you are being or have been exposed. Once you make this decision, you can try to avoid many obvious known sources of chemicals in your everyday contacts. This can cause some inconvenience but you can certainly make strides, for example, to stop the use of pesticides known to cause cancer, brain, reproductive and genetic changes in and around your own personal home and work areas or in your child's school. *(Get Set: 800.221.6188)* You can try to stop buying or using personal body products that contain chemicals. You can grow some of your own foods, buy organic produce or find a nearby organic farmer. You can install quality air and water purifiers. *(PARF: 800.787.8780.)* You can build up your nutrition so you will have less trouble from the chemicals that you cannot avoid. You can check your blood, urine and breast milk and then take steps to rid your body of some of the harmful stored chemicals using some of the many methods available for natural detoxification. *(See Chapter 3.)* This should help to reduce the potential for future medical problems.

If you can make a few simple changes, this can lead to increased wellness for you and your loved ones. You can help those who fortunately cross your path because you now have more knowledge and insight to share with others. We must all seriously try to do more to help each other, as well as ourselves.

CHAPTER 6 REFERENCES:

1a "Community and Children's Advocate Against Pesticide Poisoning," P.O. Box 5388, Ventura, CA 93005, 805.654.4186, e-mail: CCAAPP4a@aol.com.

1b Our Toxic Times, September 2001, pp. 24-5.

2a Our Toxic Times, September 1998: 9 (9) 1-7, 13-15

2b "Multiple Chemical Sensitivity," A 1999 Census Archives of Environmental Health, (International Journal) May/June 1999: 54 (3) 147. www.heldref.org/html/Consensus.html.

2c www.salon.com.

2d BBC on line August 2002, "GMT Pesticide Threat to Health." www.news.bbc.co.uk/1/hi/health/medical_notes/449303.stm

3 "Deadly Birth Defects Defy Modern Medicine - Hoosier Environmental Council," USA Today, April 12, 2000.

4a Ban Dursban® www.epa.gov/pesticides (March 28, 2000).

4b www.safe2use.com/ca-ipm/00-03-30.htm, "Ban Dursban®".

4c www.nrdc.org/health/pesticides/bdursban.asp.

5 NCAP, December 1999: 20 (3) 7. P.O. Box 1393, Eugene, OR 97440-1393. 541.344.5044.

5a Marquardt, Sandra, "Toxic Secrets: Inert Ingredients in Pesticides, 1987-1997," www.pesticide.org (*Publications & Info., Special Reports.*)

5b Cox, Caroline, "Masculinity at Risk," Journal of Pesticide Reform, 16 (2) 2-7.

5c Journal of Pesticide Reform, Fall 2000: 20 (3) 7.

5d Feldman, Jay, "New EPA Truck Banner Campaign Misleads Public on Pesticide Safety as It's Unveiled in Washington, DC," Beyond Pesticides, December 4, 2000. 202.543.5450.

6a Porter, Warren, M.D., "Lecture on Endocrine, Immune and Behavioral Effects of Pesticides, Herbicides, and Fertilizer Mixtures at Groundwater Concentrations," Toxicology and Industrial Health, 1999, pp. 15, 133-150.University of Wisconsin Foundation, 1848 University Ave., Madison, WI 53706.

6b Hamm, Keith, "What's in the Mix," Santa Barbara Independent, April 15, 1999. pg. 21. Interview with Dr. Warren Porter. http: /www.independent.com/007/001/003.html.

7. NCAP: 541.344.5044. Journal of Pesticide Reform, Winter 1995: 15 (4).

8 National Health and Nutrition Examination Survey, 1988-1999. Trouble on the Farm, Chapter 6, "Confirming Exposure: Pesticides in Blood and Urine." www.epa.gov/pesticides

9 Federal Center for Disease Control National Resources Defense Council, "Beyond Pesticides," Archiv. of Envir. Medicine, March 1993: 48 (2) 89-93.

10a Deuble, L, et al., "Environmental Pollutants in Meconium in Townsville, Australia, Study of First Bowel Movement of Babies," Pesticides and You, Spring 2000: 20, 8. Department of Neonatology, Kirwan Hospital for Women, Dept. of Pediatrics, Wayne State University, Michigan.

10b www.gsenet.org/library/11gsn/2000/gs00423-htm.

11a Adgate, J. L., et al., "Measurement of Children's Exposure to Pesticides: Analysis of Urinary Metabolite Levels in a Probability-Based Sample," Environmental Health Perspective, June 2001: 109 (6).

11b http://ehpnet1.niehs.gov/docs/2001/109p583- 590adgate/abstract.html)

12 Chensheng, Dr. Lu, et al., "Biological Monitoring Survey of Organophosphate Pesticide Exposure Among Preschool Children in Seattle Metropolitan Area," Environmental Health Perspective, March 2001:109 (3) 299-303. http://ehpnet1.niehs.gov/docs/2001/109p299-303lu/abstract.html.

13a Rogers, Sherry, M.D., Depression "Cured at Last," 1997. Cost $24.95.

13b Newsletter: "Total Wellness," 1999 to present, July 2000, May 2001. Annual Fee: $39.95 (plus S&H).

14 Spyker, Joan, "Assessing the Impact of Low-Level Chemicals on Development: Behavioral and Latent Effects," Current Status of Behavioral Pharmacology, Federation Proceedings, August 1975: 34 (9) 1835.

15 "An Association Between Air Pollution and Mortality in Six US Cities," New England Journal of Medicine, December 9, 1993: 329 (24).

16 Williams, Rose Marie, "Dioxin, The Universal Toxin, Part 1," Townsend Letter, April 2001, pp. 158-60.

17 National Academy of Science, September 7, 2000. MSNBC, "National Environmental Trust Physicians for Social Responsibility and the Learning Disabilities Association of America." (*Larry Silver, Georgetown University Medical Center*).

18a Durnil, Gordon, The Making of a Conservative Environmentalist, 1995, Indiana University Press, Indianapolis, IN. $19.95. Chapter 5.

18b pg. 85.

18c pp. 52-4.

19 Curl, Cynthia, MSNBC News, "New Reasons for Eating Organic?" December 2002.

20a Pesticide Action Network North America (PANNA), www.panna.org.

20b www.epa.gov/seahome/groundwater/src/quality1.htm.

20c www.epa.gov/pesticides/food or www.nfm-online.com.

21a "Tap Blues: H_2O Herbicides in Drinking Water." EWG (Environmental Working Group and Physicians for Social Responsibility). 202.667.6982. 1718 Connecticut Ave NW, Suite 600, Washington, DC 20009. October 18, 1994.

21b www.epa.gov/ogwdw000/protect/cirguide.html.

21c www.ewg.org.

22 Weiss, Bernard, "Pesticides as a Source of Developmental Disabilities," Research Reviews 1997: 3, 246-256.
23 www.ige.apc.org/pesticides/etc.
24 Mekdeci, Betty, "The National Vietnam Veterans Birth Defects/ Learning Disabilities Registry," 1995. Written Statement for the Committee on Veterans Affairs.
25a The Maryland Public Interest Research Group, 3121 St. Paul St., Suite 26, Baltimore, MD 21218. 410.467.0439. www.pirg.org/marypirg
25b Pesticides and You, 1998-99: 18 (3) 24.
26 www.emagazine.com/november-december2000/1100lbpest.html.
27a "How Safe is Our Produce?" Consumer Report, March 1999, pg. 29.
27b Consumer Report, March 2001.
27c www.consumersunion.org and www.ecologic-ipm.com.
27d www.mercola.com/1999/feb/21/pesticide residue.htm.
28 Allergy Hotline 407.628.1377.
29 "Do You Know What You Are Eating?" An Analysis of US Government Residues in Foods. www.consumer.org. February 1999
30a "The Food Quality Protection Act (FQP) Background." A Visit the EPA's Office of Pesticide Programs. www.epa.gov/opppsps1/fopa/backgrnd.htm
30b www.parentcenter.com/refcap/health/food/29644.html.
31 "Farmers Use More Chemicals," L.A. Times, March 29, 2000.
32 Personal Communication.
33 "America's Children and Environment," EPA, December 2000, EPA R-00-006 pg. 29.
34 www.ecologic-ipm.com
35 U.S. Food and Drug Administration: "Pesticide Program: Residues in Foods," J. Assoc. Off. Anal. Chem, 1990: 74, 121A-142A.
36 Consumer Report, February 18, 1999.
37 American Chemical Society. 202.872.4065. www.acs.org
38 Solomon, Gary, "Food Watch," July 8, 1998.
39 Hamm, Keith, "Interview with Dr. Warren Porter of U. of Wisconsin," Santa Barbara Independent, April 15, 1999. See: cdansereau@watoxic.org.
40a AmeriScan, March 20, 2000. www.ens.lycos.com/ens/mar2000/2000L-03-20-09.
40b Gertrud, S., et al., "Exposure to Indoor Pesticides During Pregnancy in a Multiethnic, Urban Cohort," Environmental Health Perspectives, January 2003: 111(1) 79-84.
41 www.theatlantic.com/issues/99jun/9906am.htm.
42 "Californians for Pesticide Reform," February 1998 (3). 415.495.1149. www.organicconsumers.org/Toxic/kidsPois.html).
43 Terrance Gray, "Ag-Culture Media Project," 502.244.9444; "Green Blood—Red Tears," 1999, 87 minute video, $55.00.
44 Bosweg, Ritzema, "Environmental and Occupational Health", P.O. Box 238, 6700 AE Wageninen, The Netherlands.
45 US Food and Drug Administration. "Residues in Food, 1990," September/October 1991, pg. 16-17.f

46 US General Accounting Office, "Pesticides: Need to Enhance FDA's Ability to Protect the Public from Illegal Residues," October 1986.
47 US EPA, "Chlorpyrifos (Dursban®): HED Preliminary Risk Assessment for Re-Registration Eligibility Decision Document," October 18, 1999.
48 "In Harm's Way: Toxic Threats to Child Development," Greater Boston Physicians for Social Responsibility with Clean Water, 2000. 11 Garden St, Cambridge, MA 02138. $10.00.

48a pg. 54.

48b Chapter 6.

49a Rachel's Environment and Health News #250.

49b Hayes, H.M. et al., "Case-Control Study of Canine Malignant Lymphoma Positive Association With Dog Owner's Use of 2,4 Dichlorophenoxyacetic Acid Herbicides," J Natl. Cancer Inst. 1991:83, 1226-1231. 468.783.1209.

49c Rachel's Environment and Health News, "Here We Go Again," September 14, 2000 (708).

50 www.txinfinet.com/ban-gef/00/5/5-11.html
51a Crinnion, Walter J., N.D., "Environmental Medicine, Part 1: The Human Burden of Environmental Toxins and Their Health Effects," Alternative Medicine Review, February 2000: 5 (1). www.thorne.com/altmedrev/fulltext/med5-1.html.

51b Crinnion, Walter J., N.D., "Indoor Air Quality as a Factor in the Genesis of Chemical Sensitivity and Environmental Illness," Issues in Naturopathic Medicine Anthology (11) 19.

52 Personal communication.
53 www.orionsociety.org/pages/om/01-4/steingraber.html.
54 "Risks to Fetuses and Nursing Infants from Breast Milk and Mother's Food," EPA, ww.epa.gov/children/food/milk-breast.htm.
55 Personal Communication.
56 Personal Communication.
57 Carson, Rachel, Silent Spring. 1962.
58 http://www.safe2use.com/ca-ipm/00-03-put25.htm
59 Hawkins, Lyndon, "Ban Pesticides." www.panna.org
60a Blondell, J., Health Effects Div., to L. Probst, Special Review and Re-registration Div. Washington, D.C.

60b Sherman, J., 1996, "Chlorpyrifos (Dursban®)- Associated Birth Defects: Report of Four Cases," Arch. Environ. Health, 51(1) 5-8.

60c U.S. Environmental Protection Agency, "Prevention, Pesticides and Toxic Substances, Chlorpyrifos Revised Risk Assessment and Agreement with Registrants," June 2000, Washington, DC.

61 Feldman, Jay, "The Lowdown on Dursban® MOEd Down by EPA," Pesticides and You, Spring 2000: 20 (1) 1 - 18.
62 Sherman, Janette, M.D., "Endocrine Disrupting Chemicals in Food and

the Environment- Public Health Risks and Societal Concerns," Deutsche Forschungsgemeinschaft, 1998, Wiley-VCH, Germany, pp. 240-252.
63 C. G. Campbell, et al., "Chlorpyrifos (Dursban®) Interferes With Cell Development in Rat Brain Regions." Brain Res Bull., 1998: 43, 179-189.
64a Avakian, Maureen D. Research Brief 80: "Mechanisms of Chlorpyrifos (Dursban®) Developmental Neurotoxicity." (*Release Date: August 01, 2002*) Dept. of Pharmacology & Cancer Biology: Duke University.

64b Jett, D.A., et al., "Cognitive Function and Cholinergic Neurochemistry in Weaning Rats Exposed to Chlorpyrifos (Dursban®)," Toxico. Appl. Pharm., July 15, 2001: 174(2) 89-98. Dept. of Environ. Health Science, Johns Hopkins Univ. School of Public Health, Baltimore, MD 21205.

65 Chanda, S.M. and C. N. Pope, "Neurochemical and Neurobehavioral Effects of Repeated Gestational Exposure to Chlorpyrifos (Dursban®) in Maternal and Developing Rats," Pharmacol Biochem Behav 1996: 53(4) 771-776.
66 Personal communication.
67a Get Set, The Bug Stops Here, downloadable free book. Get Set, Inc., www.getipm.com 800.221.6188

67b www.motherearthnews.com/energy/energy184.pesticides.shtml.

68 Starr, H., et al., "Contribution of Household Dust to the Human Exposure to Pesticides." Pest. Monit. J., 1974: 8:209-12.
69 American J. of Industrial Med., 1996: 29(5) 501- 506.
70 Cantor, Kenneth and Warren Silberman, "Mortality Among Aerial Pesticide Applicators and Flight Instructors," Am J Indust. Med., 1999: 36 (2) 239-247.
71 Personal Communication.
72 AAEM, 7701 E. Kellogg, Suite 625, Wichita, KS 67207, 316.684.5500, fax: 316.684.5709.
73a Hill, R. H., et al., "Residues of Chlorinated Phenols and Phenoxy Acid Herbicides in the Urine of Arkansas Children," Arch Environ. Contam. Toxicol., 1989: 18, 469-474.

73b Hill, R. H., et al., "Pesticide Residues in Urine of Adults Living in the United States: Reference Range Concentrations," Environ Research. 1995: 71, 99-108.

73c Hill, R. H. Jr., et al. "p-Dichlorobenzene Exposure Among 1,000 Adults in the United States," Arch Environ Health, 1995: 50, 277-280

74 National Health and Nutrition Examination Survey 1988-1999. Trouble on the Farm, Chapter 6. "Confirming Exposure: Pesticides in Blood and Urine." www.epa.gov/pesticides
75 Science News, April 1, 2000; and Vol. 160, November 3, 2001.
76 www.epa.gov/esd/chemistry/anal-env-chem.htm.
77 http://enn.com/news/wire-stories/2002/03/0312002/ap_46656.asp.

78 "Pesticide Residues Seen Too High in Children's Food" (*Excerpts*), Reuters - Washington, June 7, 2000.
www.ecologic-ipm.com/seen_too_high.html.
79 Nowak-Wegrzyn, Dr. Anna, Mt. Sinai School of Medicine, November 26, 2001, Archives of Ped. and Adolesc. Med.
80 USDA Marketing Service, Science and Technology, 1998, 2000, "Pesticide Data Program Annual Summary for calendar 1997, 1999," pp. 15-17.
81 www.worldwidehealthcenter.net/article7.htm.
82 "Is Milk Safe to Drink?"
www.panix.com/-levner/nygreens/issues/biotech/rbgh.htm.
83 www.mercola.com/2001/dec/15/irradiated_food.htm
84 "Despite Toxic History, Residents Return to Love Canal."
http://www.cnn.com/us/9808/07/love.canal
85a Colborn, Theo, Dianne Dumanski and John Peterson Myers, Our Stolen Future: Are We Threatening Our Fertility, Intelligence, and Survival? 1996. Penguin Books, Inc. New York, NY. Cost: $15.64.

85b pg.190-7.

85c www.ourstolenfuture.org.

85d pg. 59.

86 Johnson, Christine, "Endocrine Disrupting Chemicals and Transexualism," 2001. http://antijen.org/pol.html
87 Moses, Marion, M.D., Designer Poisons, 1995, Pesticide Education Center, P.O. 420870, San Francisco, CA.

87a pp. 85, 98

87b www.SaveOurPlanet.org_ June 19, 2002.

88a National Resources Defense Council, "New Studies Confirm Dangers of Atrazine, a Widely Used Agricultural Weed-Killer." http://www.nrdc.org/health/pesticides/natrazine.asp

88b Hayes, T.B. et. al., "Hermaphroditic Demasculinized Frogs after Exposure to Atrazine at Low, Ecologically Relevant Doses," PBNAS, 2002: 99, 5476-5480.

88c www.SaveOurEnvironment.org Action Center.

89 The Delicate Balance, 1991: IV (3-4)18. 609.429.5358.
90 Emmett, A., 1080. "The Sperm Scare," The Week-Seattle's News Magazine, www.seattlenewsmagazine.com
91 http://ems.org/pesticides/childrens_exposures.html.
92a Loewenherz, C, et al., "Biological Monitoring of Organophosphorus Pesticide Exposure Among Children of Agricultural Workers in Central Washington State," Environ Health Persp. 1997: 105, 13441353.

92b www.nrdc.org/health/kids/farm/farminx.asp, ref. #12).

93Website: www.nrdc.org/health/kids/farm/chap6.asp.
94 Z. Tretjak, et. al., Human and Experimental Toxicology, Vol. 9 (1990), pp. 235-441.
95 EPA, Office of Toxic Substances, EPA-560/5-886-035, "Broad Scan Analysis of the FY82, National Human Adipose Tissue Survey Tissue Survey Specimens."

96 Adeshina, F. and E. Todd, "Organochlorine Compounds in Human Adipose Tissue From North Texas," Journal Tox. Env. Health, 1990: 29, 147-156.
97 "Common Pesticide Ending up in Semen of Farmers," May 27, 2002. CBC News, www.cbc.co/stories/2002/05/27/consumers/weedkiller.
98a "Teratogenesis, Carcinogenesis and Mutagenesis," 1987: 7, 527-540.
98b www.chem-tox.com/immunesystem/pesticide/pesticides.htm.
99a Rapp, Doris J., M.D., Is This Your Child's World? 1996, Environmental Research Foundation (Formerly PARF), Buffalo, New York. 800.787.8780, 1.716.875.0398. Cost: $15.00 (plus S&H). www.drrapp.com
99b "Environmentally Sick Schools," 85 minute video. Cost: $25.00 (plus S&H) Spanish video available.
100 "The Inside Story: A Guide to Indoor Air Quality," September 1988, EPA/400/1-88-004.
101 Cox, Carolyn, "More Hazards of Pesticides for Children's Health," J. of Pesticide Reform, summer 2001: 22 (2). NCAP.
102a Padungtod, C., "Low Level Exposure to Pesticides Impairs Sperm Quality," Harvard School of Public Health, Journal of Occup. Enviro.Med., 2000: 42, 981-992
102bwww.medscape.com/reuters/prof/2000/10/10.12/20001011epid001.html
103a Spears, Tom, "Weedkiller Targeted by City Poses Risks," The Ottawa Citizen, May 26, 2002.
103b Arbuckle, Tye, "Study: Herbicide Residues Found In Semen," Farm Family Health, Fall 1999: 7 (2).
103c www.dlrm.org Doctors and Lawyers for Responsible Medicine.
104 Northwest Coalition for Alternatives to Pesticides, Winter 2001: 21 (4) 4, 54, 344, 5044.
105 Organic Lawn Guide 2002, www.neighborhood.network.org. 516.541.4321.
106a Vincent, "Pesticide Appliers, Biocides and Birth Defects in Rural Minnesota," Arch Environ. Health 1996: 51 (1): 5-8; Environmental Health Perspectives 1996: 104, 394-399,.
106b Garry, V. F., et al., "Birth Defects, Season of Conception, and Sex of Children Born to Pesticide Applicators Living in the Red River Valley in Minnesota, USA," Environ. Health Persp. 2001:110 (3, supple.) 441-49.
107 Randolph, Theron, Human Ecology and the Susceptibility to the Chemical Environment, 1967, Charles Thomas, Springfield Il.
108 Environmental News Service, April 13, 2001. www.som.tulane.edu/ecme/eehome/newsviews/whatsnew/.
109a Colette-Bouchez, Health Scout News Reporter. "Pesticide Chemical Leaves Immune System Helpless," April 9, 2002.
109b whitman.christine@epa.gov
109c Env. Health Perspec. June 1999: 107 (supple 3) 409-19.

110 www.epa.gov/ttn/atw/nata/.
111 Anderson, H.A., et al., "Unanticipated Prevalence of Symptoms Among Dairy Farmers in Michigan and Wisconsin," Environ Health Perspect., 1978: 23, 217-226.
112a Wiles, R., et al., "Overexposed: Organophosphate Insecticides in Children's Food," January 1998, Environmental Working Group, Washington, DC.

112b Cook, Sally and Joseph Amodio, "Why Buy Organic?" Healthy Living Magazine.

113 www.earthsbest.com/concernoverpesticides.asp
114a Pimentel, David, "Silent Spring Revisited," J of Royal Society of Chemistry, Pesticide Outlook, October 2002.

114b Pimentel, D. and K. Hart, 2001, "Pesticide use; ethical, environmental, and public health implications." In: New Dimensions in Bioethics: Science, Ethics and the Formulation of Public Policy, pp. 79-108. Kluwer Academic Publishers.

114c Pimentel, D. and L. Levitan. "Pesticides: Amounts Applied and Amounts Reaching Pests," BioScience, 1986. pp. 36, 86-91.

115 USA Today, June 29, 2001.
116 Stephens, Francine, "Lawn and Garden Pesticides," Children's Health Environmental Coalition.
www.checnet.org/healthehouse/education/articles-detail.asp?Main_ID=427
117a Access-Pesticides. "2,4-D: A New Lease on Life," February 1996: XXI (2). University of Arizona.

117b "The 2,4-D One-Day Status Report," November 2, 1995, in Chicago, ILL; "Assessment of Potential 2,4-D Carcinogenicity: Review of the Epidemiological and Other Data on Potential Carcinogenicity of 2,4-D." March 1994. SAB/SAP Joint Committee, "2,4-D: 45 Years of Effective Use." 1995. Down to Earth. DowElanco.

117c Green, Emily, "Growing Health Worries Sprout Weed-Killer Study," L.A. Times, June 2, 2002.

118 Knopper, Melissa, "Water is Becoming a Dangerous Drug," E Magazine, December 2002. http://www.emagazine.com/january-february_2003/0103gl_health.html
119 Environmental Science and Technology, March 15, 2001.
120 Jensen, A.A., "PCBs, PCDDs and PCDFs in Human Milk, Blood and Adipose Tissue," Sci. Total Envir., 1987: 64(3) 259-93.
121 Park, D., et al., "Endosulfan Exposure Disrupts Pheromonal Systems in the Red-Spotted Newt: A Mechanism for Subtle Effects of Environmental Chemicals," Env. Health, Persp., 109, 669-683.
122 www.earthbest.com/concernoverpesticides.asp.
123a Press Release: "Latest Pesticide Results Bad News for Children," March 14, 2002 [found at: http://www.foe.co.uk/pubsinfo/infoteam/pressrel/2002/20020314113031.html]

123b www.pesticides.gov.uk

124 "Into the Mouths of Babes," FOE (Friends of the Earth), 26-28 Underwood St., London, Ontario, N1 7JQ. Tel: 020 7490 1555, Fax: 020 7490 0881. e-mail: info@foe.co.uk. http://www.foe.co.uk
125 Indoor Air Quality, http://comfortclean.com/cleaning_duct_air.html.
126 Robb, JoAnne, "Toddler Feeding and Nutrition: Pesticides in Your Children's Food," http://www.babycenter.com/refcap/toddler/toddlerfeeding/5054.html.
127 Rappoport, Jon, "A Miracle in Wisconsin," October 14, 2002. StratiaWire, 800.558.3535.
128 Reed, Barbara, Food, Teens and Behavior, 1983, Natural Press, P.O. Box 2107, Manitowoc, WI 54220.
129 Pall, Martin, The Federation of American Societies of Experimental Biology Journal, September 2002. www.fasebj.org/cgi/content-nw/full/16/11/1407/T1
130 Personal Communication.
131 Pesticide Data Program from 1944 to 1998.
132 Journal of Pesticide Reform, Winter 2001: 21 (4).
133 Giuliano, Jackie, Ph.D., Healing Our World: Weekly Comment: "Biological and Chemical Warfare Are Here Now," September 30, 2001. jackie@ deepteaching.com.
134 Ott, Wayne R. and John W. Roberts, "Everyday Exposure to Toxic Pollutants," Scientific American, February 1998.
135 Immerman, F. and J. Schaum, "Final Report of the Nonoccupational Pesticide Exposure Study," U.S. EPA, Research Triangle Park, January 23, 1990.
136 Feldman, Jay, "Hidden Pesticide Hazards Lurk in Newly Built Homes," Beyond Pesticides, National Coalition Against the Misuse of Pesticides. www.beyondpesticides.org.
137 Lazaroff, Cat, "Polluters Sully US Waters Despite Federal Regulations," Environment News Service, February 17, 2001.
138 EPA's OP Risk Assessment, "Technical Report: Beyond Pesticides," July-August-September 2002: 17 (7) 8-9.
139 Wallace, A., et al., "Personal Exposure, Indoor-Outdoor Relationships, and Breath Levels of Toxic Air Pollutants Measured for 355 Persons in New Jersey." EPA 0589.
140 Wallace, L. A., et al., "Personal Exposures, Outdoor Concentrations, and Breath Levels of Toxic Air Pollutants Measured for 425 Persons in Urban, Suburban and Rural Areas." EPA 0589 Presented at annual meeting of Air Pollution Control Association. June 25, 1984. San Francisco, CA.
141 www.epa.gov/epaoswer/hazwaste/recycle/fertiliz/risk/index.htm
142 Environmental Working Group (EWG). "One Million Kids a Day Exposed to Unsafe Levels of Toxic Pesticides in Fruit, Vegetables, and Baby Food: Report Urges Ban on Dangerous Insecticides Download Overexposed." 1998, Washington, DC. www.ewg.org.

143 Alternate Food and Pesticide Reference: "Pesticides Residues in Food," 1996, Joint FAO/WHO Meeting on Pesticide Residues (JMPR), Evaluations 1996, Part II-Toxicological, pp.45-96, Rome 16-25 September 1996, WHO Geneva 1997.
144 Cavieres, M., et al., "Developmental Toxicity of a Commercial Herbicide Mixture in Mice: I. Effects on Embryo Implantation and Litter Size." Environmental Health Perspectives. November 2002: 110 (11).
145 Ashford, N. and C. Miller, Chemical Exposures; Low Levels and High Stakes, 1998, Van Nostrand Reinhold, NY. $52.50.
146 Williams, W. Martin, et al., "Pesticides in Groundwater Base," December 1988, pg. 4. See: National Library of Medicine (1992). Hazardous Substances Databank. TOXNET, Medlars Management Section, Bethesda, MD, citing Williams, W. Martin, et al., 1988 Interim Report, US EPA, Office of Pesticide Programs, Environmental Fate and Effects Division.
147 Fagin, Dan and Marianne Lavelle, Toxic Deception, Center for Public Integrity, Birch Lane Press Book. 1996. Chapter 2.
148 Environmental Working Group, "How Bout Them Apples? Pesticides in Children's Foods 10 Years After," Alar. Washington DC, October 18, 1999.
149a www.care2.com
149b www.nrdc.org/legislation/rollbacks.pdf
149c http://enn.com/news/wire- stories/2002/10/1012002/ap_48678.asp
150 Pesticide News, Pesticide Trust, December 1994, pg. 22.
151 www.sustainablecotton.org/PESTICIDES/sttstcsS.html
152 U.S. Geological Survey National Water Summary 1984, Water Supply Paper 2275, 1985, pg. 120.
153 Bogo, Jennifer, "Children at Risk- Widespread Chemical Exposure Threatens Our Most Vulnerable Population," E Magazine October 3, 2001.
154 Environmental Health Perspectives, October 2001:109 (10) 1063-1070.
155 American Assoc. of Suicide. 202-237-2280. www.suicidology.org www.my.webmd/content/article/1728.68576
156 Razak, Dzulkifli Abdul, "Poison Control: Agent Orange – A Deadly Legacy Continues to Devastate." www.prn.usm.my/bulletin/nst/2000/nst19.html
157 www.metroke.gov/hazw-aste/teachers/california.htm
158 Mercola, Newsletter, January 16, 2002.
159 Vedantam, Shankar, "Report Shows Big Rise in Treatment for Depression," Washington Post Staff Writer, January 9, 2002; pg. A01.
160 http://www.ADHD-biofeedback.com/alternate.html
161a Food Allergy News, June-July 2001, pg. 9.
161b JAMA, Vol. 235, #13.
161c www.foodallergy.org
162 http://www.ewg.org/reports/bodyburden/es.php

163 Simcox, N., et al., "Pesticides in Household Dust and Soil: Exposure Pathways for Children of Agricultural Families," Dept. of Env. Health, Univ. of Washington, Seattle, WA 98195, Envir. Health Persp., 1995: 103 (13) 1126-1134. 103:1126-1134, Vol. 103, No. 13.
164 Wong, Brad, "Pesticide Traces Found in Kids Here," Seattle Times, August 10, 2001.
165 Tilson, H., et al., "Polychlorinated Biphenyls and the Developing Nervous System: Cross Species Comparisons," Neurotoxicology and Teratology 1990: 12, 239-48.
166 Fenski, Richard A., et al., "Children's Exposure to Chlorpyrifos and Parathion in an Agricultural Community in Central Washington State," Environmental Health Perspectives, May 2002: 110 (5).
167 Shealy, D., et al., "Correlation of Environmental Carbaryl Measurements With Serum and Urinary 1-Naphthol Measurements in a Farmer Applicator and His Family," Environ Health Persp., 1997: 105, 510-513.
168 Richter, E., et al., "Sequential Cholinesterase Tests and Symptoms for Monitoring Organophosphate Absorption in Field Workers and Persons Exposed to Pesticide Spray Drift," Tox. Lett., 1986: 33, 25-35.
169 Brucker-Davis, Francoise, et al., "Significant Effects of Mild Endogenous Hormonal Changes in Humans: Considerations for Low-Dose Testing," Environmental Health Perspectives, March 2001: 109 (Supplement 1).
170 "Paracelsus Revisited - Part 2," Rachel's Environment and Health News, October 31, 2002 (755).
171 http://www.ourstolenfuture.org/NewScience/broadtrends.htm
172 "Why Do You Think They Call Them DIE-oxins?" Teen Source Endometriosis Association Newsletter, Spring 2002.
173 Rea, William J., M.D., CRC Press, Inc., Corporate Blvd., NW, Boca Raton, FL 33431. 214.368.4132, or call American Health Environmental Center. 800.428.2343.
173a Chemical Sensitivities, Vols. 1-4, 1992-1997.
173b Optimum Environment for Optimum Health and Creativity, 2002. Cost: $39.95.
174 Rogers, Sherry, M.D., Prestige Press, P.O. Box 3068, 3500 Brewerton Rd., Syracuse, NY 13220. 800.846.6687; 315.468.4417. Fax: 315.468.8119. www.prestigepublishing.com
174a Wellness Against All Odds, 1994. Cost: $17.95 (plus S&H).
174b No More Heartburn, 2000. Cost: $15.00 (plus S&H).
174c Depression Cured at Last, 1997. Cost $24.95 (plus S&H).
174d Detoxify or Die, The Ultimate Healing Plan, 2002. $22.95 (plus S&H).

175 U.S. Environmental Protection Agency, "Estimating Exposure to Dioxin-like Compounds," Vol. II, Properties, Sources, Occurrence and Background Exposures [EPA/600/6-88/005Cb June 1994 External Review Draft] (Washington, D.C.: U.S. Environmental Protection Agency, 1994), (Table 3-18 on pp. 3-58).
176a http://www.epa.gov/envirohealth/children/ace_2003.pdf
176b http://yosemite.epa.gov/ochp/ochpweb.nsf/content/index.htm
177 "Warning on Male Reproductive Health," Rachel's Environment and Health Newsletter, April 20, 1995 (438). P.O. Box 5036, Annapolis. MD 21402-7036. 410.463.1584. Fax: 410.263.4894. www.rachel.org.
178 Colborn, Theo, Ph.D. and Coralie Clement, "Environmental Estrogens: Health Implications for Humans and Wildlife," Environmental Health Perspectives, 1995: 103 (Suppl 7) 135-136.
179 J. Auger, et al., "Decline in Semen Quality Among Fertile Men in Paris During the Past 20 Years," New England Journal of Medicine, 1995: 332 (5) 281-85.
180 Holloway, Marguerite, "Toxic Reduction: Dioxin Indictment," Scientific American, January 1994: 270, 25.
181 Padungtod, Chantana, Harvard School of Public Health, J Occup Environ Med., 2000: 42, 982-992.
182 "Airline Passengers Are Sprayed for Bugs," PANUPS, March 17, 2003. www.panna.org.
183a Daly, H., "Laboratory Rat Experiments Show Consumption of Lake Ontario Salmon Causes Behavioral Changes," J of Great Lakes Research, 1993: 19 (4) 784-88.
183b Daly, H., "Reward Reductions Found More Aversive by Rats Fed Environmentally Contaminated Salmon," Neurotoxicology and Teratology, 1991: 13, 449-53.
183c Brenner, Loretta, "Malathion," J. of Pest. Reform, Winter 1992: 12 (4) 29-37.
183d Nature, "Health Prof. for Malathion in 2nd Generation," Malathion Health Library Index, pg. 6, November 4, 1961.
184 Regenstein, Lewis G., Cleaning Up America The Poisoned, 1993, Acropolis Books LTD. 2311 Calvert Street, N.W., Washington, D.C. 20008. Chapter 8. Cost: $14.95.
185a "EPA Issues Powerful Indictment of Chemicals in Teflon." http://www.ewg.org/policymemo/20021113/20030328.php
185b Alexander, B., "Mortality study of workers employed at the 3M Cottage Grove facility. Final Report," April 26, 2001, Division of Environmental and Occupational Health, School of Public Health, University of Minnesota. Reviewed in U.S. EPA Administrative Record AR226-1137 (pp. 143-146; PDF pp.40-43).

185c Gilliland, F.D. and J.S. Mandel, "Mortality Among Employees of a Perfluorooctanoic Acid Production Plant," J. Occup. Med., 1993: 35(9): 950-4.
185d Olsen, G. W., et al., "An Epidemiologic Analysis of Episodes of Care of 3M Decatur Chemical and Film Plant Employees, 1993-1998." 2001.Reviewed in U.S. Environmental Protection Agency Administrative Record AR 226-1137 (pp. 156-159; PDF pp. 53-56).
186 Environmental Working Group, "Warning: Teflon Can Cause Birth Defects and Infertility," March 2003.
187 Woolf, Norma Bennett, "Canine Thyroid Disease Can Be Tough to Diagnose," Dog Owner's Guide Online Magazine. http://www.canismajor.com/dog/thyroid.html
188 Scott-Clark, Cathy and Adrian Levy, "Spectre Orange – Nearly 30 Years after the Vietnam War, a Chemical Weapon Used by US Troops is Still Exacting a Hideous Toll on Each New Generation," Guardian Unlimited © Guardian Newspapers Limited 2003. March 2003.

CHAPTER 7

How Helpful Are Pesticides and Are We Protected?

How Effective Are Pesticides, Herbicides and Fungicides?

In the previous chapters you have read how extensive the potentially harmful health effects of pesticide chemicals can be in animals, children and adults. As you read the following, consider that some 60 million pounds of organophosphate pesticides are applied annually to 60 million acres of cropland and another 17 million pounds are used for insect control and lawn and home care.[13] There is no doubt we are using plenty of chemicals.

However, before we consider health safety factors, let us review how effective pesticides have been in eradicating pests. It is an acknowledged fact that in 1972 pest damage to crops was 7%. By 1998, after using millions of tons of stronger and stronger pesticides, the loss had almost doubled to 13%. If our government is aware of this, why do they not encourage the safer methods of pest control that are already known and why do they not allocate more money to find new and safer pest control measures?[6, 27, 68a-c]

Unfortunately, humans appear to adapt less well than pests to pesticides and herbicides. The brains, nervous systems and bodies of children and adults are being increasingly damaged by the extensive use of these toxic chemicals. We must keep asking why we do this when safer, equally effective and less expensive pest control measures are available.[1a,b]

The bottom line is that in spite of spending billions of dollars on ever-increasing amounts of progressively more potent pesticides, chemicals have failed to control insects. Maybe it is time to evaluate what we are doing and why.

Are We Informed Adequately by MSD (Material Safety Data) Sheets?[2, 5a, 18, 32, 61]

When you wonder about the safety of a product, you can legally ask for and must be given an MSD sheet. This is true for any product you use or those used by others in or near your home, work or school areas. One would logically assume that MSD sheets, which are designed to tell us about the safety of the contents of products, would do exactly that. They do not. The MSD sheets do not have to reveal all ingredients, even when certain products contain toxic "registered" poisons known to pose an unreasonable risk to our health or environment. In addition, they do not have to reveal "trade secrets", for example, in relation to the chemicals used in cosmetics. This means MSD sheets provide only partial information. It is virtually impossible to find out the specific exact needed information about the contents of many products.

Let's examine further how and why these sheets, that should assist and inform the consumer, can be incomplete, deceptive and misleading. Although they provide information about the *key* component of a product, this is not necessarily the *major* component. The key portion pertains to the part for which an item is purchased and is certainly specified but it might comprise only 1% to 5% of the total product. The other 95% to 99% can contain well-studied, well-known registered toxic substances, which do *not* need to be specified on the label. Even worse, these are often deceptively lumped into a so called "inert" category so they do not have to be revealed or listed. That means potentially or proven registered poison portions, such as the solvents benzene, toluene or xylene, do not need to be listed. At least 200 chemicals, referred to as "inert" on MSD sheets, are classified as environmental pollutants, hazardous to our health under certain federal environmental statutes.[2, 3a,b] *(Someone, somewhere must still be celebrating the creation of the term "inert" as a successful, most clever ploy of deception.)* For these reasons, our MSD sheets are a mockery. We must ask why this is allowed to continue. *(See Chapters 1, 6, 8, 10.)*

One Typical Example

Let us look at just one example. Here are the unspecified "inerts" found in one herbicide called Triclopyr:[4]

- Ethoxylated sorbitan monooleate: It can cause an elevation of blood pressure in dogs and adrenal tumors in rats.

- Ethylenediamine tetraacetic acid: It is known to cause skin, eye and lung irritation in humans and birth defects in rats.

- Kerosene: It can cause eye and respiratory irritation, fatigue, headache, dizziness, poor coordination, a burning sensation, disorientation, drowsiness and euphoria.

- Petroleum solvent: It appears to cause irreversible damage to the kidney and nervous systems in exposed workers. This is a form of hydrocarbon and can cause all types of allergies.

- Triethyamine: It can cause irreversible damage to eyes and vision and can harm the skin and respiratory system. It causes coughing, wheezing, headache and nausea.

What Type of Information Should MSD Sheets Contain?

We want and need MSD information about every ingredient in every product, as indicated in the previous sector. We need to know the possible acute and chronic health and toxic effects of each ingredient. It should clearly specify if a chemical is a suspect or known cause of cancer or some other particularly incapacitating or deadly illness. It should provide pertinent resources for additional in-depth information concerning both animal and human research studies, if this is desired for some reason. There should be detailed reference resources which tell where and how every ingredient enters a body and where each one tends to accumulate or be stored. Data on how much exposure to what concentration is thought possibly to cause serious harm and how long each chemical ingredient will remain in the environment and body should be available.

Are We Protected by Our Laws, Legislators and EPA (Environmental Protection Agency)? [5-7]

The Toxic Substances Control Act of 1976 allows chemicals to be sold and used *unless they are proven to be a risk.* The EPA, however, does *not* conduct its own safety tests, but relies on research conducted by manufacturers. Yes, you read it correctly. Is the fox in charge of designing the chicken coop?

How Certain Can the EPA Be of Manufacturer Data?

How well is the act of faith, integrity and honesty justified in relation to the safety and scientific data supplied by chemical companies? Surprisingly, we absolutely know the answer. In 1991-2, the EPA offered amnesty to chemical manufacturers if they would turn in their studies showing their products caused harmful health or environmental effects. Ten thousand were quickly turned in! [5a,b, 7]

At the present time, the safety data submitted by chemical companies to the EPA for registration of pesticides does not have to be published and access to this data is very limited. This means there can be no chance of a critical, impartial, outside scientific review. If a chemical is claimed to be safe by a manufacturer, why are knowledgeable non-EPA or outside scientists not allowed to scrutinize, evaluate and critique the data? We are obviously protecting the manufacturers but we surely need a better system to ensure the safety of the American public.

A Review of Some Reports of Our Government's Administrative Record after 2000

How well is our government protecting our land, air, water wildlife and us? Here are some reports of decisions made by legislators during the previous and current administrations.[35, 36a,b]

- In January 2001, under the Clinton administration, there were efforts to control raw sewage overflows and to maintain the sewers. The proposals were placed in limbo during the Bush Administration. This will potentially allow some 400 sewer systems to overflow and this means 400,000 basement backups of untreated sewage each year. This sewage can contaminate homes and eventually, our waterways.[36a,b]

- In January 2001, they legislated to use wetlands for landfills and boosted logging on public lands and national forests. This put some migratory birds and even some salmon on a direct path to extinction.[36b]

- In March 2001, drilling for oil and gas in Artic Wildlife Refuge was proposed and supported by legislation. Over two million acres of land in Utah is also in danger with gas and oil leases.

- In April 2001, environmental protection budgets and programs were cut.

- In June 2001 reintroduction of protection of certain endangered species was stopped.

- In August 2001, known environmental offenders received government contracts.

- In February 2002, superfund funding was cut. This enabled more loopholes in relation to stored nuclear wastes under the Nevada Enforcement Act. It "grandfathered" in some factories or allowed them to increase their emissions, with fewer modern pollution controls. Consideration of such issues was reported to contribute to the resignation of the director of the Office of Regulatory Enforcement of the EPA in July 2002.[35]

- In December 2002, the Clean Water Act was weakened again so pesticide spraying would allow known harmful chemicals to be put into our water, under certain circumstances, without permits.

Roads now destroy the natural character of many pristine public forests. Logging, drilling and mining are becoming more evident because of the total disregard of our watersheds, animal and marine wildlife habitat and recreation areas in favor of developers and big business. Federal agencies do not protect our water, and state and local agencies do not hold polluters accountable for violations. The Bush Administration has been accused of refusing to go to court to defend our present environment against legal assaults by groups who are violating the federal laws and mandates that were previously passed to protect our water, air, wildlife and national preserves.

Outside pressures, however, can and do help. It was reported that the Bush administration was about to raise the allowed amount of arsenic to increase from 10 to 50 ppb (parts per billion) in our drinking water. This was prevented when the National Academy of Sciences concluded that even the standard of 10 ppb carried an increased cancer risk. After they intervened, the Bush administration fortunately backed off and did not allow an increased unsafe level of arsenic in our water.[36, 67]

Since President George W. Bush took office, air pollution restrictions have been weakened so it is easier for older power plants, factories and refineries to pollute. In addition, it is easier for developers and homebuilders to pollute the wetlands and waterways. It is now easier to log in National forests and refuges and numerous forms of wildlife and nature are no longer protected.

A Review of the Chemical Industry Conclusions

The following are a couple of reported research studies and decisions made by the chemical industry that illustrate what happens in the real world.[18]

- In 1964 Dow Chemical dipped dogs in different concentrations of Dursban® solutions to check the safety of their product. Twelve of the 40 dogs were pregnant at the time of the dip. The cumulative mortality of the pups was 62%. One third of the young died at or shortly after birth. With this information the chemical industry researchers concluded an emulsified 0.1% Dursban® solution was safe to use as a dip on pregnant bitches, their offspring and adult dogs of any size. We must ask why research scientists in the chemical industry did not reach obvious valid conclusions. From their own data how could they conclude this chemical was safe for the offspring of pregnant bitches?

- In a second study, during a four-year period, Dow Chemical ascertained that humans who sprayed with Dursban® (chlorpyrifos) had decreases in their cholinesterase levels. This lack means the normal transmission of nerve impulses through their bodies was impaired. It was reported that they concluded, in the absence of an epidemic, this chemical should not be used and stated this pesticide was not acceptable for use inside premises as a larvacide to kill developing pests. This time the industry reached the correct conclusion, but proper action was not taken to protect the public. In spite of the above, thousands of gallons of Dursban® have been and continue to be used in the foundations of millions of homes for termite control and inside and outside buildings for pest and weed control. *(See Chapter 10 about the disastrous effects this product had on one family's health and future.)* We must again ask why?

A Brief Review of a Few of EPA's and FDA's Decisions [5a,b, 14, 16a,b, 17]

The evidence of mistakes goes way back and continues to the present.

- In 1950, the FDA (Food and Drug Administration) approved cyclamates as a sweetener in everything from children's vitamins to canned ham. In 1939 The Secretary of Health, Education and Welfare announced a ban on cyclamates because of complaints about birth defects, tumors and other serious health effects. It took 20 more years before the FDA reviewed the ignored evidence of its own original research.[79, 80, 81]

- For nearly 20 years before the FDA declared a moratorium on silicone breast implants, the manufacturer knew the risks. One Dow Corning executive was reported to have resigned in protest because no one listened to warnings that the implants could rupture and leak. In spite of this, the FDA did not investigate or regulate silicone implants until more than 2 million had been inserted into women.[55, 82]

- In 1993, FDA, Department of Agriculture and the Environmental Protection Agency pledged to curtail pesticide use by promoting sustainable agriculture and the development of safer chemicals. In the next three years, pesticide use rose 20 %. At the same time, the agricultural research budget designated to evaluate or find better alternative agricultural methods of pest control was reduced to less than 1%.[6, 68a-c]

- In 1995, the EPA determined that evaluation techniques originally used to register many pesticides were outdated from both the health and safety viewpoints. For example, four previously deemed safe chemicals were eventually reevaluated and recognized to cause cancer after more appropriate laboratory tests. [14]

For example:

In 1997, the EPA concluded 2,4-D was "non-carcinogenic (not a cause of cancer), non-teratogenic (not a cause of birth defects) and non-mutagenic (not a cause of genetic abnormalities)".[8a, 37, 41a-c] This information now appears to be seriously in question.[41d] Later studies suggest this chemical is a cause of lymphomas in both humans and dogs, a cause of birth defects and a link to cancer in a variety of organs in those who are exposed. For example, these problems are more evident in wheat-growing areas where this chemical is used extensively on crops.[37, 41b,c] *(See Chapter 6.)*

- In 1999, the EPA finally banned the use of methyl parathion on certain foods, making peaches, for example, safer, but this toxic chemical is still present and allowed on other foods. Why?

- About 66% of other chemicals found on foods, have not had their dietary risk evaluated.[16b, 21] Many more continue to wait for reevaluation and in the meantime, the health of your family and you can be in jeopardy. This should be given a higher priority.

- In 1996, the EPA decided to implement improved safety measures under the Food Quality Protection Act. The EPA was requested to eventually assess some 9,000 agricultural pesticides in common use to ascertain the level of pesticides on foods. The improved safety measures were recommended because of definite concerns about the safety of chemicals, in particular, in relation to vulnerable infants and children, and the need to study possible health effects from the interaction of multiple chemicals.[15, 16a,b, 17, 32, 54] Initially, the government mandated no less than about 400 of the highest risk pesticide chemicals be tested for their effects on the nervous, endocrine and immune systems. Three years later, by August 1999, only eight organophosphate reviews had been finalized although about 15 were to have been tested by that deadline. From 1996 to September 1999, they had only put restrictions on two of 125 of the highest risk pesticides.[19a,b]

- In August 1999, the authorities were also advised to place a limit on the amount of pesticide residue allowed on foods according to new standards. To protect children, the margin of safety for chemicals was to be increased 10 fold, rather than the usual 3 fold. The higher level of protection was to be used whenever available data was insufficient to make a valid decision.

- In February 2001, Consumer's Union's evaluated the EPA's performance and stated that they had failed to do their job. The EPA had failed in 84% of its decisions to raise the margin of safety by the 10 fold level. In addition, only a third of food residues were evaluated to determine how much should be considered safe, based upon new scientific data.

- In July 2002, an independent panel of scientists seriously questioned the EPA again because they concluded 28 of 30 pesticides were safe for fetuses, infants and children.[20a,b]

They were reported to have continued to use the three-fold, not the 10-fold safety factor required by the Food Quality Protection Act.

Table 7
How EPA Banning Really Works

1. The banned chemical in stores is not immediately recalled.
2. Numerous products incorporating the banned substance can continue to be sold.
3. The chemical typically can be stockpiled for several years.
4. If the stockpiles are not fully eliminated by the original designated deadline, generous extensions are typically granted, sometimes repeatedly, for many years.
5. Negotiations and compromises with the manufacturer allow for incredible, even implausible exceptions and exclusions. For example, tons of certain poison pesticides can be allowed to be used indefinitely on freeway medians or golf courses, for insect control, on certain crops or foods etc.
6. Obvious polluting factories are "grandfathered" in so they are not required to meet current pollution standards.
7. When a chemical is considered too toxic to be sold in this country, manufacturers can continue to sell it to third world countries.

- In addition, the EPA had industry-based data on only six of 30 pesticides in relation to their effects on the developing nervous systems of animals.
- In August 2002, Bayer Crop Science agreed with the EPA to slowly "phase out" the insecticide called Guthion®

(azinphos-methyl) on 30 crops. For other fruits, vegetables and nuts it will be stopped or allowed with registration permits until December 31, 2005. If it is safe, why is its use not allowed; if it is unsafe why a delay of years before it is stopped entirely without exceptions? [84]

Loopholes starting with the 1976 Toxins Substance Control Act appear to obviously allow the EPA to give greater consideration to the chemical industry's economic status than to the health and welfare of the American public. The EPA was supposed to weigh the costs to the chemical industry against the benefits to the public in relation to all proposed actions concerning toxic substances. Their record for the next 20 years speaks for itself. In that period of time, the EPA's ability to issue decisive regulations has been so thwarted and delayed, that they only mustered adequate proof to overcome the cost/benefit ratio in relation to nine of some 75,000 chemicals.[19a]

We must ask why the EPA does not have adequate help to review the effects of many more of the potentially toxic chemicals more efficiently. Why do they not have adequate funding and staff so they can protect the public in a timely and proper manner?

Let's Look At How the EPA Typically Bans Toxins

Table 7 is one general example of how the system typically works after the government *finally* makes the decision that some product is so toxic that it must be banned.

Problems When Toxic Chemicals Are Sold to Foreign Countries

By continuing to sell third world countries our toxic chemicals, their inhabitants become ill and their soil, water, air and produce also become contaminated. Ironically, there is a bit of fairness in all this. Their exported pesticided produce eventually is sold and purchased for use in the United States so we are again exposed to the poison we knowingly produced and sold to them. If a foreign country objects to importing our toxic chemicals, is it possible for political pressure to be exerted? Is it possible that benefits received in the past or promised in the future from our government can be denied unless they accept certain known toxic substances for use in their country?

The EPA "Bans" Dursban® in June 2000[75]

The EPA has stated that 30% of insecticides, 60% herbicides and 90% of fungicides can cause cancer. They are well aware of the dangers to the public.[22] Once they know for sure how toxic a chemical is and go forth to protect us, let us examine exactly what they actually do and how effective their actions are. You decide if the degree to which the EPA appeared to compromise adequately protected the American public when it finally concluded that Dursban® could be dangerous and should be banned.[23]

1.
You Can Buy It for 18 Months

Why were retail sales and home use of Dursban® allowed from 2000 to 2002 (an additional 18 months) after they knew and finally acknowledged how bad it was?

2.
You Are Not Informed It Is a Banned Product

Why do they not have to tell home users that it is a banned item? *(See Chapter 10 about how one family's life was decimated by this chemical.)*

3.
You Can Stockpile It and Use It Later On

Anyone can stockpile this chemical and use it indefinitely. Years from now people will wonder why Dursban® is still in the blood and urine of the newborn, children and adults when it was "banned" in 2000. This is because for years after known toxic chemicals are banned, they can legally continue to be used to further contaminate the air, water, soil and homes. Once the soil is contaminated, it may take many years before crops grown on it do not contain the toxic chemical. This happens because of many exceptions, extensions and industry-favoring loopholes in the pesticide laws. Although DDT was banned in the 1970s, for example, some form of it continues to be found in most people's blood, in uterine fluid, women's breast milk and even the first bowel movement of newborn infants.

4.
Banned Dursban® Can Be Used In Home Foundations for Five More Years

Why can Dursban® be used in home foundations until December 31, 2005? For example, in Phoenix, AZ it has been noted that builders routinely put 300 to 500 gallons in the foundations of new houses (depending on the size) and this has been done for many years. This chemical can gradually seep up the walls and through floor cracks and holes, into the air of the buildings. This can cause some occupants to gradually become ill. Many will never know or understand why they are sick or what caused their symptoms. Most people, and some in the health profession, might not suspect this chemical could be the cause of chronic asthma, fatigue, muscle aches, arthritis, heart disease, depression, cancer or behavior, mood or memory problems. For many years, I personally would certainly not have believed it was possible because this type of medical information is not always taught to doctors in training. It is understandable that real estate agents and/or bankers insist on termite inspection and insect control, if it is indicated, but who decides on which pesticides to use? Who looks the other way when toxic chemicals are used even though safer, less expensive and more effective pest control measures are available?[27] Who allows this type of pollution to continue?

5.
Dursban® Is Only On Some Fruits and Vegetables[75]

Some 13 million pounds of Dursban® are applied to corn, grain, fruits, nuts and vegetables each year. The public has no way of knowing which food items contain this chemical and which do not. For example, why is the use of this pesticide limited mainly to a few selected fruits, such as grapes and apples? Is there a good reason why some fruits can legally continue to contain this harmful chemical, while others are not?

What about the equally contaminated and potentially dangerous vegetables? Why are tomatoes, for example, selected as one product on which this pesticide cannot be used as of December 12, 2000? Are tomatoes more permeable to the pesticide because of their thin skin? How does the EPA decide which vegetables are allowed to be polluted with a dangerous toxic chemical and which are not?

6.
Dursban® Allowed Indefinitely on Golf Courses for Insect Control and Agriculture[31]

Spraying with Dursban® on non-resident golf courses, for mosquitos and on agriculture is to be allowed indefinitely.[24] Do they dislike golfers or maybe think they are stronger than the rest of us. Golfers beware. Maybe your sporadic bad game or chronic ill health are due to toxic sprays used on the courses that are known to adversely affect the brain, muscles, nervous and reproductive systems of humans, as well as animals. The fairways and greens can look fine but there is a price. If you chose to live within breathing distance from a golf course, you could be inhaling toxic dangerous pesticides on a regular basis. Also read about cancer in golf course superintendents.[31] If you are an avid golfer you might want to think about having your blood and urine checked for chemicals, so you can take proper precautions *before* you develop any symptoms of some serious illness. (*Accu-Chem: 972.234.5412 ImmunoScience: 800.950.4686.*)

Were the above decisions of where and for how long Dursban® can be used determined by the EPA with the safety of the public in mind or was it a compromise so the manufacturer, Dow Agrosciences, lost less money? Threats of lengthy litigation should not be the reason for half-hearted banning. If federal laws bar the EPA from issuing a pesticide recall except in an emergency situation, change the laws. Is it not an imminent hazard when the brains of innocent children can be permanently damaged or we knowingly allow one more chemical on the market that can contribute to the present obvious epidemics of cancer, learning problems and attention deficit disorder in humans?[13 *]

Not Much Better with Dioxin[52, 63]

It took from 1985 to May 2001 before a Science Advisory Committee finally voted to send the long stalled report to federal regulators that concluded that dioxin probably causes birth defects, miscarriages and cancer in laboratory animals and probably in humans. They acknowledged that dairy, beef, pork, chicken and fish were major sources of this contamination. This unwanted chemical can be a byproduct of pesticide production. It is released as industrial pollution from factories related to paper pulp, dyes, municipal waste, burning plastic, sewage and medical waste products that contain chlorine. It can contaminate future generations because it has been found in human breast milk in many areas of the world and because of its persistence in the environment.[37, 63*]

---

* *Can Chemicals Cause Epidemics?*, Doris J. Rapp, M.D. ERF, P. O. Box 60, Buffalo, NY 14223-0060, 800.787.8780, www.drrapp.com.

What Has Gone Wrong?[38, 39]

The following are sensible and practical suggestions to improve the protection of the American public. The apparent dilemma of our government is a realistic need to choose between the economy and the health of the public. There are times for compromise but this should not be a factor when one considers the efficiency in controlling pests versus cancer and brain damage in children and adults. In addition, there is really no need for compromise when safer methods of pest and weed control are proven and possible.[27] If foreign countries can reduce pesticide use by 50% and not reduce crop yields, why can't we?[68a-c]

Challenges for Federal Agencies and Legislators

- In some situations the solution appears to be blatantly obvious. Why does our government, on a federal or state level, not simply mandate that no school be allowed to use toxic chemicals for pest control or cleaning if these contain ingredients (this includes the "inerts") known to damage the brain and nervous system, interfere with learning or cause cancer in animals? [26a,b] We should insist schools implement Integrated Pest Management (IPM) because it is not only safer, but more effective and less expensive.[27] This is simply common sense. An increasing number of progressive states such as Maine, New Jersey, New York and Pennsylvania already have or are presently implementing these sensible measures.

- We need a change in our government's attitude and priorities. Drugs or medications are typically carefully controlled and monitored by the FDA but there is no similar control or monitoring for certain other exposures. For example, in 1947 the government passed FIFRA, (Federal Insecticide, Fungicide and Rodenticide Act). This was not designed to assure the public that pesticides were safe, but rather to assure farmers that certain products were sufficiently lethal to control or kill insects and weeds. [5] When the law was amended in 1972, the chemical industry still did not have to prove human safety. Instead, the government was required to show that a chemical was dangerous. Does the public want industry or public protection?

Most European countries have adopted the so-called Precautionary Principle" Their manufacturers must prove their products are safe "before" release. Why is this not our philosophy?

- In Europe, 40 to 60 agricultural chemicals are to be withdrawn because of safety concerns. European regulators are presently reassessing another 800 agricultural products for safety.[9] They have adopted a "Precautionary Principle" in relation to chemicals. Chemicals must be proven safe *before* they are released, not as is done in our country, *after* they have been proven, over and over again, to be harmful. Does it not seem reasonable that until there is well-documented proof that a chemical is safe, it should not be used? The message to the public should be one of reassurance that all chemicals have been proven safe before they are released.

- In May 2003, the European Union took their attitude one step further and created REACH (Registration, Evaluation, and Authorization of Chemicals). Their new strict regulatory policy would require industrial chemical manufacturers to test their products before they are sold to determine their effects on the environment and human health. Europe is becoming increasingly protected from harmful chemicals in contrast to the United States.

The Public Must Recognize the Following Possible Political Realities [76]

1. Repeated budget cuts have lead to markedly reduced staffing problems in relation to various key positions in the EPA. The end result is the EPA, in spite of the extraordinary expertise and dedication of many of its scientists, appears to be understaffed and unable to effectively or properly evaluate or ban the multitude of chemicals that potentially can make us ill. We must ask why politicians have allowed the EPA funding to be decreased to such a level that they do not have adequate numbers of scientists to do the research evaluations that have been recommended or mandated to protect us. If we are to continue to allow progressively more pollution, we need more, not fewer scientists to evaluate the effects on humans. They need more funding, not less, to responsibly protect us.

2. Legislators must see that our EPA officials and scientists are not threatened with less funding if they do not delay or avoid evaluating sensitive areas that might negatively impact select vested interest groups or the personal priorities of powerful legislators. Is it possible that common sense has been obstructed by a gigantic maze of politically vested interest groups? Can the realistic potential of expensive red tape, legal delaying maneuvers and well-directed political contributions indirectly lead to inertia in EPA evaluations? Is the bottom line to significantly prevent potential economic losses to pesticide manufacturers or to protect the public? The EPA needs to be staunchly sheltered from all political and chemical industry persuasive pressures. They cannot possibly do their job effectively and honestly if this is not done.

3. The EPA's union's leader, William Hirzy, Ph.D., asked for the EPA to enforce the Principles of Scientific Integrity Policy. This action was precipitated when an employee man-

ager complained to the union that he was told, "It is your job to support my decisions, even if I say 2+2=7." Pressuring employees to craft spurious scientific data to support deceptive invalid management decisions is hardly the way to go. After grievances in this regard were submitted by the union, the EPA denied the request by the union to enforce the Principle's Policy because it was said to be impractical or not possible.

Glaring Potential Red Flags within Governmental Agencies[76]

The following show we need to be on guard. There are apparently many with possible vested interests in key positions.

- It has been reported that some former executives in the chemical industry are presently or were previously placed in key pesticide control positions within the EPA. It has been reported that some former EPA employees, who worked in the area of chemical pollution, eventually become highly paid consultants for the chemical industry after they left the EPA.

- It was reported early in August 2002 that a United States District court ruled that the United States Department of Agriculture and Department of Health and Human Services violated federal laws when they selected individuals with known financial ties to various food industries to serve as members of the Dietary Guidelines Advisory Committee. This same group makes decisions related to federally funded food programs. This certainly can create obvious conflicts of interest in key areas if decision makers lack integrity.

- Similarly, decisions can occur in relation to which types of children's vaccines are to be approved by the Food and Drug Administration. Their recommendations are passed on to the Center for Disease Control and eventually mandated by the Advisory Committee on Immunization Practices. Ultimately this committee endorses and provides federal funds to buy the vaccines. Each individual state then also decides how many of which vaccines must be given. All these agencies must have immense integrity because of tempting potentials for conflicts of interest. It has been reported that more than half of the decision makers who determine which, how many and how often vaccines are to be given, have financial ties to the vaccine industry. Provisions for special waivers allowed during "secret" deliberations make it very difficult for public scrutiny. For example, even after copious evidence of health dangers from vaccines containing mercury was presented on June 18, 2000, they were not immediately recalled. Some well-conducted studies showed that it was possible for some children to receive 40 times the amount of mercury considered to be safe according to the EPA guidelines during routine immunization protocols.[22, 69a,b] *(It is of interest to note that veterinarians recognized the mercury problem and removed it from dog vaccines in 1996. They also believe pets do not need all the vaccines they presently receive and that some vaccines are being administered more often that necessary.)*[70]

Is it possible that some harmful vaccines can continue to be given to babies for years so the manufacturers have the opportunity to use up their stock of vaccines? If they remove the mercury, have they removed enough so the infants are truly safe? *(They apparently still contain some mercury.)*[69] How can they do long term follow up safety studies unless they take the time to do this? Without this, how can they say the vaccines are safe?

4. And the final straw was the report that a provision was slipped into the Homeland Security Bill in December 2002 that granted immunity to the manufacturer of certain vaccines if they caused illness in children.

We must ask: why were faulty tires quickly recalled when they were dangerous while infant vaccines are not when there are so many claims they appear to cause autism and brain damage? If they are safe, use them. If they are not, stop using them. And if there is serious doubt about their safety, err on the side of caution. We should not allow the present autism epidemic to continue. [69a,b *]

The bottom line is:

- Decisions by federal or state agencies for either vaccines or the use of drugs such as Ritalin® should be recommended and suggested but not compulsory or mandatory.
- Legal action should be possible when vaccines are proven to be dangerous.[38f]
- Parents should have the final say and religious, medical and philosophical exemptions should be possible. Non-compliant parents should not be threatened with Child Protective Services, foster care for their children or jail. We live in the United States.

More Illogical Thinking of Health Issues

- Why are mercury fillings not allowed in pregnant women or young children but allowed to be used in filling dental cavities in everyone else? California implemented regulations concerning this early in 2003, and lawsuits in relation to this and similar issues are pending in Georgia, Ohio, Texas, Maryland, New York and California. Mercury and other dental metals are toxic.[40a-c] It appears the proof of

* *Can Chemicals Cause Epidemics?*, Doris J. Rapp, M.D. ERF, P. O. Box 60, Buffalo, NY 14223-0060, 800.787.8780, www.drrapp.com.

mercury toxicity danger, in animals and humans, certainly can no longer be denied.[44-48] A study in spring 2003, showed the risks of neurodevelopment and heart disease rose with increased mercury exposures. It also showed strong evidence that the mercury in children's vaccines was linked to neurodevelopmental problems.[85] Why is the American Dental Association so reluctant to admit they have made a serious error in judgment?

- Why is swallowing a pea sized amount of fluoridated toothpaste considered to be unsafe for children under six years of age, but all right if you are over seven or an adult? Read your toothpaste label. Switch to natural brands. The amount of fluoride in water combined with that in toothpaste and from fertilizers and pesticides found in and on foods and beverages is reported to be excessive for children.[49, 67]

- Why are so few concerned about reports that 1.5 to 3.4 million children use drugs such as Prozac for depression when there is so little research data about this drug, especially in young children?[55, 56] The liquid form of this drug has had no studies on the effects on young children, even though many are presently using this drug. Why are long term studies not conducted before such a drug is released? If there are no studies on young children, why is it not forbidden to prescribe it for children under seven years of age? *(Call 800.249.9576 for latest information.)*

Challenges for EPA Officials[86]

- The EPA certainly has many well-qualified scientists who are typically and rightfully very cautious. They want all the facts and could never be accused about making hasty decisions. In general, however, the EPA is aware of the many dangers of a product for many years or for excessively long periods of time before any definitive action is finally taken to protect the public.

- We should inquire in depth to determine why the EPA would accept incomplete research data from a chemical industry or not allow outsiders to see the data they use to make decisions. Anyone in science knows you can deceptively design a study to have the outcome you desire by clever omissions and deletions, by the selection, number or type of study patients, by changes in the amounts or types of exposure or by limitations in the length of a study so the effects of what is being studied will not have time to become apparent. The EPA needs to insist on having adequate staff to properly evaluate all research for quality. They should have so much confidence in their judgment that they encourage outside critiques of their decisions.

- State and federal health scientists should have the right to strongly disagree with their department's decision. This happened in July 2002. Consideration of measures to weaken the enforcement of the Clean Air Act are reported to have contributed to the resignation of the director of the Office of Regulatory Enforcement of the EPA.[35]

- In the past other exemplary conscientious scientists, who had the temerity to "blow the whistle" in relation to some toxic exposures, appeared to have experienced unwarranted difficulties. It has been claimed that if the pesticide industry is threatened in some way or a scientist is too critical of a pesticide product or its use, there can be "gag" orders with threats of various repercussions. It is possible for some kind of personal attacks to take place to question the ability, integrity or character of that scientist, for his research funding to be withdrawn and for warnings about dire consequences, such as embarrassing dismissal, to be carried out.[71a,b]

- One veteran scientist, an author of more than 300 published papers, showed how cancer developed in mice and rats when they were fed chemicals over a lifetime. It was reported that he was warned not to send letters, emails or other communications critical of the NIEHS (National Institute of Environmental Sciences) as an Institute, or its scientific work to the media, scientific organizations, scientists, administrative organizations or individuals outside the NIEHS. If he violated the agreement or negotiation, it was stated he must retire or resign voluntarily within a week.[42] Is this a new version of American freedom? *(For more scientist battering, see reports in Chapter 8 about Dr. Shafey and in Chapter 9 about Dr. Pusztai.)* [71a,b]

Should Implementation of Laws Be Monitored More Closely?

We must ask why the government passes laws and does not establish mandatory follow through methods of implementation. EPA officials, who are dedicated and highly qualified, can do their part but it is of little value if powerful industries get a mere slap on the wrist for flagrant wrong doings. The public needs effective implementation and enforcement of sensible regulations and recommendations. How much longer will the public tolerate delays in relation to unfulfilled essential mandates?

As an example, consider the fact that OSHA (Occupational Health and Safety Administration) estimates 32 million workers are exposed to harmful substances in more than 3.5 million workplaces. Yet, in over 30 years, OSHA is said to have issued citations to only 170 employers for not properly protecting their employees against toxic substances.[43]

Even laws that have more possibility of truly protecting the public have large gaping loopholes in regards to state and federal regulations. They tend to have so many built in exceptions and delays that there is no way to adequately notify, inform or protect those who are being exposed. Too many laws lack any means of effective enforcement. When there is evidence of non-compliance, shrewd industry lobbyists leak draft rule changes to undermine potential lawsuits. Even when the evidence is irrefutable, the chemical industry tends to slip by with barely the need for a whimper. The present system has so many holes it is challenging and difficult to plug the leaks.

The public should know who sponsors legislation that protects the public and environment so those legislators can be encouraged and re-elected. They also need to know which ones appear to have vested interests. This type of information should be highly publicized. For example, how much money for campaign re-elections and paid recreational/work trips have specific members of the Senate and House subcommittees on Agriculture received from the chemical industry? [6]

Can We Learn From Certain States?

Some states are better than the federal government, but others are still favoring pollution.

On the good side:

- California has signs on the doors of some public buildings warning and clearly stating that chemicals within these building are known to cause cancer, birth defects, developmental delays in children and reproductive problems.

- California has the best monitoring protective groups in the country. They monitor changes in animals and they have documented, for example, that the incidence of mice having both male and female sexual organs in a certain areas has increased from 3% in 1995 to 25% in 1999.[50] *(In other places where similar sexual changes have occurred in various forms of wildlife (frogs and fish), it is claimed that chemical exposures could be the major suspect cause of such changes.[2,62]) (See Chapter 5.)*

On the bad side:

- In California it is reported that certain farmers were legally exempted from complying with the state's clean water laws. The farmers were given a special waiver in December 2002 so they can continue to pollute the water in that state. This happened in spite of the fact that the EPA declared that 500 miles of rivers and streams, as well as 480,000 acres in the Sacramento River Delta were contaminated with pesticides. The California Water Quality Board is said to have ignored all the evidence of contamination and danger to humans and wildlife.[67] We must ask why.[33a,b]

Can We Learn From Canada?

Quebec announced new pesticide laws in the late summer of 2002. It is reported that no pesticides will be mixed with fertilizers or used in schools, daycare centers or on public lands including hospitals, clinics, etc. However, they too have built-in-delays and exceptions. Until 2004, certain pesticides are said to be allowed on store shelves but only qualified licensed personnel can continue to sell them. By 2005, several pesticides will be totally banned. Fines will be large if the mandates are ignored and mass education and government ads will warn all of pesticide dangers.[25, 51]

The Final Straw in the Abominable Tragedies of Chemical Wars[77,78]

It is 30 years later and the tragedy of the Viet Nam War is not going away because of the immensity of the errors in judgment and cover up and because proper and fair resolutions of the wrongs have never been forthcoming. It all started when the Kennedy administration sanctioned the use of defoliants in the Viet Nam war. The Nixon administration supplied the South Vietnam regime with herbicides until 1974. Viet Nam was contaminated with 70 million liters of chemicals of which 66% was the infamous Agent Orange which contained a most virulent poison strain of dioxin called TCCD. About 170 Kg of this chemical was reported to have been widely scattered over 10%

of the country for ten years. *(It is estimated that 80 grams could kill the eight million in NYC.*[75-77]*)* It was said to have been applied in concentrations exceeding the guidelines by 25 times. From 2.5 to 4.8 million people were directly sprayed.[77] It remains in the food, soil, water and bodies of the Vietnamese 28 years later. It also continues to be evident in the American soldiers who were exposed. In addition, the effects are evident in the Vietnamese and American offspring. And finally, as impossible as it seems, it is even worse. It appears the terrible effects of this chemical are present in the third generation of deformed children born to the Vietnamese people. Alarming levels of dioxin have been found in the blood of individuals who were not alive at the time of the war or who lived in areas that were not directly sprayed. It is obvious that their contaminated soil, water and food continue to pollute their breast milk and bodies—and harm their unborn children.

What has it specifically done to the health of the Vietnamese people and American veterans who were exposed? About 500,000 Vietnamese have already died. Of the 650,000 or more Vietnamese who remain ill but alive, the major complaints include rashes, asthma, cancer, gastrointestinal, muscular, skeletal, neurological, endocrine, reproductive and psychological illnesses. Many Vietnamese families have four or five seriously disabled suffering children. These same symptoms continue to plague many of our exposed Viet Nam veterans. Too many of the children born to those who were exposed are deformed, paralyzed and suffer from many of the same illnesses as their parents.

Did we know it would be this harmful? Unfortunately, we did. The National Institute of Health reported that mice exposed to Agent Orange gave birth to stillborn or deformed litters. The EPA at one time reportedly concluded that dioxin was a class-l human carcinogen. An admiral's son, who was later reported to have died of two forms of cancer from his exposures in Vietnam, provided military documents that the government knew what they were doing. From the time of the herbicide program's conception in the 1960s, it was reported to be known that dioxin was being used in too high a concentration.

At one point a group of over 5000 members of the Federation of American Scientists signed a petition against the use "of chemical and biological weapons in Vietnam." They were aware of the potentially grave danger. In April 2002, another group of the world's leading environmental scientists concluded, at a conference at Yale, that the Viet Nam war was the largest chemical warfare campaign in history—and we were the ones who did it. Our shame should be immense.

A Tragic Example of a "Straw" that is Even Closer to Home

Probable Misdiagnosis and Miscarriage of Justice

The following story is true. As you will see, there can be tragic results. It is everyone's responsibility to become more aware of what can happen, and whenever possible, to take action to protect those who are in danger. It could happen to you.

Meet Chrissy[10]

It all started with a chicken farm near a school that attracted flies. To combat the flies, a nearby school installed insect sprayers to dispense chemicals in the classrooms throughout the school. Every 15 minutes gushes of potentially poison insect killing chemicals filled the air, to such a degree that a residue had to be removed each day from the tabletops in the dining room. This happened every single day. Every child in that school was breathing and ingesting this insecticide for years. The parents of Chrissy and her brother had no idea that, along with many other students and teachers, their children were being exposed to potentially harmful chemicals. At that time, Chrissy's only symptoms were a repeated bloody nose and severe headaches. She appeared to be a very healthy child and a gifted athlete.

**First Collapse:
An Outside Chemical Exposure**

While Chrissy was playing softball at a local park in June 1993, she collapsed. The diagnosis was "heat stroke". Later it was reportedly discovered that the grass had been sprayed with a mixture of pesticide chemicals. As a pitcher, her hands repeatedly touched the polluted softball.

**Second Collapse:
An Inside Chemical Exposure**

Chrissy collapsed again in her school in the spring of 1995. This time the episode was called epilepsy, even though she had no twitching. Later on, her parents found out Dursban®, Tempo and other chemicals had been used in the school for insect control.

**Third Collapse:
An Inside Exposure**

Her next episode occurred in the fall of1995, again in school. This time it was diagnosed as hypoglycemia. The same types of chemicals were routinely and repeatedly being applied inside or outside the school. When she was evaluated in the hospital, they found a heart irregularity but her parents apparently were not informed about a possible cardiac weakness.

**Fourth Collapse:
Another Outside Chemical Exposure**

The fourth collapse occurred in June 1997 after pitching on the mound at the same playground where she had collapsed before and where another child was said to have also collapsed and died. Again, Chrissy had to be rushed to the hospital. This time she did not live. She died in a coma six days later. The diagnosis at this time was a heart problem. Her electrocardiogram showed a prolonged QT abnormality, similar to the EKG taken in 1995 when she had collapsed at school.

Could Chemicals Be the Culprit?

As explained in the introduction of Chrissy's story, while she was a student in elementary school an automatic sprayer spread pesticides in the air every 15 minutes throughout the school. When she entered middle school, they were said to have used Dursban® Tempo, Diazinon and other chemicals to control pests. *(Both Dursban® and Diazinon have been "banned" since then.)* As an 8th grader, she frequently was seen in the nurse's office complaining about intense headaches, nosebleeds, nausea and dizziness. She had these same symptoms previously in elementary school, but they became more frequent and intense in her middle school. At that time, some thought she had a psychosomatic illness. (*Many children continue to be similarly and incorrectly diagnosed when they have various forms of chemical sensitivities.*)

Investigation of the health effects of organophosphate pesticides indicated that her medical complaints could have been due to the chemicals to which she was repeatedly exposed in each of her schools and also when she was in the ballpark. These chemicals are reported to include Roundup®, diazinon, chlorpyrifos (Dursban®, cyclotron, cypermethrin, Tempo, 2,4-D and Fumiti to control gophers). Many of these organophosphates are thought to possibly damage the heart and the nervous system of some individuals.[29a-d, 30, 58, 64]

Summary of Chrissy

It is certainly possible that Chrissy, along with many other children, had been sensitized to chemicals by exposures over the years to the repetitive spurts of insecticide and other chemi-

---

** Chrissy G. Foundation, 40485 Murrieta Hot Springs, #381, Murrieta, CA 92563. 909.679.3900. To assist other families who have had similar, possible chemically-related tragedies.

cals used inside the school and to those used outside on the lawns, ballparks or playgrounds. It is possible for some of these chemicals to cause irregular heartbeats and an abnormal electrocardiogram.[57-60, 72-74] Her headaches were possibly due to chemically-associated brain swelling or brain blood vessel changes. These were her personal major vulnerable, target organs probably hurt or damaged by chemical exposures. Much literature confirms this type of possibility. [29a-d, 30 **]

Why Are So Many Young Physically Fit Athletes Dying?

One must also wonder why we keep reading about young, strong football and baseball players or golfers suddenly dying. Their deaths are attributed to "heat stroke", "dehydration" or "unknown causes". Is the weather hotter? This is unlikely. Are children and adult athletes weaker? Are they more prone to heat for some inexplicable reason than they were in the past? Might they not have been similarly affected by unsuspected exposures to toxic chemicals used on or near the grass on the playing fields? Are their hearts being affected by chemicals?[57-60] Maybe toxic pesticides, herbicides and fungicides used in the play areas can be unsuspected factors that need more serious consideration. We must keep asking if the blood and urine of all athletes who have unexplained deaths have been checked thoroughly for chemicals. Remember, there can be economic and legal reasons for not checking the right way for all the right chemicals in all body fluids. (Accu-Chem: 972.234.5412 and ImmunoScience: 800.950.4686.) For legal reasons authorities may be reluctant to provide accurate information about when, where and what was used inside and outside schools or play areas.

Chrissy's Brother, Matthew

Unfortunately this family's sad tale has only begun. Chrissy's brother, Matthew also attended kindergarten at the same school and was similarly sprayed for years with chemicals to control flies every 15 minutes. From August 1994 to May 1995 his perplexing medical complaints included rashes, blisters, coughing, diarrhea, bed-wetting, abdominal pain and difficulty breathing. Because of his sister's death in 1997, Matthew's heart was thoroughly evaluated to ascertain if there was a genetic defect. There was no hereditary problem but his EKG did show a heart irregularity similar to his sister's and of the type sometimes associated with exposure to pesticides or certain medications. He, however, was not on any drugs. His medical complaints were compatible with those attributed to a group of chemicals called pyrethrins. This chemical was part of the spray dispenser pesticide (Purge 111) to which he had been exposed for years. One other major component, an "inert" substance 1, 1,1-trichloroethane, was also emitted from the spray dispenser. It is known to cause dizziness, lightheadedness, skin rashes, breathing and nervous system problems. His heart irregularity fortunately appeared to subside when the family moved and he attended another school.

Other students were ill with symptoms similar to Matthew's. The parents of these children, however, were said to have settled out of court with the pesticide company with the gag proviso so they could never discuss what happened to their children. Chrissy and Matthew's parents, however, refused the money offered in return for signing away their right to speak out to help others.

For several years Matthew was not able to attend school or play ball regularly without careful monitoring. Because of the heart condition, he was in special jeopardy on a daily basis if he was near pesticides or other possible toxic chemicals. On several occasions, when toxic pesticides were being used on the playing fields, the official response was that, "our pesticide company says these are safe." When that happened, his parents would not allow him to continue to play with his team or he had to change schools. They could not take a chance that they were not given correct information.

At the present time Matthew is older and he is usually able to actively engage in sports activities without obvious difficulty, *but he must, always be alert and avoid contact with chemicals.* His parents must continue to check carefully for any exposure to chemicals.

His First Close Call

In May 2000, Matt attended a Christian camp in which some of the campers used an insect repellant which contained Deet®.[66] This exposure appears to be a factor in Matt being rushed to a hospital emergency room. He was ashen, cold, too weak to stand and very lethargic. His appearance was very similar to his sister's when she collapsed. When his heart was checked, no abnormality was found. No one examined his blood for chemicals but his recovery was fortunately uneventful.

Second More Serious Close Call

In March 2003, when Matt was 13 years old, the inside of his school was sprayed by an extermination company with a time-released form of pyrethrum. His blood pressure became elevated, and he developed a severe headache, nausea, and appeared to be cold, clammy and pale. He could barely stand up and was unresponsive for several minutes. His appearance again was strikingly similar to his sister's. However, the doctor in the emergency room would not believe his mother's concerns so his heart was not immediately evaluated. When his EKG was finally taken, it showed no abnormality. His heart was subsequently monitored over a period of several weeks and he developed heart abnormalities approximately five times a day, mainly when he was in school.

At the present time, in view of his recent exposure and probable chemical reaction, Matthew needs to have his body carefully detoxed so he has fewer chemicals stored in his tissues. This will need to be supervised because of the degree of his sensitivity and the potential severity of his response. For emergencies, the medications that appear to possibly help individuals with this type of serious chemical sensitivities include intravenous and oral vitamin C, an alkali such as Alka Aid, glutathione, heparin under his tongue and oxygen at the rate of 4-6 liters per minute.

Results of His Court Trial

When Matthew was 10 years old, the court had to decide if his exposures and illnesses could be related to his chemical exposures. His parents said that the legal system would not allow the family to discuss their daughter's cardiac problem or death or share important information about her autopsy report. They said the cardiologist was not allowed to show the EKG similarities between the heart irregularities of Chrissy and her brother. They were not allowed to mention about another young women who lived and died under unusual circumstances in the vicinity of the same ballpark where Chrissy died. They were said to be forbidden to mention that other children in the school had symptoms similar to their son's or that some other children had EKG changes similar to Chrissy's and Matt's. The parents said the plaintiff was not allowed to present medical records of similarly sick classmates provided by expert physicians and a toxicologist.

The school refused to provide health office records of student visits before and after pesticide spraying, or to make comparison to other schools where certain chemical pesticides were not sprayed in the air every 15 minutes for years. The parents said the defendants could present hearsay evidence but the plaintiff was denied this opportunity.

The Verdict

The jury decided in favor of the pesticide company and

Matthew was ordered to pay them $132,276. As can happen in these types of cases, the family paid the lawyers thousands of dollars, but the injured person and family received little or nothing. In addition, they were left with the loss of one dearly loved child, a massive debt to the pesticide company and the fear that their remaining sick child will never be normal and like his sister, could conceivably die, at any time, from some unanticipated chemical exposure. They feel the chemicals used in their children's schools and city parks took the life of their one child and has placed their remaining child in possible jeopardy.

The Irony of It All

Similar to the movie, Class Action, the evidence came too late. Only two days after the above verdict, the CDC published a new report of 90 incidents showing injury from "Automatic Insecticide Dispense Units" (June 9, 2000). These contained the same chemicals to which both Chrissy and Matthew, and many other students, had been exposed for several years.[12] In spite of this, a motion for a new trial was denied.

Matthew, at the age of 13 years, had to file for bankruptcy. Was this justice? Can an ordinary citizen win against powerful corporations and unscrupulous lawyers? This appears to be a challenge. Terrible wrongs can sometimes override what is obviously right and fair. This family could have easily accepted "hush" money and been much more secure financially. They are to be commended for doing what was right.

We must live by a higher than ordinary standard of principles if our world is to survive. Americans are worried about possible chemical warfare in the Middle East. Realistically we need to be at least equally worried about the everyday toxic chemical exposures that are present and allowed in our own air, water, foods, homes and schools.[26a,67]

Samuel Epstein, M.D. Puts It All Together[32]

Dr. Epstein succinctly summarizes what he believes has

happened and why, in his "must read" book, The Politics of Cancer Revisited.[32] His summary says it all. "The pattern of industry-sponsored fraudulent scientific research, supported by bribed government officials and corporate-controlled mass media is so common that it can be considered 'business as usual' in the United States." He provides more than enough the data to support his statements. I believe we all have to take off the blinders.

Summary

We are using toxic chemicals on everything in sight, and not in sight, and while doing so, we are creating stronger and more chemically-resistant pests and weeds and weaker and more unhealthy humans. Our government's Material Safety Data sheets are of little use for they do not have to reveal the dangerous poisonous ingredients in the products we use. In fact, it is illegal for the public to be given certain known source material so they can be fully informed. Although our federal protective agencies have slowly made important needed decisions and regulations, they tend to fail miserably with implementation. By compromising on enforcement and not following through with needed restrictions, laws and limitations, they have allowed the American public to be needlessly hurt by what appears to be blatant loopholes, exceptions and unnecessarily prolonged delays.

The EPA's action, or lack of action, in relation to environmental issues gives the impression that they are much more of an agency for the protection of big business and personal vested political interests than for the protection of the American public. The EPA must be made totally free of subtle and overt coercion by politicians and various vested interest groups. They urgently need adequate funding so they have the staff and money to properly protect us.

In addition, our government should certainly learn to err on the side of caution, as is exemplified in the Precautionary Principle adopted by many European countries. Let the chemical manufacturers prove their products are safe before they are released; not force the public to prove they are unsafe after the damage is done. What happened to Chrissy and Matthew is a warning of how bad it can get. Let us hope that many will listen before it happens to someone in their families.

CHAPTER 7 REFERENCES:

1a www.safe2use.com/ca-ipm/00-04-14a.htm-

1b www.epa.gov/pesticides.

2 Colborn, Theo, et al., Our Stolen Future: Are We Threatening Our Fertility, Intelligence, and Survival? 1996. Penguin Books, Inc. New York, NY. Cost: $15.64, pg. 217.

3a www.safe2use.com/ca-ipm/00-03-30.htm, "Ban Dursban®".

3b www.safe2use.com/ca-ipm-00-08-25b-htm.

4 Herbicide Factsheet, Triclopyr, Journal of Pesticide Reform, 2000: 20 (4) 12-19.

5a Fagin, Dan and Marianne Lavelle, Toxic Deception, 1996, Center for Public Integrity, Birch Lane Press Book. Pp. 11-14.

5b pp. 12-14, 137-142.

6 Interview with Dr. Warren Porter by Carol Dansereau, Washington, Toxics, Coalition, Fax: 206.632.8661.

7 www.publicintegrity.org/toxic-deception.

8 http://www.24d.org/Rev4.pdf.

9 New York Times, November 4, 2000. www.nytimes.com.

10 "Adding Insult to Injury, Young Victim Ordered to Pay Company Court Costs," Journal of Pesticide Reform, Fall 2000: 20 (3) 4.

11 Rea, William J., M.D., Chemical Sensitivities, Vols. 1-4, 1992-1997, CRC Press, Inc., 2000 Corporate Blvd., NW, Boca Raton, FL 33431. 214.368.4132. Cost: $75.00.

12 Shafey, O., "Illnesses Associated With Automatic Insecticide Dispensers Use," CDC News Report Mortality and Morbidity Weekly Report, June 9, 2000: 49 (22) 492-5.

13 www.motherearthnews.com/energy/energy184.pesticides.html

14 NCAP winter 1995.

15 "Tap H2O Blues," Environmental Working Group and Physicians for Social Responsibility. 202/667-6982, 1718 Connecticut Ave., NW, Suite 600, Washington, DC 20009, www.ewg.org.

16a "How Safe is Our Produce?" Consumer Report, March 1999, pg. 29.

16b Consumer Report, March 2001.

17 "The Food Quality Protection Act (FQP) Background. A Visit to the EPA's Office of Pesticide Programs. Consider the 1995 survey of 76 jars of brand name baby foods."
www.epa.gov/opppsps1/fopa/backgrnd.htm

18 Sherman, Janette, M.D., Chemical Exposure and Disease, 1994, Princeton Scientific Publishing, Princeton, NJ, Cost: $35.00, pp. 162-3.

19a www.consumersunion.org/food/epade899.htm.

19b www.mercola.com/2001/feb/28/epa_pesticides.htm

20a www.abcnews.com: "EPA's Review of Pesticides Faulted," July 24, 2002

20b www.epa.gov/pesticides/cumulative

21 www.ecologic.ipm.com/pdp/updaate-childrens-foods.pdf. June 8, 2000.

22 www.txinfinet.com/ban-gef/00/5/5-11.html.
23 Feldman, Jay, "The Low Down on Dursban®; MOEd* Down By EPA: Do EPA Negotiations with Pesticide Manufacturers Compromise Public Health?" Pesticides and You, 2000: 20 (1).
24 http://www.emagazine.com/november-december_2000/1100ib_pest.html.
25 www.pestlaw.com/x/news/2002/20020630.htm.
26 Environmental Medical Research Foundation (ERF - Formerly: PARF), P. O. Box 60, Buffalo, NY 14223. 800.787.8780 www.drrapp.com.

26a Rapp, Doris J., M.D., Is This Your Child's World? 1996, ERF (*formerly PARF*), Buffalo, NY.
800.787.8780. Cost: $15.00 (plus S& H).

26b Video: Environmentally Sick Schools, 90 min. Cost: $25.00 (plus S&H).

27 Steve Tvedten, Get Set, The Bug Stops Here, download free book. 800.221.6188, www.getipm.com
28 Carson, Rachel, Silent Spring. 1962, Mariner Books, Cost: $11.20 (*Amazon.com*).
29a Heuser, G., P. Axelrod, and S. Heuser, "Defining Chemical Injury: A Diagnostic Protocol and Profile of Chemically Injured Civilians, Industrial Workers and Gulf War Veterans," International Perspectives of Public Health, 2000. http://www.iicph.org/docs/ipph_Defining_Chemical_Injury.htm

29b Heuser,G., and I. Mena, "NeuroSPECT in Neurotoxic Chemical Exposure Demonstration of Long Term Functional Abnormalities," Toxicology and Industrial Health, 1998: 14 (6) 813-827.

29c Bartha, L., et al., "Multiple Chemical Sensitivity: A 1999 Consensus," Arch. Environ Health, 1999: 54, 147-149.

29d Heuser, G. "Indoor Air Pollution l. A Medical-Legal Analysis." In: Legal Neurology and Malingering, 1993, Warren F. Gorfman, M.D., ed. Warren H. Green, Inc., St. Louis, MO. Pp.310-326.

30 McGovern, J.J., et al., "Food and Chemical Sensitivity," Archives of Otolaryngology, 1983: 109, 292-297.
31 "Golf Course Superintendents Face Higher Cancer Rates," Am. J. Industrial Med., 1996: 29 (5) 501-6.
32 Epstein, Samuel S., M.D., et al., "The Politics of Cancer Revisited," 1998, East Ridge Press, USA. Cost: $34.95 (plus S & H). (*An exceptional book.*)
33a www.cleanframscleanwater.org/action.htm

33b "California Farmers Allowed to Pollute," PANUPS (Pesticide Action Network Updates Service) December 16, 2002. 415.981.3939.

34 www.nfm-online.com
35 www.msnbc.com
36a www.care2.com

36b www.nrdc.org/legislation/rollbacks.pdf

37 www.epa.gov/sab
38 www.mercola.com/2001/mar/14/drugs_children.htm
39 www.rense.com/general131/working.htm
40a Kranhold, Kathryn, "The Beginning and the End of Amalgam in the US," www.mercola.com/2001/may/19/amalgam.htm

40b "Proposition 65, Safe Drinking Water and Toxic Enforcement Act," (Health and Safety Code 25249.6)

40c Shawn Khorrami, 818.947.5111.

41a "2,4 D: A New Lease on Life," Access- Pesticides, Feb 1996: XXI (2) University of Arizona.

41b Green, Emily, "Growing Health Worries Sprout Weed-Killer Study," L.A. Times, June 2, 2002.

41c Arch Environ. Health, 1996: 51 (1): 5-8; and Garry Vincent, "Pesticide Appliers, Biocides and Birth Defects in Rural Minnesota," Environmental Health Perspectives, 1996: 104, 394-399.

41d U.S. Environmental Protection Agency, "Estimating Exposure to Dioxin-like Compounds," Vol. II, Properties, Sources, Occurrence and Background Exposures [EPA/600/6-88/005Cb June 1994 External Review Draft] (Washington, D.C.: U.S. Environmental Protection Agency, 1994), Table 3-18 on pg. 3-58)

42 Ferber, D., "NIEHS Toxicologist Receives a Gag Order," Science, August 9, 2002: 297 (5583) 915-6.
43 Giuliano, Jackie, Ph.D., "Biological and Chemical Warfare Are Here Now." www.healingourworld.com
44 Laidler, James R. M.D., "Mercury Detoxification of Autistic Children: Consensus Position Paper." (*Three part article found at www.mercola.com/2001/jun/2/mercury_autism.htm*)
45 www.mercola.com. Has many articles on dangers of mercury.
46 "Defeat Autism Now! (DAN) Mercury Detoxification Institute, 4182 Adams Avenue, San Diego, CA 92116. www.autismresearchinstitute.com
47 Ericsson, Yngve and Britta Forsman, "Fluoride Retained from Mouth Rinses and Dentifrices in Preschool Children," Caries Research, 1969: 3, 290-299.
48 Augenstein, W. L., et al., "Fluoride Ingestion In Children: A Review of 87 Cases," Pediatrics. 1991: 88, 907-912.
49 IFIN (International Fluoride Information Network Bulletin). No. 627. June 16, 2002. ggvideo@northnet.org
50 Earth Island Journal, "Mickey/Minnie," Fall 1999: 14 (3). Gary Santolo of the Sacramento consulting firm of C2HMHill, headed the Kesterson field study.
51 Personal communication with Rohini Peris. Peris.gaudet@videotron.ca
52 PVC and Me, Endometriosis Association, 414.355.2200.
53 Davis, Adelle, Let's Have Healthy Children, 1985, New American Library. This book is out of print. pp. 206-208.

54 Abou-Donia, M.B., et al., "Locomotor and Sensorimotor Performance Deficit in Rats Following Exposure to Pyridostigmine Bromide, DEET, and Permethrin, Alone and in Combination," Toxicology Science, April 2000: 60(2) 305-14.
55 Thomas, Karen, "Behavioral Drugs Should Be Researched First," USA Today, July 14, 2002.
56 Snowbeck, Christopher, "Children on Prozac," Post-Gazette Staff Writer, March 3, 1998.
57 Journal of Pesticide Reform, Summer 1986.
58 Zoltani, C.K. and B.J.Baskin, "Simulation of Acetylcholine Cardiac Overload Caused by Soman, a Cholinesterase Inhibitor." http://cinc.mit.edu/Program/s52-4.htm
59 Baughman, Fred, Jr., "Alert Regarding Ritalin Amphetamine/Psych Drug- Heart Deaths," April 21, 2000. www.adhdfraud.org/alert_regarding_ritalin.htm
60 Solomon, Dr., "Heart Defects in Fish from Low Levels of Malathion," Teratology, 1979: 19, 51-62.
61 Moses, Marion, M.D., Designer Poisons, 1995, Pesticide Education Center, P.O. Box 420870, San Francisco, CA 94142. 415.391.8511. Cost $19.95.
62 Durnil, Gordon, The Making of a Conservative Environmentalist, 1995, Indiana University Press, Bloomington, Indianapolis, IN. Cost: $19.95 (plus S&H).
63 "Healthy Milk, Healthy Baby Chemical Pollution and Mother's Milk. Chemicals: Dioxins and Furans," Natural Resources Defense Council. www.nrdc.org/breastmilk/chem9.asp
64 http://Yosemite.epa.gov/ochp/ochpweb.nsf/content/index.htm pg. 117.
65 The New England Journal of Medicine, July 4, 2002:347, 2-3, 13-18.
66 "Chemical Watch Fact Sheet, DEET, Pesticides and You," Summer 2002: 22 (2) 9-10.
67 The Pure Water Place, Inc, 3347 Longview Blvd., Longmont, CO 80504. 888.776.0056. www.purewaterplace.com
68a Pimentel, David, "Silent Spring Revisited," J of Royal Society of Chemistry, Pesticide Outlook, October 2002.

68b Pimentel, D. and K. Hart, 2001. "Pesticide use; ethical, environmental, and public health implications." In: New Dimensions in Bioethics: Science, Ethics and the Formulation of Public Policy, Kluwer Academic Publishers, pp. 79-108.

68c Pimentel, D. and L. Levitan, "Pesticides: Amounts Applied and Amounts Reaching Pests," BioScience, 1986, pp. 36, 86-91.

69a Tenpenny, Sherri J., D.O., 14761 Pearl Road, #263, Strongville, OH 44136. Audiotape series and video on vaccines. 440.268. 0897; 440.572.2195.

69b Cave, Stephanie F., M.D., What Your Doctor May Not Tell You About Children's Vaccinations, September 2001, Time Warner Bookmark, www.twbookmark.com

70 "Annual Dog Vaccines May Not be Necessary," Journal American Animal Hospital Association, March-April 2003: 39(2) 119. www.mercola.com/2003/apr/2/dog_vaccines.htm
71a Shafey, Omar, "Interoffice Memorandum, 1/3/9 to Brian Hughes from Omar Shafey," MMWR Nov 12,99 48 (44): pp. 1015-1018, 1027.
71b J. Mercola, "Dangers of Genetically Altered Foods," www.mercola.com/2001/jul/14/gm_foods.htm
72 http://www.chem-tox.com/malathion/research/index.htm
73 Ludomirsky, A., H.O. Klein, P. Sarelli, "Q-T prolongation and polymorphous ("torsade de pointes") ventricular arrhythmias associated with organophosphorus insecticide poisoning," Am J Cardiol., May 1982: 49(7)1654-8.
74 "Pesticides Linked to Infant Heart Defect," American Journal of Epidemiology, 2001: 153, 529-536.
75 Pesticide Action Network Updates Service, "New York Sues Dow for Calling Dursban® Safe," April 18, 2003. www.www.panna.org.
76 "The Revolving Door, U.S. Government Workers and University Researchers Go Biotech…and Back Again, A Question of Ethics." http://www.mindfully.org/GE/Revo
77 Scott-Clark, Cathy and Adrian Levy, "Spectre Orange – Nearly 30 Years after the Vietnam War, a Chemical Weapon Used by US Troops is Still Exacting a Hideous Toll on Each New Generation," March 2003, Guardian Unlimited © Guardian Newspapers Limited 2003.
78 Pesticide Action Network Updates Service, "More Were Exposed to Agent Orange," April 25, 2003. www.www.panna.org
79 Gibbs, Gary, Deadly Dining, The Food That Would Last Forever, 1993, Avery.
80 Turner, S., The Chemical Feast, 1970, Grossman Publishers, New York, NY. Pp. 12-13.
81 Remington, Dennis W. and Barbara W. Higa. The Bitter Truth About Artificial Sweeteners, 1986, Vitality House International, 3707 N. Canyon Road, #8C, Provo, UT 84604.
82 Podolsky, D. and R.J. Newman, "A Ban on Silicone," U.S. News and World Report, January 1992, pp. 61-62.
83 Greater Boston Physicians for Social Responsibility, In HARM'S Way: Toxic Threats to Child Development, January 2001. 11 Garden St., Cambridge, MA 02138. 617.497.7440.
84 www.essential.org/cchw
85 Geier, Mark R., M.D., "Thimerosal in Childhood Vaccines, Neurodevelopment Disorders, and Heart Disease in the United States," Journal of American Physicians and Surgeons, Spring 2003: 8 (1).
86 http://www.gristmagazine.com/muck/muck/052103.asp

CHAPTER 8

Why And How To Protect Your Home And Town

What You Must Know to Protect Your Home Town[1, 2, 5a, 19a, 64, 78, 79, 84, 85, 92]

Can a New York City type of chemical pesticide spraying occur in your city?[79a,b, 128] Politicians in many cities make decisions, which can directly impact your future, personal health and welfare. Because of misunderstandings, poor communication and a lack of unbiased information, some decisions made by your politicians and health officials are not always prudent. It is also sometimes possible for those who have been given the position to serve, honor and protect to have vested interests that can sway their choices. At times you may have to critically look at who stands to gain from local and city health decisions. You can be given reasons that appear to be sound and responsible, but these may not always be the real reasons. There are those who rationalize their actions as a way to "prevent panic", but when your present and future health are at stake, you should have the right to be fully informed. Repeated reassurances that "all is safe" do not make it true. At times, you may not be informed at all. Your best recourse is to personally become more aware of the pros and cons of issues that impact your health and the lives of your loved ones. One good example of this is the repeated spraying of toxic malathion and other chemicals over a city to decrease the chances of a non-existent epidemic.

This chapter discusses the issues related to New York City's (NYC) 1999 to 2001 extensive and repeated chemical spraying to prevent encephalitis from the West Nile virus. The possible harmful health effects of this decision are potentially far greater than most would ever imagine, not from encephalitis, but from the malathion and other toxic chemicals that were used. As others have pointed out, the real epidemic is not the West Nile Virus, but the many illnesses potentially caused by the multiple chemical exposures used to handle the problem. In the past the West Nile viral disease, in general, has been a mild illness.[64,79, 80] Was the chemical spraying a tragic example of extremely poor judgment? In time we shall find out. What occurred there demonstrates how easily this same situation could happen in your hometown since many cities are being or have been sprayed with the same or similar types of toxic chemicals and the residents are often misinformed, partially informed and, at times, totally uninformed.

To add to the repeated chemical poisoning, New Yorkers were also exposed to the monumental amount of pollution associated with the September 11, 2001 tragedy. This can greatly compound the immediate and potential long term, serious health concerns for all who were exposed.

Pesticide Spraying to Kill Insects[65]

It is impossible to fully comprehend the health and economic splatter effect on humans, wildlife and the environment due to the spraying of the New York City area. The major chemicals sprayed over a two-year period included the organophosphate, malathion, and other toxic chemicals such as the synthetic pyrethroids combined with piperonyl butoxide.[3a, 5a,b, 84] At the same time as the New Yorkers were sprayed, many of those who live along the east coast were similarly sprayed with these same toxic chemicals. This chapter will give you some needed information so you can decide if the use of malathion, in particular, was potentially worse than the disease for which it was used to prevent. You may need to have this information if officials in your town decide to do similar spraying at some time in the future.

If the aim were to kill the adult mosquitos with spray, this treatment would be considered to be highly ineffective.[24b] The chances of enough spray actually hitting and killing a mosquito was negligible. It is estimated that for every million drops of pesticide spray only one would land on a mosquito, and it takes two to three drops to kill a mosquito.[3a] Humans realistically were much more apt to be hit or hurt with the spray.

When malathion was used to diminish the mosquito breeding grounds, it made more sense but there certainly are known safer and better ways to control the mosquito population.[71a] We must ask why anyone would even consider the use of toxic chemicals that are potentially harmful to humans, wildlife, birds, fish, amphibians and plants when safer, more effective forms of preventing insect-related health problems are available.[65, 71a,b] In time, the full extent of the impact of the medical decisions made in NYC and in other areas of the country will gradually become apparent to many who presently have no idea why they are ill. Some will never know. The information in this chapter will enable you to anticipate and be better prepared if the air you breathe is destined for "legislated pollution". *(If you have already been sprayed and are ill, Chapter 3 explains how you can possibly recognize and confirm the diagnosis and find appropriate helpful treatment.)*

What Are Some Reasons for Concern[19a]

Organophosphates such as malathion can be human poisons. Documents released in a lawsuit in 1996 against the manufacturer reported that high temperatures caused malathion to break down to an even more toxic substance called isomalathion or malaoxin. This chemical is 40 times more toxic than malathion.[2, 3a-e, 4a, 5a,b]

Reports state this pesticide, used over NYC, was stored improperly and at temperatures that were excessive allowing

TABLE 8A
Possible Symptoms from Malathion or Pyrethroid Pesticides

Insomnia	Changes in heart beat
Weakness	Fatigue
Asthma, coughing	Headaches
Problems breathing	Loss of memory
Small pupils	Unclear thinking
Nausea	Skin irritation and rashes
Stomach ulcers	Diarrhea
Twitching	A bad mouth taste
Dizziness	Loss of hair
Hemorrhages	Loss of coordination
Pain	Increased salivation
Convulsions	Increased urination
Encephalitis[70]	Anxiety
Sexual difficulties	Tingling in fingertips
Blurred vision	Depression
Myopia (near-sightedness)	Testicular shrinkage
Watery and burning eyes	Excessive mucus, drooling

malaoxin to form before the spray was applied.[19] The EPA also required Cheminova, the manufacturer, to provide information to users of malathion (Fyfanon ULV) not to spray it over bodies of water, near foods, directly on people or in places where humans would return within 12 hours. Reports state that many of these suggested rules were broken when the NYC areas and people were sprayed. *(The lobster industry was almost destroyed because of the pollution.)*

(The rules of the game can also change. It is of interest to know that in October 2002 the EPA altered the rules to stem the rapid spread of the West Nile virus. It is now easier to spray over water with toxic substances to kill mosquitos without a permit as previously required by the Clean Water Act.[13, 80] It appears to be possible to make exceptions to laws that were specifically designed to protect the public.)

Later on, pyrethroid products such as Scourge and Anvil 10+10® were also used to control the mosquitos in the NYC area. These pyrethroids disrupt hormones and can mimic estrogens. They are reported to be linked to breast cancer in females, decreased sperm counts in males and possibly brain tumors in children.[5b, 65]

In addition, malathion and the above formulations typically contain some solvents in the form of xylene, benzene or toluene.[2] Even though these are known to be exceedingly toxic and are registered poisons, they do not have to be specified on the Material Safety Data Sheets.[5a] They can be legally included in a deceptive lump category referred to as "inert" ingredients.[5b, 19] *(See Chapters 1, 6, 7, 10.)*

What Are the Known Acute and Chronic Symptoms from Malathion Exposures? [1, 2, 4a, 6, 19a, 101]

The initial complaints after exposure to malathion spray are typically the sudden onset of a prolonged flu-like illness, an upper respiratory infection or breathing problems such as coughing and asthma. How many who were exposed, however, are also aware that this chemical is known to cause the array of symptoms listed in Table 8A?[19a]

No, not every symptom or all individuals will be affected, but all these medical conditions can and do arise in some individuals after exposure to organophosphate chemicals, such as malathion or pyrethroids. The effects from inhaling the chemicals can be different from those caused by eating the chemicals on or in a food, for example.

Although the above medical complaints tend to occur three to 15 days after exposure, those who have been sensitized to chemicals become ill while indoors and even worse, in seconds, from merely walking outside and breathing air that is slightly more contaminated with traces of chemicals such as pesticides.[116] Headaches, difficulty thinking clearly and problems walking can quickly become evident. After one significant exposure, such symptoms might last hours to days but for a few, the harmful effects last for months or possibly a lifetime. For many, from then on, *future minute exposures to many different unrelated chemicals can cause symptoms similar to those that were originally experienced.* This is called the "spreading" phenomenon. *(See Chapters 1, 8, 10.)*

What about the Other Sprayed Pesticide Chemicals or Ingredients? [5a, 7, 19 a,c,d, 30a]

Pyrethrums and pyrethrins (from chrysanthemums) and synthetic forms called pyrethroids, including Anvil 10+10® (sumithrin) and Scourge (resmethrin) were sprayed from trucks in Manhattan, Brooklyn, Bronx, Queens and Staten Island. Pyrethrins, in general, are considered to have a low toxicity and to be one of the safest forms of insecticides. These chemicals, however, have been associated with increased respiratory illness, asthma, burning of the eyes, nose and skin, increased saliva, an increased sensitivity to sound and touch, lowered sperm counts, sexual difficulties, thyroid damage, miscarriages, preterm deliveries and toxic damage to the liver, kidneys, intestines, skin and nervous system.[1, 2, 5a,b, 6, 19] These are hardly low toxicity. In addition, severe reactions or deaths are uncommon but have been reported in extremely ragweed-sensitive individuals or those who have had contact with a pyrethrum-containing shampoo, for example.[124]

Some of the other chemicals such as piperonyl butoxide are also suspect causes of cancer in the breast, prostate and brain.[7] This substance is also reported to combine with pyrethroid chemicals to prevent the liver from filtering and eliminating toxins allowing potentially harmful poisons or pollution to remain in the body.[5a,b, 19a-d]

Who Is Most Vulnerable to the Chemically Polluted Air? [19]

- Fetuses, infants, children, pregnant women, the elderly and those who have a depressed immune system (for example, from cancer therapy), are the most likely to be adversely affected by pesticides and other toxic chemicals.[85] It appears that chemicals can be found in pregnant women and their offspring. Women exposed to chemicals have more birth injured children than normal.[8] *(See Chapter 5.)* One study, however, showed that the exposure of pregnant women to indoor pesticides was considerable and one study showed no effect.[121a,b] Their urine showed excessive levels of break-down products from several toxic pesticides. Further studies are needed urgently to determine the effects these chemicals can have on the developing fetus and infant.[107]

- Pesticide truck sprayers are also an increased jeopardy. Some of the men who sprayed in NYC claim that they were saturated with the chemicals after they applied it and they subsequently became ill.[19, 80, 133] They were diagnosed as having pesticide poisoning and for some, it caused severe sexual problems.

- Pesticide chemicals can suppress the immune system in both humans and animals.[3a] Initially this can lead to repeated infections and allergies, and in time it can cause reproductive and learning problems, as well as blood disorders. Late or end stage effects can lead to cancer and degenerative diseases such as rheumatoid arthritis, lupus erythematosis and multiple sclerosis.[2, 65]

You Need to Ask Yourself

If your family or you were exposed to malathion or other chemical sprays, how would the above symptoms affect your child's school performance and your own ability to think, act, behave or function well at work? The answers might not be known right away, but eventually most of those who were seriously harmed will find out. Some NYC residents have already seen changes in their children and themselves but relatively few suspect the sprays. Unfortunately, the full effects of toxic poison sprays might not be evident initially at the time of exposure. Some medical effects might not be recognized for years. Once you are aware of the possible cause of any symptoms you have, there are some ways you can try to credibly document and treat your medical complaints. (*See Chapter 3.)*

What Does Malathion Do to Wildlife? [2, 11, 19a,c, 30, 41, 65, 66, 80]

- Bees, waterfowl, freshwater fish, lobsters, shrimp, clams, snails, worms, butterflies, dragonflies (that eat mosquitos) and other beneficial insects, as well as frogs and birds, can be seriously damaged by malathion or various types of pesticide sprays.[2, 80, 19] The economic impact can decimate entire businesses, such as the Long Island lobster industry in New York and Connecticut. There are reports some have been almost destroyed from the obligatory spraying.[30, 65, 80]

- Both domestic and laboratory animals have been reported to show evidence of genetic, immune and reproductive system damage after malathion exposure.[65]

In Rats

- Male and female rats have different types of toxic responses due to variations in their metabolism, storage and excretion of chemicals such as malathion.[19c, 41] In general, however, female animals appear to be more susceptible to pesticides than males.[41] *(In humans, females also appear to be more sensitive to chemicals.)* There are some studies that show tumor development in both sexes.[2, 41, 67]

- In one rat study, it was claimed that ingested insecticides diminish rat growth by 25%, but if rats were also given vitamin C, the decrease was only 10%.[20] *(We do not know if this would also help humans who are sprayed with toxic insecticides.)*

- Rat studies also have suggested they can have difficulty remembering after exposure to malathion.[2, 19] *(Human studies also have shown decreases in intellectual function, such as abstract or flexible thinking after exposure to certain pesticide poisons.)*[21a,b] *(See Chapter 4.)*

- The results of one study suggests breast tumors develop in about 11% of rats given parathion, and 24% of those given malathion.[25] *(It might take years before some of these types of changes become evident in humans. What happens will depend, in part, upon the genetics of each person and the degree, duration and exact type of adverse exposures.)*

- One single oral dose of malathion was shown to cause a reduction in lung cells in rats.[104] This only occurred in relation to the "technical grade" malathion which has more impurities in contrast to the more pure form.[19a,c] Some of the malathion used in NYC was said to be technical grade.

In Mice and Rats

- Low doses of pyrethroids have been reported to cause irreversible brain changes in mice and thyroid suppression in rats.[19c, 65]

In Mice and Lizards

- Mice are reported to develop liver cancer and tumors in the thyroid and breast from malathion; so do lizards.[2, 19a,b] In some studies of rats, the evidence is inconclusive.[25, 41]

In Fish

- Studies indicate that fish exposed to low level concentrations of malathion develop damaged and deformed gills.[2, 19, 22, 23] Very low concentrations (one to five parts per million) also are said to cause heart defects in fish, especially if the exposure is to more than one pesticide.[19, 23]

In Turtles

- Turtles are reported to develop birth defects after malathion exposure.[19]

In Frogs

- Frogs injected with DDT, malathion or the chemical cyclophosphamide are reported to have decreased immune function. This can cause antibody production to decrease to only 1% to 2% of normal.[68] This type of change would make the frogs much more sensitive to infections of various types.

- Minute doses of chemicals in less than one part per million are said to cause a variety of deleterious effects in frogs.[19a, 68] Frogs exposed to pesticides such as malathion or atrazine are likely to have weakened immune systems and limb deformities.[69] Tadpoles are reported to be have unusual swimming patterns because of malformed tails and heads from such malathion exposures.[19a]

In Hens

- Hens fed malathion and carbaryl are reported to develop a number of health problems which increase as the dose of pesticide in their mash is increased. Studies indicated they had defective eggs, decreased hatchability and more birth defects. The liver and kidney of the affected chicks stored more malathion than usual.[19a]

Pregnant Animals

- One study in pregnant animals showed no problems in the offspring until they were mature and had their own offspring. This second generation, however, weighed less, grew more slowly and had excessive infections.[19a, 71a]

What Does Malathion Do to Humans?[19]

- In 1979 isomalathion was misapplied on agriculture during a malaria eradication program. Of the 2800 who became ill, five died.[19a,d, 28a]

- It has been reported that infants born to pregnant mothers who were exposed in California to malathion sprays in the second trimester had more than twice the amount of intestinal disorders when compared to those who were not exposed.[2, 9]

- One study in India showed malathion causes chromosome defects or DNA abnormalities in all doses tested in human white blood cells.[19] This type of effect could lead to birth defects and developmental abnormalities.[19c]

- In another study of white blood cells, chromosome loss was reported in humans after malathion exposure. This could weaken or alter the human immune system's ability to fight disease and cause genetic defects.[19]

- One child born to a mother who was exposed to malathion in a lice shampoo when she was three months pregnant developed serious muscle and birth defects.[19] *(One cannot conclude much from one report of one child but it does suggest we must be more aware of all kinds of possible effects from chemical exposures that occur during pregnancy. We must ask, how safe are lice shampoos that contain malathion? Safe shampoos are available.)*[71a]

Cancer Studies in Humans

- In one report, seven children developed leukemia and aplastic anemia after exposures to malathion and other pesticides.[19]

- A Nebraska study in 1988 showed increases in cancer in farmers after malathion exposure.[87]

- Another study in 1992 showed that malathion exposed farmers in Iowa and Minnesota had an increased risk of non-Hodgkin's lymphoma.[2, 5, 24-27, 65, 87]

- Similarly, employees in flour mills where malathion was used to control insects were said to more frequently develop cancer.[2]

- Reports indicate apple growers exposed to organophosphates, such as malathion, have an increased incidence of leukemia in comparison to a controlled population.[86]

Why Is There Confusion About Malathion and Cancer in Humans? [2, 19, 24-27, 86]

We do know there is quite a bit of evidence, as indicated above, in exposed mice and rats that pesticides can cause cancerous tumors in the brain, liver, lungs, blood and endocrine glands, such as the thyroid.[2, 26, 41, 109] We also know that pesticides depress the immune system and that alone can lead to increased infections but, in addition, these two factors are thought to make women more prone to breast cancer because chemicals tend to be stored in these fatty tissues. We know malathion can cause chromosome changes in human blood cells and this can lead to both birth defects and developmental problems.[10, 19a, 30a, 129]

There are conflicting opinions, however, about the development of cancer in humans related to malathion exposure.[2, 3] As indicated previously, several studies do suggest such a relationship exists.[14, 19, 26, 27, 86] The skeptics stress these are not large studies, and this makes it difficult to fairly interpret any conflicting or sparse data. When negative scientific reports involve economics, however, it is sometimes of value to know exactly who paid for and was involved in such studies.[109] For example the lead attorney for Cheminova (a company producing toxic chemicals) was reported to have been a former EPA attorney who worked on malathion issues for the EPA. It has been stated that he disagreed strongly with pathologists who believed malathion was a "likely human carcinogen".[39a,b] We obviously need more research by totally impartial scientists so we know if malathion poses a significant cancer danger in humans.

Did the EPA Change its Report About Cancer?[28a-c]

An anonymous source stated that EPA scientists had concluded and were about to report that malathion was a "suspect" carcinogen. One day before the report was to be released on May 10, 2000, however, their risk assessment was revised. The EPA's final report was reversed overnight after it was suddenly decided to use the interpretation of the data supplied by the chemical industry rather than that of the EPA scientists. Just prior to the announcement, the pesticide's manufacturer had supposedly requested another interpretation of the EPA's data.[28] At that point it was decided to re-classify malathion to a "lower level carcinogen". By changing the level of risk from "suspect" to "lower level", it meant that measures to monitor and protect the public were markedly diminished. The final published report concluded there was "insufficient evidence" to decide about its carcinogenicity. Who decides to let the fox design the hen house? Why did they do it?

One major challenge in this type of research is that it can take years after an exposure before cancer becomes evident, although at times it can happen in a year or two. This makes it more difficult to prove a cause and effect relationship. In animal research, you must always ask how long the animals were studied *after* a possible cancer-causing exposure or a false conclusion can easily be reached. Even when an inordinate number of animals develop this illness, those who are pro-chemicals will say that humans are not rats, so the information is of little value. Disregard of this type of evidence in the past, however, has proven animal illnesses do indeed warn us — if we will only listen.[113, 114]

Which Laboratory Tests Confirm a Possible Harmful Pesticide Exposure?[17]

Organophosphate pesticides are no longer in the blood after 24 to 48 hours so tests to document exposures should be done as soon as possible. Some of the characteristic breakdown products, however, can be measured after a longer period of time. The most helpful laboratory test to confirm a possible organophosphate poisoning is the CD 26 or Ta1 antigen memory test. In addition, an autoantibody test, especially to antimyelin, would suggest damage to the sheath that covers nerves. This type of antibody is associated with symptoms in the nervous system and/or brain. You can check with your doctor about available laboratory tests to examine your own blood or body fluids.[89, 90] *(Accu-Chem: 972.234.5412; ImmunoScience: 800.950.4686 and see Chapter 3.)*

In some patients there are also measurable decreases in levels of acetyl-cholinesterase. This lack can greatly impede normal nerve impulse transmission. *(See Chapter 3.)* Call 316.684.5500 to contact an environmental medical specialist who is knowledgeable about how to recognize, diagnose and treat these types of illnesses.[88]

What Is the Antidote for Malathion?[4a]

The antidote for organophosphate poisoning, such as malathion, is 2 PAM or Protopam. It must be given within 24 to 48 hours to be effective. This should be available in most emergency rooms. This will not help poisoning due to the class of pesticides called carbamates. For malathion or toxic carbamates, atropine is helpful.

Before Pesticide Spraying, What Should the Public Know?[19a, 30a, 64, 78, 79a, 103]

You should be aware of the common medical problems listed in Table 8A. *(See Chapter 6.)*

In Relation to Mosquitos:

- Even the CDC (Center for Disease Control) says that daytime aerial spraying is the least effective method of insect (mosquito) control.[70]

- Studies have shown chemical sprays from planes have been found 22 miles from targeted areas. They may not hit a mosquito, but they potentially can travel long distances and find human targets.[24b]

- Spraying wipes out the natural predators to mosquitos and also is reported to create mosquitos that are more pesticide-resistant.[24,b,30]

- One report indicated malathion makes some mosquitos more aggressive for up to two hours after spraying.[78] This could make them more apt to bite.

In Relation to Animals:

- Birth defects have been noted in animals exposed to malathion or its breakdown products.[2, 14]

- Exposed pregnant ewes produced stillborn, aborted fetuses and their offspring weighed less than normal.[108]

- In other animals, ulcers, testicular atrophy and blood sugar increases have been noted, as well as kidney, liver, adrenal and intestinal changes.[2, 3a, 19a-d]

- The neurotoxic effects of malathion may not begin to be evident for one year after exposure. See Table 8A for changes related to the nervous system.

In Relation to Humans:

- Many do not realize that sudden uncontrollable aggression, hyperactivity or an inability to think, speak, or walk normally can be manifested in some children or adults after pesticide or chemical exposures.[17]

- Many aspects of a child's future health, sexuality, development or learning ability might be adversely affected by repeated toxic exposures to organophosphate pesticides.[2, 4b, 19a, 30a, 92] Even chronic debilitating illnesses such as multiple sclerosis and Parkinson's disease have been linked to chemical exposures.

- Toxic chemicals might possibly genetically damage unborn children.[2, 10, 11, 12] It is known that mothers working in cotton fields exposed to malathion and other pesticides had children with chromosome breaks. This means that there is damage to the gene or cellular structure of exposed children.[2] Proven genetic damage to mosquitos has also been reported from malathion.[3b]

- There are critical, brief periods of time during pregnancy when unborn infants (and the young of wildlife) are in jeopardy because their mothers breathed pesticide-contaminated air.[117] Those who want to increase their chances of conceiving a normal child should select a time when the air is not heavily polluted with chemicals.[110]

- In the San Francisco Bay area, there was a correlation between ear and bone anomalies associated with malathion exposure.[91]

- According to Alfredo Sudan M.D., Ph.D., an authority on malathion, "It should not be used in the home."[15]

- Omar Shafey M.P.H., Ph.D. was the health department official in Florida who recommended that the use of the organophosphate pesticide, malathion, be stopped. He suggested that Florida should compensate injured residents and provide shelter for those who wished to evacuate if spraying was to be continued. He has stated malathion was responsible for adverse health effects and had no direct health benefits. It is reported that when he refused to alter his report, he was suddenly dismissed and the reason given was an alleged overcharge of $12.50 on a travel claim for reimbursement. Is it likely that the real reason was his refusal to alter his Health Department Report that recommended malathion spraying for medflies be stopped and suggested that those who might be hurt, be protected?[16a-d]

- In a previous article in November, 1999 the CDC conducted a phone survey after malathion was used to control a problem with medflies. They reported that 123 residents appeared to have possible or probable illness from the spraying. Of this group, 72% were females, 7% were children, 16% were elderly and 3% were work-related. They developed intestinal, respiratory, nervous system, skin, and eye symptoms.[16b]

- In April 2003, the CDC reported on medfly eradication using malathion sprayed from fogger trucks. They concluded that mosquito spraying did not increase pesticide levels or harm humans. They claimed the doses used were enough to kill mosquitos and not hurt humans.[125] How did they select their patients and how sensitive were their detection methods in the blood and urine for pesticides? Who conducted and paid for the studies. *(Many chemically sensitive patients were extremely ill in seconds and could not think clearly or breathe normally from simply walking outside shortly after the malathion spraying took place in NYC.)*[116]

How High Is Your Risk of Becoming Ill with West Nile Encephalitis? [3a, 29]

What you should know:

- In Africa, where the West Nile Virus has been evident for 60 years, there have been very few epidemics.[3]

- Less than 1% of mosquitos exposed to the virus are infected but later reports say it is over 1%.[5b, 81, 84] Even if you are bitten by an infected mosquito less than 1% will become severely ill, and of those who become ill, the vast majority will not be sick enough to know they are infected.[3b, 64, 84]

- It has been reported that more than 80% of Egyptians were previously or are presently infected with the West Nile virus but, in general, only the very young, the elderly or those with weak immune systems are considered to be seriously at risk.[29]

- The majority of those who were killed by the virus in a recorded Israeli outbreak were over 80 years old.[29]

- Human mortality varies from 3% to 15%, mainly in the elderly. Other studies predict much lower rates.[84]

- In 1999, however, in Bucharest, Romania, an outbreak of West Nile fever implicated a flavovirus that affected about 500 people with more than 50 dying. The strain of virus in Romania appears to have been different than the one found in the NYC area.[29] There also were some sanitation, water, and nutrition problems in Romania that could have contributed to weakening their immune systems. Under these types of circumstances, epidemics obviously can be serious.

- As of September 10, 2002, there were 113 cases of West Nile illnesses in the United States and five people unfortunately died.[80, 81] At that time, it was estimated your chances of dying from the illness was one in a million. There was some reason for concern, however, because by December 2002 the statistics were 3,852 cases of West Nile virus in the USA and 241 deaths. These occurred mainly in Illinois, Mississippi, and Louisiana, each with about 50 cases. Most of the remaining states had one to ten cases.[79d] Again those who died were older and they had weakened immune systems.

If an Epidemic Is Imminent, What Can You Do?

We hardly have an epidemic at this time but it is imperative that safe ways to control this problem, without chemicals that hurt humans, be in place before your city officials decide how to handle any mosquito problem that might occur during the next few years.[77, 127] Is your city ready? Will they spray with malathion or other harmful chemicals without informing you?

Was NYC at Risk from West Nile Viral Encephalitis?[3a,f]

In NYC in 1999, with a population of about 10 million, 62 people were reported ill with the West Nile virus, or about six persons per million. A high estimate suggested if you were bitten by an infected mosquito, less than 1 in 300 would show mild signs of a flu-like illness.[3a, 30] Based on current information on casualties, the odds of anyone in the United States dying from this virus is roughly one in a million.[3a] Was there really such a high risk of a deadly epidemic that such drastic action as repeated extensive spraying with toxic chemicals was justified – especially when safer, equally effective and less expensive methods of insect control measures were available?[71a,b, 80]

- In NYC, one in a million or seven, who were all between 68 and 87 years old, died. Three of these were on drugs to suppress their immunity. In the year 2000, one person died in New York and New Jersey, although 17 did become ill.
- Outside the New York area, there are some statistics. There were six birds positive for the West Nile virus in New Hampshire and 448 birds in Massachusetts in the year 2000, but no human cases of encephalitis in either state.[30]

Those in favor of spraying believe their prophylactic spraying measures helped prevent an epidemic. Weigh this possibility against the more probable one. In time, if and when all the facts are known, it may be determined that the health of an immense number of humans was temporarily or permanently hurt because they developed a chemical sensitivity type of illness due to the exposure. Major basic questions remain unanswered. Were millions needlessly exposed to toxic malathion? Was the treatment much worse than the disease? Did the treatment make the illness worse?[3b] (*For example, in Brevard County in Florida a mosquito problem was treated with the chemical Dibrom® over an 11 year period. They found it not only did not help, but it was reported that it caused a 15 fold increase in the number of encephalitis-carrying mosquitos.*)

The true benefit/risk ratio in relation to the malathion spraying in NYC will be difficult to assess. Patients called their doctors for help but the NYC officials did not initially create a NYC "hotline" and sick people complained they were rebuffed by officials when they attempted to convey information about their immediate health-related complaints that appeared to be directly related to the pesticide spraying.[116] Why would those who tried to communicate their illness to authorities be met with so little success?

The final conclusion is: Toxic chemicals can be used, allegedly to protect the public from epidemics that do not exist. If, in fact, there are mosquito problems, safer, more effective and less expensive alternative control measures are known and readily available.[71a,b, 80]

Additional Comments of Interest and Value

In Humans

- We must ask: Why was some of the mosquito spraying done in the daytime when mosquitos are nocturnal? Even at night, the city streets and playgrounds were not breeding grounds. Were humans needlessly exposed?[32]

- In California, Florida and Japan, thousands of gallons of toxic malathion were used in recent years to control med-flies or fruit flies. Each group eventually concluded that there were safer and better ways to control these insects.[9, 15, 16a-d, 36-39, 120]

- Most people in Florida and Alabama are not aware that without any public warning, trucks or planes regularly spray toxic chemicals, such as malathion, around and in buildings and on beaches for insects, weeds and fungi. This sometimes is done in the daytime.

- In 1969, 98% of children in an agricultural area in Japan, where malathion was applied regularly, had well-documented reduced visual acuity and myopia.[40a,b, 106] This was not evident during the years this chemical was not applied.

- Malathion spraying can contaminate the air, water and soil. In one California study, five out of 28 county water systems were contaminated.[2] In one river, 30% of the malathion continued to be present in the water one month later.[2, 88] Vast kills of fish occurred in Staten Island's Clove Lake, Queens Alley Pond Park and other waterways after malathion was sprayed over the water.[5b] It is reported that if water is contaminated, it lasts for about one to six weeks depending on the type of water (fresh, distilled, pond, etc.).[41] If soil is contaminated with malathion, the half life is one to 25 days.[2, 3b,41] You might want to determine how many chemicals are in your drinking water or soil.* [88, 89] *(Accu-Chem: 972.234.5412 or ImmunoScience: 800.950.4686.)*

- The Food and Drug Administration has detected malathion in about one in five food items. The EPA has a report stating malathion residues were 1100% in excess of the amount considered safe for children and 500% in excess for adults.[2] How high are the levels now in foods presently grown in the NYC area? How much malathion is in the foods you or your children are eating where you live?

- A secret memo issued by the NYC Police Department at the time of the spraying warned officers to stay at least 25 feet from the spray, put their air-conditioning vents on recirculate, wear protective clothing, keep the patrol car windows tightly shut and avoid all contact with the spray. [5, 42] Why weren't the New York residents similarly warned? If malathion is really as safe as the politicians claimed, why should the NYC police be warned to be so cautious? [5, 43a,b]

In Wildlife

- Birds are the original carriers of viral encephalitis. The mosquitos become infected after they bite infected birds and then we are infected when these mosquitos bite us. Of the thousands of mosquitos who bite and infect birds, only one or two of them develop the illness. Up to 70%, however, can become infected with the virus.[31] *(Most illnesses typically affect a relatively small proportion of those exposed, except when an epidemic occurs. Those who are genetically strong are the least apt to be affected.)*

- There is some research that noted a strong correlation between petrochemical refinery pollution and the death of birds from the West Nile virus. One must ask if full spectrum toxicological studies are being done on either the humans or the birds that died from this illness. Could some of them have died from chemical pollution unrelated to or secondary to infected mosquito or malathion exposure? If the proper testing was not done, who would know?[126a,b]

- It appears that a weakened blood brain-barrier enables viruses, for example, to enter the brain more readily. The barrier apparently can be weakened by insect repellents, pesticides or exposures to inhaled or injected anesthetics in laboratory mice studies.[132]

- It is theorized by some that an inordinate number of crows have died from the West Nile Virus because of exposure to chemicals.[130-132] More crows have died, for example, near oil refineries or contact with MTBE *(methyl tertiary butyl ether)* than crows in areas that are less polluted.[134]

- Other studies suggest high ozone levels are correlated with increased viral deaths in crows.[134] It is known that high ozone levels can damage the brain, lungs and immune system. If these observations are validated this would have great implications in humans because it suggests that the development of West Nile encephalitis is indirectly related to toxic environmental chemical exposures, and not simply contact with an infected mosquito.

- There is one controlled laboratory report indicating the West Nile virus causing encephalitis spread from bird to bird without any interaction with mosquitos.[31b, 33] If this were true, mosquito control would certainly not be the total answer to control this virus.[29, 34a,b]

- More crows died from pesticides, along with many beneficial birds, than from the West Nile virus from July 1, 2000 to March 31, 2001.[35]

- It is evident that crows and horses are more sensitive to this virus than humans but there is some question as to whether this is the same virus.[5b]

- Dogs, cats and horses can become infected with the West Nile virus but, like humans, they usually recover. [2, 11, 18, 30a, 65, 66] Horses need vaccines, however, to control this illness. [66]

- There is one anecdotal single controlled observation that might be of great interest. In the group treated with a dietary supplement of edible diatomaceous earth and garlic, the flies and mosquitos did not bother the horses. This was not true for the control group and in addition, that group had more infections. In this one farm, some of the horses who did not receive these supplements developed the West Nile Disease.[5b, 71a] Is it not of interest that these preparations helped and did not hurt? We need studies to determine if these food supplements would help protect humans who lived in areas where they was grave concern.

What About the Additional Health Impact of the World Trade Center Attack? [93a-c]

In spite of the initial assurance that there was no immediate danger from the many contaminants polluting the NYC air after the September 11, 2001 attack, there is much that needs serious consideration. The environmental impact of this additional, ongoing pollution, added to the years of extensive and repeated aerial spraying with malathion and other chemicals, can greatly increase the potential health concerns of all those living in the vicinity of NYC for many years.

The destruction of the Twin Towers caused toxic fumes and smoke to be released which contained dust particles, pulverized cement, glass, fiberglass, sheetrock, germs, molds, carbon monoxide, solvents such as benzene, toluene, xylene and volatile, gaseous organic compounds. Chemical fires released highly carcinogenic forms of aromatic hydrocarbons. These exposures can irritate the eyes, nose and throat but more importantly, they can potentially damage the lungs, liver, heart, kidneys and nervous system. Some are suspect or definite carcinogens.

Specific released toxic chemicals included dioxins (industrial waste), construction materials from wood, natural gas, phenols (resins, adhesives), phthalates (plastics) and PCBs (polychlorinated biphenols, found in paper, plasticizers, compressors, heat transfer systems, etc.). To this list must be added the toxic jet fuels, the toxic metals, such as asbestos and mercury, and a multitude of infectious germs and fungi. Many of these materials or inhaled substances are known to damage the immune, nervous, endocrine and reproductive systems. These types of exposures can lead to birth defects and developmental delays in children and chronic debilitating disease or even cancer in children or adults. As time passes, the full impact of this environmental catastrophe will become evident in ways that are presently not fully evident, understood or appreciated.

By October 2001, more than half the students and the schools' staffs on the edge of the Ground Zero area suffered from respiratory symptoms (shortness of breath and persistent coughing). At the present time, fortunately, the respiratory symptoms, anxiety and depression are said to be diminishing. It has been reported, however, that some of the diligent workers who tirelessly helped for days, weeks and months at the time of the tragedy, have lung problems, in particular, bronchitis or asthma. Residents in the Ground Zero area have reported similar problems. All these individuals should be medically monitored for any other future illnesses and assisted indefinitely if that is required.[93a-c] It is of interest that both the EPA and the National Institute of Occupational Safety and Health continue to issue reports that the Ground Zero area was and is safe.

The effects of the individual role of the West Nile mosquito and the associated malathion and other chemical exposures plus the massive air pollution from the World Trade tragedy cannot be fairly determined. We have insufficient data, for example, to fairly evaluate the incidence and types of physical and emotional complaints before and after the malathion spraying. Is there an overlap of those who became ill after malathion or other chemical spraying and those who developed serious illness after exposures from the 9/11 Trade Center collapse? I would be surprised if this were not true.[44, 72] Theoretically, malathion or similar chemical exposures would be expected to increase the number of those affected by chemical sensitivities, and these individuals in turn would be more prone to be more seriously affected by inhaling the additional air pollution from the 9/11 disaster. Those who had allergies, also, would be more prone to chronic health effects from either exposure.

The Department of Health and Human Services was supposed to be given funds ($90 million) to make a registry to monitor the health of 100,000 to 200,000 New Yorkers who were exposed in the ground zero vicinity of the World Trade Center.[73, 93a-d]

It was disappointing to read a report that President Bush did not sign the appropriation bill with the result that the money designated to provide care for those who were made ill, did not become a reality. It was reported that *spending restraints were needed and the money was supposedly not to be used for pressing needs and priorities, but for emergencies.* Hillary Clinton recognized that those who became so ill and incapacitated from helping with the rescue work deserved more than a medal and praise. Some will need ongoing specialized medical care. It is certainly possible that more than a few will develop perplexing chronic illnesses because of their exposures and need the expertise of environmental medical specialists. *(316.684.5500.)* We should provide long term medical care for every single worker who so diligently helped to save lives and clean up the ground zero area. We also should medically evaluate and monitor the health of the aerial and ground pesticide spray applicators.[30a, 80, 94]

In time, hopefully there eventually will be some studies about the effects from the repeated malathion exposures in NYC and elsewhere. This should include studies to determine if there is a significant increase in the number of children who need to wear glasses in NYC, as happened in Japan.[40b, 106] In the next few years, do the rates of cancer, lupus, multiple sclerosis, Parkinson's or Alzheimer's disease increase more than anticipated or elsewhere? Does the number of eligible sperm donors decrease more than in the past or than in other countries? Eventually, we should have some definitive answers. If the highly exposed individuals are given appropriate nutrients, urged to avoid chemicals in all forms in their air, water, foods and clothing and taught methods to detoxify their bodies to help eliminate the chemicals and toxic metals stored in them, they should be much less likely to develop serious dreaded diseases, now or in the future.[46b]

How Can New Yorkers Help Diminish the Effects of the Malathion and the Twin Tower Pollution?

In essence, one major challenge is to get rid of the chemicals stored in the body. [17] *(See Chapter 3.)*

- Nutrients will help in many ways. Antioxidants, including vitamins B_2, C and E, essential fatty acids, superoxide dismutase, N acetyl cysteine, L cysteine, folic acid, selenium and garlic would help to strengthen the immune system. L glutathione is needed and helpful because this is a major component in the human body's antioxidant defense system. *(Ask your doctor about the new under the tongue form available from College Pharmacy: 800.888.9358.)* N-acetylcysteine, alpha lipoic acid, CoQ 10, vitamins C and E, taurine and glutamine have all been suggested to help to increase the body's glutathione levels and help sustain healthier cardiac function. These substances might be combined in some products and should aid in reducing the total load of toxic burdens in the human body.[77, 95-96]

- Additional natural ways to detoxify exposures to biological toxins include green tea, garlic, oregano oil , melatonin, iron-binding chelators and Huperzine A (Chinese club moss).[46c, 77, 95, 96, 97a-f] Check with your physician or an environmental medical physician if you want to use any of these.[90]

- Inhaled asbestos fiber exposure is particularly toxic, and for this the flavonoids in green tea are said to be helpful.[74]

- To evaluate for heavy metal poisoning, a hair analysis would be helpful.[46a,b, 47]

- Detoxifying homeopathics or herbal remedies, often administered under the tongue as drops, and organic cleansing teas might be beneficial.[45, 46b] *(See Chapter 3 and Appendix D.4)*

- Dry or wet saunas are both said to eliminate toxic chemicals and metals.[119a,b] *(See Chapter 3.)*

- Improved lymphatic drainage and appropriate massage unquestionably will help eliminate toxins from the body.[75a,b, 119a,b, 122a,b] Some new mechanical devices are thought to be helpful in this regard.[122a,b]

- Various types of liver, kidney and bowel cleanses are claimed to be helpful.[45, 46a-c, 76a,b] Some of these methods require more patient studies and more solid scientific evaluation but they have been used by different cultures for many years. They all appear to help some excrete some of the chemicals or toxic metals stored in their bodies.

- Research is presently being conducted to evaluate the Life Vessel. Very preliminary information suggests it can possibly be helpful for some individuals who have chemical sensitivities.[75b]

- If you are concerned about prevention in relation to some global or local emergency situation, there are kits available with detailed instructions about what is needed and how to protect yourself if there is another devastating public health disaster. The necessary information is contained in the First Response Kit.[77, 96, 127] *(Klaire Laboratory: 800.533.7255 or*

The Center for Occupational and Environmental Medicine: 843.572.1600, www.coem.com.)

What Can You Do to Prevent or Treat West Nile Encephalitis? [43a,c]

There is no cure for West Nile encephalitis. Symptomatic treatment with liquids or antibiotics is available, if needed. Remember, if you are bitten but in normal good health, your chance of developing this serious illness is truly remote.

- The development of a West Nile genetically altered strain of vaccine called OroVax has been in progress for some time.[3b, 43a, 60, 98] It uses the technology of ChimeriVax, which is a subsidiary of the United Kingdom biotech company called Peptide Therapeutics. It is being designed for use in an impending epidemic but was not available as of 2002. The big questions remain. Can the genes in this vaccine derived from yellow fever be incorporated into your own DNA? What can they do to you as time passes? *(See Chapter 9 regarding genetic engineering.)*

- A drug called Intron-A, a cloned version of interferon, has been developed by Schering-Plough Corporation *(908.298.4000)*, to fight viruses and stimulate the immune system.[61] This will be tried only on those patients who have developed encephalitis or inflammation of their brain from this infection. This same vaccine is supposed to help those patients with Hepatitis C, which is in the same class of viruses as the West Nile.

THE MOSQUITO CHALLENGE[71a,b, 80, 105]

The remainder of this chapter discusses how you can protect yourself against infected mosquitos without being hurt from the treatment. See if you can urge your local health officials to consider safer methods of insect control. There are effective ways to target mainly the mosquito and not harm other insects, humans or the balance of nature.

How Are Mosquitos Claimed to Be Safely and Effectively Eradicated?[71a,b, 80]

NYC officials claim that pesticide spraying lowers the mosquito count by 85%; but others report this method helps control 60% to 80%. In Florida, where they have had extensive accurate mosquito-control experience, they state they found only a 30% reduction using trap studies. As indicated earlier, after extensive pesticide spraying in California, Florida and Japan, all three concluded that there were more efficient and safer ways to control insects than the use of malathion. *(Get Set: 800.221.6188.)*

Even more surprising, one 11 year research project found evidence that encephalitis infected mosquitos initially decreased after spraying, but after repetitive pesticide use there was as much as a 15-fold increase in their numbers.[3b] Does this mean we were making the situation worse by spraying with pesticides? Does spraying cause "super" pests to develop because only the strong ones survive and reproduce? Will this eventually make certain mosquitos increasingly difficult to control? This type of information should have been known long before sprays were used.

Points to Consider in Mosquito Control

- Does malathion kill the natural predators of mosquitos? The answer is yes.[71a,b]

- Malathion spray has been observed to make some mosquitos more aggressive than normal.[78]

- Research has indicated toxic pesticides damage the immune system and genetic structure of mosquitos making them more prone to illness from the virus.[3b, 49] There is also evidence that chemicals damage the stomach of the mosquitos. Similar effects or gastrointestinal damage also have been reported to occur in humans.[14, 21] Some have written about their serious concerns related to a possible increased risk of bacterial or viral infections, especially because very low levels malathion appears to have the potential to harm the immune system more than previously recognized.[19a,c]

- The environmental and economic splatter effect and drift of the NYC malathion and pyrethroid insecticide spraying is immense. The total ecology and balance of the marine environment (including fisheries, lobster, shrimp and shellfish) and the economy of these industries, appears to be in jeopardy. This might be just one more unanticipated splatter effect of the malathion spray.

- It appears that mosquitos may not be as sensitive to pesticide sprays as other forms of life. For example, it is estimated that more than 10 million lobsters died in the western part of Long Island Sound.[30]

- The West Nile virus spread across the country in the late summer of 2002.[79c] *(It is expected also to be a possible problem in 2004.)* The fear of encephalitis created a varied response. Some community leaders petitioned for no spraying and others insisted on it be done as soon as possible. Most need to become more informed before they make decisions in this regard. Dr. L. Horowitz's book, Death In The Air would be worth reading for anyone who is more fearful of mosquitos than of pesticide sprays.[79a,b, 118]

How Can You Personally Prevent Mosquito Bites?[80]

- **Wear long sleeved pants, shirts, hats and high socks.**
- **Do not wear dark clothing.**
- **Keep away from dark, damp areas, shrubs and bushes.**
- **Mosquitos are attracted to beer.**[71a]
- **Do not wear scented fragrances, perfumes or shampoos.**
- **Do not smell of body odor, perspiration or fabric softener.**
- **Apply insect repellents to clothing, not your skin.**

Skin Preparations to Prevent Mosquito Bites

There are a number of herbal repellants to ward off mosquitos. (*Similar to bees, mosquitos tend to prefer some people more than others.*) The following might be helpful:

- "Do it yourself" non-toxic repellents can be created providing you are not sensitive to the aroma of the product used.[80] Some essential oils, can be combined into natural mixtures containing some mix of peppermint, eucalyptus, lemongrass, citronella and catnip. Try to use only natural, therapeutic grade essential oils. Ten drops of the essential oils can be mixed with two tablespoons of non-rancid vegetable oil. Mix and dab on clothing. *(Pregnant women and anyone who is allergic or chemically sensitive to fragrances should always check first with their doctor or an environmental medical specialist before these are used.)*[90]

- Mosquitos do not like the following herb aromas: garlic, cedar wood, lemongrass, frankincense, cinnamon, geranium, eucalyptus, basil, rosemary, cloves, peppermint, lemon balm (citronella), onions, feverfew, thyme and marigold.[80]

- Naturale Ltd., a vapor wristband that is said to give insect protection up to 60 hours.[56]

- Bite Blocker™ is said to provide 97% insect protection.[57]

- Natrapel, a citronella-based lotion reported to be 84% effective against mosquitos.[58]

- Avon Skin-So-Soft™, another citronella-based repellent, is said to provide about 40% protection.[59]

- Neem oil, used as a mosquito repellent cream, is reported to be highly effective against 75% of certain mosquitos.[80]

- Herbal Armour™ proved as effective and safer than certain forms of DEET-containing products.**[30c,d, 83, 99]

- Some believe that Vitamin B_1 or thiamine hydrochloride, and ultrasonic and electronic repellents are not helpful.

> **Caution: Do not use products that contain DEET as repellents in concentrations over 30% because they have been reported to cause very serious illness in some children.[30a-d ,83] The EPA says it is illegal to label such products "safe for children" but it is possible for lower percentages of DEET containing products to be legally sold in stores and labeled as safe. It has been reported that under certain circumstances some products with old labels, which are not considered to be safe for children, can be sold for four additional years because the manufacturer was given a special "grace" period.[30b] Again, read all labels and keep asking why.[30a-d.]**

What Are Safe Mosquito Control Measures to Discourage Mosquitos Inside and Around Your Home?[43a,c, 48a,b, 71a,b, 80]

Inside Your Home

- Use a fly swatter.
- Use fans indoors because mosquitos do not like drafts of moving or circulating air.
- Repair screens.
- Close outside doors tightly, use door closers.
- Use natural aromas of herbs that mosquitos dislike.

Outside Your Home

- Use "yellow" bug lights at night.
- Avoid outside nighttime walks in damp or wooded areas.
- Keep grass cut short.
- Clean up clutter, debris and remove garbage.

- Trim landscape, bushes, vines, etc. near buildings.
- Clear vegetation from pool and stream edges.
- Turn over any containers or furniture that can accumulate water.
- Fill empty ditches or natural tree cavities.

How to Prevent Mosquitos from Maturing [43a,c, 80]

- Eliminate breeding sites of standing water such as swamp areas, irrigation ditches, basements and sump pump areas, etc. near buildings. This will help diminish breeding grounds with larvae and immature insects.

- Empty water from containers such as old tires, buckets, cans, swimming pool covers, etc. that can serve as breeding areas.

- Drain water from birdbaths, fountains, wading pools, plant pots and drip pans twice a week.

- Eliminate drips from air conditioners, water in gutters or standing on flat roofs.

- Diatomaceous earth comes in different forms and the pure type, without piperonyl butoxide or pyrethrums, is said to be safe and used as an insecticide on grains and to control crawling insects in schools. That pure form is apparently so safe it can be used to treat parasites in animals and humans. Although this helps control cockroaches, crickets, etc., it is not said not to be helpful for mosquitos.[71b, 123]

- If the combination of the food supplements of edible diatomaceous earth and garlic helps protect horses from mosquitos and flies, we need studies to see if it is effective and safe for humans.[5b]

What Are Specific Safer, More Effective Mosquito Control Measures To Use Outside? [44, 55-59, 80]

The following are said to be examples of potentially better and safer ways to control mosquito infestations outside your home. The aim is to eliminate the larvae, not the adult mosquito.

- Bacillus sphaericus makes a toxin that can kill when it is ingested by the mosquito larvae during the first initial two stages of their development. It lasts for about 32 days. Bacillus thuringiensis and israelensis are powerful and highly selective in controlling insects. Unlike malathion, these products are toxic but only to a very narrow range of organisms.[50, 51a,b] In moderate to high concentrations they eliminate half the test population of some mosquitos in 15 minutes and the rest in about an hour. Some mosquitos die in five minutes.[51]

- Methoprene (Altosid®) is helpful for the more mature larvae in stage three to four. The effect lasts for 150 days.[80] It is toxic to fish and possibly to frogs.

- Try Arosurf. It forms a film on standing water and clogs the breathing apparatus of mosquitos.[52, 80]

- Vegetable-based oils can be used to cover mosquito-breeding areas such as the surface of stagnant water. The oil will smother the mosquito eggs and larvae.

- Trypsin Modulating Oostatic Factor (TMOF) is an insect hormone that stops the digestive protease enzymes from functioning so the target insect dies of starvation. Normally mosquito larvae eat chlorella green algae. If TMOF is added to the chlorella, the larvae quickly die because they cannot digest the algae.[53, 100]

- A microsporidium called Edhazardia aedis is said to be helpful.[54]

- The water fungus or mold called Lagendium giganteum is said to control mosquitos. It is sold as Laginex in California.[55]

- There are some mosquito eating fish in the Gambusia genus.[80]

- A red food dye preparation called SureDye is said to be effective to control fruit flies but not mosquitos. Once a fruit fly ingests it and is then exposed to sunlight, it dies. This product is claimed to be safe for beneficial insects and wildlife and appears to be at least as effective as malathion. [11,19a, 120]

(For more general information about safe insect control contact Get Set at 800.221.6188 or 202.543.5450 or www.beyondpesticides.org.)

Spraying to Kill Mosquitos [80]

Much more research is needed but studies indicate that the health effects of mixes of chemicals can be much more toxic than individual single exposures.[19, 83]

- Aerial spraying is the least effective means of mosquito control.[19a, 80] For this to be effective in controlling mosquito-transmitted illness, it must be used about a month before an illness is expected to occur. Symptoms do not typically occur for two to 10 days after an infected bite and it takes another two to three weeks before the blood test confirms the presence of the virus. Sick chickens and ducks, not dead birds, can provide the first and best clues that there is a need for concern.[80] Birds fly so they may not be sighted near the original sources of mosquito infestation while chickens tend to stay near the area of potential concern.

- Spraying from vehicles requires trained professional certified applicators who know exactly how to prepare the spray and when and where to apply it.[30a] Proper application with protective clothing and equipment is imperative. It has been reported that applicators need an 11th-grade education to read the directions and properly mix and apply the spray.[111, 115a,b]

- In this regard, consider the following. In NYC the company that owned the hired pesticide trucks was reported to be paid $650 per hour to spray up to 16 hours a day over a three-year period. Some of the $11 per hour employees became ill and were reported to be both untrained and unsupervised.[31a, 94, 115a,b]

- The selection of which pesticideis used is critical. The synthetic pyrethroids as resmethrin (Scourge) and sumithrin (Anvil 10+10®) are commonly thought to be less dangerous to humans and the environment than organophosphates such as malathion.[82, 84] Others strongly disagree and state the pyrethroids are different, but equally dangerous. They also have been linked to breast cancer and hormonal disruptions. There are even some reported fatal reactions so they are certainly not as innocuous as some would like the public to believe.[82,124]

- One ingredient in the pesticide Dibrom® (naled) called trichlorofon is used for mosquito control. Studies show that exposing unborn guinea pigs during the critical period in the uterus while the brain is developing, can cause a severe reduction in the weight and shape of their brains. Can this happen to the offspring of exposed pregnant women? We do not know but this needs to be investigated.

- Dursban® is highly toxic and should be avoided. *(See Chapter 10.)*

What Should You Know Before Pesticide Spraying?[80]

- Those who can be made ill should be informed 72 hours in advance of the spraying. The young, pregnant and those with weak immune systems or allergies might have to leave town or at least seal their windows and doors and stay inside.

- To be safer, close all windows and turn off intakes on air conditioners.
- Drinking water sources must be protected against contamination. *(Recent legislation allows for more legal water pollution in emergencies.)*[13,80]
- Cover swimming pools.
- Keep children away from trucks that are spraying pesticides.
- Bathe pets after outside exposures or whenever foliage has been sprayed.
- Do not wear outside shoes in home.
- Remove outside lawn furniture and toys or wash them thoroughly if they have been sprayed.
- There should be a hotline to your local health department to provide information and guidance about how to protect yourself and to report and record the incidence and type of medical problems that occur.

Remember, mosquitos do not like drafts so a simple fan blowing directly on you can sometimes solve a buzzing nighttime mosquito problem.

Summary

The health problems in New Yorkers, now and for the next 20 years, will be difficult to interpret because of the combination of the repeated spraying with several potentially harmful pesticides followed by the September 11th exposures. Those who were closest to the World Trade Center, who also happened to have allergies and chemical sensitivities, probably will eventually prove to be the ones who were in most jeopardy. It is highly doubtful that the splatter health effects of the NYC pesticide mosquito control will disappear as time passes. Eventually we shall be more able to judge the effects on children, adults and the planet caused by the toxic chemicals that were used so liberally.

We must learn from previous poorly conceived medical decisions to use much more caution because all possible harmful effects will not be evident immediately. *(See Chapters 4, 5.)* We need more research to answer basic questions before we further pollute large sectors of our country with toxic chemicals such as malathion. [19a, 85] We must keep asking over and over:

- Why would officials chose to use a known poison, toxic to humans, when safer, better and less expensive mosquito-control measures are available?

- Why would politicians continue to expose the public to toxic pesticides when the proven danger of a deadly West Nile encephalitis epidemic appeared to be minimal?[5a, 64, 78, 79a 84, 85]

The bottom line is that someone might want to check on both the decisions and the decision makers in relation to any proposed pesticide spraying. Keep asking if vested interests could possibly cloud or obscure common sense, logic and good judgment.[92] For example, one company was said to receive up to $50 million for spraying NYC for a three years period.[3a, 5a,b, 35b, 94] Is it possible that someone, other than the company hired to do the spraying, stood to gain from this decision?[94] New Yorkers, in general, are much too well-informed and sophisticated, on many levels, not to eventually recognize what has happened to themselves and those they love and not ask why.

Spraying with a toxic chemical to control insects of various types can happen in your city. Now is the time for you to be concerned enough to take some action to protect your hometown, those who live in your area, those you love and yourself. You need to know what to do to prevent a NYC malathion-type experience *before* it occurs in your city. Educate your city, state and county officials now so they know it is a high priority to keep safer methods of mosquito and other insect control in place *before* there is a definitive need. One potential catch exists. It has been reported that the Office of Homeland Security has urged toxic pesticide spraying of urban areas and ecosystems throughout the United States—even if there is no danger of the West Nile virus.[126a,b] *(Get Set: 800.221.6188.)* We must ascertain if this is hearsay or fact. If it is, then it is imperative that we act now to urge safer forms of insect control.

CHAPTER 8 REFERENCES:

1 Blondell, J., et al.,"Review of Chloropyrifos Poisoning Data, Office of Prevention, Pesticides and Toxic Substances," U.S.E.P.A., January 14, 1997, pg. 70.
2 Brenner, Loretta, "Malathion," J. of Pest. Reform, Winter 1992:12 (4) 29-37.
3a www.meepi.org.
3b Howard, J. J. Oliver, NYS Dept. Health, SUNY, Syracuse, 13210; J of Am. Mosq, Control Assoc. Vol. 13 (4) pp. 316-25, 1997 USA.
3c www.chem-tox.com/brevard/index.htm.
3d http://baltech.org/lederman/spray/
3e Envirographic 100, BADGER.
4a Moses, Marion, Designer Poisons: How to Protect Your Health and Home from Toxic Pesticides. 1995, Pesticide Education Center, San Francisco, CA, pg. 45, 415.665.4722.
4b Phelliker@cdpr.ca.gov.
5a Cohen, Mitchel, No Spray Coalition, P.O. Box 334, Peck Slip Station, NYC 10272-0334. No Spray Hotline: 718.670.7110. www.nospray.org
5b Cohen, Mitchel, personal communication: mitchelcohen@mindspring.com
5c Swan, Cathryn, cathrynbe@earthlink.net.
6 Sherman, Janette, M.D., Chemical Exposure and Disease, pp.158-60. 1994, Princeton Scientific Publishing, Princeton, NJ. Cost: $35.00.
7 Good, Dr. Dennis, Dept Biology, U of Maryland, College Park, MD 20742, 301.405.6917. dgO@umail.umd.edu.
8 Interview with Dr. Warren Porter by Carol Dansreau, Washington, Toxics Coalition. Fax: 206.632.8661.
9 "Intestinal Disorders in Children Born after California Spraying," Epidemiology, January 1992:3 (1):31-39.
10 Balaji, M., K. Sasikala, "Chromosome Damage Occurs to Human Red Blood Cells," Mutation Research, 1993:301, 13-17.
11 Cancer Research, May 15, 1996:56, 2393-2399. www.swmed.edu/homepages/epidermi/gws/9/10.
12 Genetics Laboratory, University of Vermont, Burlington, Vermont, "Human Gene 'Broken Off' DNA Molecule by Malathion," Cancer Research, May 15, 1996:56, 2393-99.
13 Heilprin, John, "EPA to Allow Pesticides Without Permits against West-Nile-Virus-Carrying Mosquitoes," Associated Press, October 11, 2002.
14 Env. Res. Foundation, Box 5036, Annapolis MD, 21403. 410.263.1584, erf@rachel.clark.net.
15 Sudan, Alfredo, M.D., Affidavit: Letter to Dr Satoshi Ishikawa, M.D. Kitasato University, Kitasato Sagamihara, Kanagawa, 228, Japan.

16a Shafey, Omar, Interoffice Memorandum, January 3, 1999 to Brian Hughes from Omar Shafey, MMWR November 12, 1999: 48 (44) 1015-1018, 1027.

16b "Surveillance for Acute Pesticide- Related Illness During the Medfly Eradication Program, Florida, 1998," Supt. of Doc., US Govt. Printing Office GPO, Washington DC 20402-9371. 202.512.1800; or MMWR Homepage.

16c "Florida Health Department Epidemiologist Fired After Refusing to Alter Malathion Study Results," Technical Report, "Beyond Pesticides," Nat. Coal. Against Misuse Pest, May 2000:15 (5).

16d www.tompainecom/features/2001/11/16/index.htm.

17 Environmental Medical Research Foundation, ERF [Formerly: PARF], Is This Your Child's World? Chapter 13. P. O. Box 60, Buffalo, NY 14223-0060. 800.787. 8780 Cost: $15.00 (plus S&H).

18 PANNA. 415.941.1771.

19a Malathion Medical Research, University of Florida and University of South Florida Medical Libraries, wwww.chem-tox.com/malathion/research/index.htm.

19b Gross, A., US, EPA Office of Pesticide Protection Programs, senior science advisor, 1984, "Carcinogenicity of Malathion, Memo" to Kevin Keaney, US Pesticide Protection Program, April 24, 1984.

19c "Brain Injury from Malaoxin at Lower Doses in Older Animals," Toxicology, 1993: 79, 157-67.

19d Aldridge, et al., "The Toxicological Properties of Impurities in Malathion," Archives in Toxicology, 1979: 42, 95-106.

20 Chakeraborty, B., et al., "Studies on L-Ascorbic acid Metabolism in Rats under Chronic Toxicity due to Organophosphorus Insecticides and Effects of Supplementation. Ascorbic acids in High Doses," J of Nutrition, 1978:108, 973-980.

21a Savage, E., et al., "Chronic Neurological Sequelae of Acute Organophosphate Pesticide Poisoning," Archives Env. Med, January/February 1988:13 (11) 37-45.

21b "Behavioral and Biochemical Effects of Malathion in Animals, Study No. 51-051-73/76," Dept. of Army, US Army Environmental Hygiene Agency, Aberdeen Proving Ground, Maryland, 21010.

22 "Bulletin of Environmental Contamination Toxicology," 1989:43, 122-130.

23 Teratology 1979:19, 51-62.

24a "The Causes of Lymph Cancers," Rachel's Environment and Health News, September 4, 1997, No. 562. erf@rachel.clark.net. 410.263.1584.

24b #710 West Nile Virus, Part 2, 11/26/00.

25 Cabello, G., et al., "A Rat Mammary Tumor Model Induced by the O Phosphorous Pesticides Parathion and Malathion," Env. Health Persp., May 2001:109, 471-9.
26 Driggers, David A., et al., "Child Leukemia and Aplastic Anemia after Malathion Exposures," Lancet, August 8, 1981, pg. 300.
27 Mayo Clinic Proc., 1978:53, 714-18,.
28a EPA Reverses Decision, Pesticides and You, 2000:20 (1).
28b Gross, A. (U.S. Office of Pesticide Programs senior science adviser), "Carcinogenicity of Malathion, memo to Kevin Kearney," April 24, 1984.
28c www.epa.gov/pesticides/op/malathion/cancer.
29 Boulder Daily Camera, September 29, 2000.
30a Sugg, William, May 20, 2001, Maine Voices, "West Nile Virus Study," Blethen Maine Newspapers; Hallowell, Maine, Maine Environmental Policy Institute.
30b www.meepi.org/wnv/overkill.htm.
30c "Health Canada to Ban Some Deet Products," Pesticides and You, Summer 2002: 22 (2), 9.
30d "Chemical Watch Fact Sheet, DEET," Pesticides and You, Summer 2002:22 (2) 9-10.
31a NCAMP, Tech. Report, December 2000:15 (12) 4. www.chemtox.com.
31b "West Nile Moves Bird to Bird in Lab," USGS Researchers: October 25, 2000. 703.648.4732.
32 Edmon, Dr. John, Center for Vector-Borne Disease, Research School of Veterinary Medicine, U of Calif., Davis, CA 95616.
33 NCAMP, Tech. Report, December 2000:15 (12), 4.
34a www.usgs.gov.
34b www.unmesc.usgs.gov/http_data/nwhc/news/westnil2.html.
35a Technical Report, NCAMP, Vol. 16, No. 7, July 2001.
35b Vol. 16, No. 3, March 2001.
36 Kahn, E. et al., "Assessment of Acute Health Effects from the Medfly Eradication Project in Santa Clara County, Calif.," Arch. Env. Health, 1992: 47, 279-84.
37 Kreutzer, R., "Citizen Illness Reports Following February to May 1994, Aerial Applications in Corona and Norco Riverside Country, CA," Emeryville, CA, California Department of Services, 1996.
38 "Florida Fiasco: Florida Medflies. Florida Health Department Epidemiologist Fired after Refusing to Alter Malathion Study Results," Pesticides and You, Spring 2000, pg. 7.
39a Hollingsworth, Jan. "A Small Increase." Letter. "Re: Florida Air Report Scathing Metro, October 4." The Tampa Tribune. Letter Response Published on October 8, 2002. 813.259.7607.
39b jhollingsworth@tampatrib.com.

40a Ishikawa, S. and M. Miyata, "Development of Myopia Following Chronic Organophosphate Pesticide Intoxication: An Epidemiological and Experimental Study," In Merigan, W.H. and B. Weiss (eds.) Neurotoxicity of the Visual System. 1980, NY: Raven Press.

40b Ishikawa, Satoshi, et al., "Evaluations of the Autonomic Nervous System Response by Pupillographical Study in the Chemically Sensitive Patient," Clinical Ecology, 1990: 7 (2).

41 NYCAP, New York Coalition for Alternatives to Pesticides. 518.426.8246.

42 NYC Police No Spray Coalition. 718.679.7110; and May 16, 2001 Operation order No. 33.

43a www.baltech.org/lederman/spray/

43b Newsday, September 4, 1999 (Guiliani).

43c www.nospray.org.

44 Aerotech Laboratories' IAQ Tech Tip # 64: "Air Sampling Strategies Following Recent Tragedies," techtips@aerotechlabs.com.

45 Krohn, Jacqueline, M.D. and Frances Taylor, Natural Detoxification, A Practical Encyclopedia: The Complete Guide to Clearing Your Body of Toxins. 2000, Hartley and Marks. Cost: $24.95 (plus S&H).

46a Rogers, Sherry, M.D., Wellness Against All Odds, 1994, Prestige Press, P.O. Box 3068, 3500 Brewerton, Syracuse, NY 13220. 800.846.6687; 315.468.4417. Fax: 315.468.8119. Cost: $17.95 (plus S&H). www.prestigepublishing.com.

46b Detoxify or Die, The Ultimate Healing Plan. 2002. $22.95 (plus S&H).

46c Newsletter: "Total Wellness." Annual Fee: $39.95 (plus S&H).

47 www.naturalhealthline.com/newsletter/15sep01/wtc.htm/

48a Mosquito Control. www.mcdef.org.htm. McHenry County Defenders, 132 Cess St. Woodstock Ill, 60098. 815.338.0393.

48b Wilkenfeld, Irene, SafeSchools, 8818 Sherman Mountain Rd., Cheyenne, WY 82009-8844. 307.772.0655 irw27@qwest.net, http://www.head-gear.com/SafeSchools.

49 "Behavioral and Biochemical Effects of Malathion in Animals," Study No. 51-051-73/76 Dept. of Army U.S. Army Environmental Hygiene Agency Aberdeen Proving Ground, Maryland 21010.

50 "Pesticides and You," June 1988:8.

51a Abbott Laboratories, Chemical & Agricultural Products, North Chicago, IL.

51b Nelson, Willie. 703.308.8682 (EPA). nelson.willie@epa.gov.

52 "Arosurf MSF Chemical Fact Sheet," William H. Miller, EPA, 703.557.2600; Pest Control Supply, 800.323.5016.

53 Borovsky, Professor Dov, Univ. of Florida, www.insectbio.com. 919.484.1429.

54 Becnel, James of USDA/ARS in Gainesville, Fl, USDA, Agricultural Research Service, Center for Medical, Agricultural and Veterinary Entomology, 1600 SW 23rd Drive, Gainesville, FL 32608. 352.374.5961. Fax: 352.374.5922.
55 AgraQuest, Inc. - USA, 1105 Kennedy Place #4, Davis California 95616-1272. 530.750.0150. www.agraquest.com. e-mail: AgraQuest@aol.com.
56 Naturale, www.au-naturale.com. P.O. Box 608, Pine Lake, GA 30072. 404.786.2947.
57 Bite Blocker, www.biteblocker.com.
58 Natrapel, Tender Corp, P.O. Box 290, Littleton, New Hampshire 03561. www.tendercorp.com.
59 Skin So Soft, Gardens Alive, 5100 Schenley Place, Lawrenceburg, IN 47025. 812.537.8650.
60 OroVax, Newsday, September 25, 1999, "Deadly Discovery."
61 Intron-A, Schering-Plough Corporation. 2000 Galloping Hill Rd., Kenilworth, NJ 07033-0530. 908.298.4000.
62 Mold Contamination Bills and Laws, Aerotech Laboratories, Inc., 800.651.4802, e-mail dated August 15, 2002.
63 www.safesolutionsinc.com.
64 Barry, John M., "Misplaced Fear of a Viral Epidemic," August 10, 2002. www.nytimes.com/2002/08/10/opinion/10BARR.html.
65 "Pesticides Used in Massachusetts to Control WNV Could Affect the Lobster Industry," www.meepi.org/wnv/overkillma.htm.
66 Cavazos, Jamie, "Dog, Cat Health Unaffected by West Nile; Horses Need Vaccine," U.S. Army Medical Department. News release August 16, 2002. http://www.armymedicine.army.mil/armymed/news/releases/petowners.htm.
67 TR-24, "Bioassay of Malathion for Possible Carcinogenicity" (CAS No. 121-75-5).
68 Mittelstaedt, Martin, "Study Finds Pesticides May Spur Disease," Globe and Mail, April 24, 2002.
69 Kiesecker, Joseph, Penn State Univ., Environmental Study, in the Proc. of the Nat. Acad. of Science, July 9, 2002.
70 Townsend Letter, May 2000.
71a www.getipm.com, Get Set, Steve Tvedten. 800.221.6188. www.thebestcontrol.com
71b The Bug Stops Here. Download free book, www.getipm.com.
72 www.nycosh.org/#anchor16234.
73 NYC Department of Health & Mental Hygiene, Office of Public Affairs, Press Release, July 8, 2002. Contact Sandra Mullin/Greg Butler, 212.788.5290.
74 Head, Kathi, N.D., www.primapublishing.com.
75a Thermal Life Far Infrared Therapy, High Tech Health, Inc. 800.794.5355.

75b Life Vessel, Dr. Valerie Donaldson and Barry McNew, 34 N. Alamos Dr., Cottonwood, AZ 86326. FVSL@wildapache.net. 602.380.3486; 412.767.9890.

76a Rockwell, Sally J, C.C.N., Ph.D., A Rotation Diet. 1998, P.O. Box 31065, Seattle, WA 98013. 206.547.1814. Fax: 206.547.7696. Cost: $ 12.95 (plus S&H).

76b Rotation Diet Game. Cost: $18.95 (plus S&H).

77 Klaire Laboratories, 800.859.8358, www.klaire.com.

78 Radek, Renata, "West Nile Virus Less Threatening Than Insecticide," August 14, 2002, www.virtualbirder.com/bmail/pabirds/200208/20/.

79a Horowitz, Leonard G., Death in the Air- Globalism, Terrorism and Toxic Warfare. 2001, Tetrahedron Publishing Group, Suite 147, 206 North 4th Ave., Sandpoint, Idaho 83864. 800.336.9266. Cost $29.95.

79 b www.tetrahedron.org.

79c Gilberti, Walter, "West Nile Fever Spreading Throughout US," August 23, 2002. World Socialist Web Site www.wsws.org.

79d United States Department of Health and Human Services, Centers for Disease Control and Prevention, Office of Communication, Division of Media Relations http://www.cdc.gov/od/oc/media/wntrend.htm

80 Pesticides and You, Summer 2002: 22 (2) 11-23.

81 Centers for Disease Control and Prevention, Office of Vector-Borne Infectious Diseases. West Nile Virus Background, 2001. www.cdc.gov/ncidod/dvbid/westnile/index.htm.

82 Go, Vera, et al., "Estrogenic Potential of Certain Pyrethroid Compounds in the MDF-7 Human Breast Carcinoma Cell Line," Env. Health Perspectives, 1999:107(3).

83 Abdel-Rahman, A., et al., "Subchronic Dermal Application of "N,N-Diethyl m-Toluamide (DEET) and Permethrin to Adult Rats, Alone or in Combination, Causes Diffuse Neuronal Cell Death and Cytoskeletal Abnormalities in the Cerebral Cortex and the Hippocampus, and Purkinje Neuron Loss in the Cerebellum," Experimental Neurology, November 2001:172.

84 Dexter, Maya, "Not Just a River in Egypt," Genexhibitionst. www.ericfrancis.com/issues/0209/0209westnile.html.

85 Press Release, "West Nile Virus Coalition Releases Letter by Physicians and Scientists: Pesticide Spraying Far More Dangerous than the West Nile," August 19, 2002, St. Bruno, Quebec, Canada.

86 Canadian Med. Society J, 1965:92, 597-602.

87 Weisenburger, D.D., et al., "A Case Control Study of Non-Hodgkin's Lymphoma and Agricultural Factors in Eastern Nebraska," American Journal Epidemiol., 1988: 128, 901.

88 Accu-Chem, Laboratories, 990 N Bowser Rd., Suite 800-880, Richardson, TX 75081. 972.234.5412.

89 ImmunoScience, Inc., 325 S. 3rd St., #1-107, Las Vegas, NV 89101. 800.950.4686.

90 American Academy of Environmental Medicine, 7701 E. Kellogg, Suite 625, Wichita, KS 67207. 316.684.5500.

91 Grether, J.K., et al., "Exposure to Aerial Malathion Application and the Occurrence of Congenital Anomalies and Low Birth Weight," AJPH77, 1987(9) 1009-1010.

92 Kempf, Mary, "Malathion and Health Risks: Who Profits," Madre Grande Monastery, Philosopher's Stone, Autumn l991: 1 (3).

93a Rubin, Rita, "WTC Firefighters Sidelined by Persistent Cough," USA Today, September 10, 2002.

93b www.nycosh.org/#anchor162347

93c Scanlon, P.D., "World Trade Center Cough: A Lingering Legacy and a Cautionary Tale," N Engl J Med., September 12, 2002: 347, 840-842.

94 Gonzalez, Juan, NY Daily News, April 3, 2001. www.nydailynews.com/2001-04-03/News_and Views/City_Beat/a-105855.asp

95 Sahley, Billy, Pain and Stress Clinic, 5282 Medical Drive, #160, San Antonio, TX 78229. 800.669.2256. www.painstresscenter.com.

96 Ross, Gerald, "Terrorism and Toxic Exposures," pg. 32 of "Practical Ways for Physicians and Patients to Reduce the Effects of Nuclear, Biological and Chemical Contamination," AAEM, 37th Annual Meeting, October 31, 2002, Hot Springs, VA. 316.684.5500.

97 "Natural Antidotes to Biological Toxins," email from Steve Tvedten, October 24, 2001.

97a "Garlic," Fitoterapia, 1984:5.

97b "Sulfur-Bearing Antioxidants," Molecular Medicine, November 1994; Immunopharmacology, January 2000; Applied Environmental Microbiology, May 1979.

97c "Melatonin. Cell Biology," Toxicology, 2000:16.

97d "Iron and Medal-Binding Chelators," Free Radical Biology Medicine, 1990:l, 8; Journal Biological Chemistry, August 25, 1987; Biochemistry Journal, September 15, 1993.

97e "Oregano," Journal Food Protection, July 2001; Phytotherapy Research, May 2000.

97f "Nerve Gas Antitoxins: Defense Technical Information Centre Review," December 1996: 2.

98 Proceedings of the National Academy of Sciences, May 2002, Issue 5.

99 Herbal Armour™ Insect Repellant, www.productsforanywhere.com/market/mkt_pages/all_terrain/all_terrain.html.

100 Insect Biotechnology, Inc., www.insectbio.com/tech.htm.

101 Turner, Jack, "Well Digger's Turnstation." www.txdirect.net/users/jeturner.

102a www.newyork.sierraclub.org – Sierra Club.

102b www.chem-tox.com/malathion/research/index.htm Behavorial Toxicology, U of So. FL.

102c www.accessone.com/~watoxics/ - Washington Toxics.

102d www.envadvocates.org – Environmental Advocates.
102e www.beyondpesticides.org – Nat'l Coalition Against Misuse of Pesticides.
102f www.americanpie.org – American PIE (Public Information on the Environment).
103 "Spraying Pesticides to Combat Mosquitoes Suspected of Carrying the West Nile Virus," Consumer Health Newsletter, July 2001: 24 (Issue 7).
104 "Lung Damage Occurs from Single Oral Dose of Malathion," Toxicology, 1983:26, 73-79.
105 McKinney, Deanna, "Meeting the Challenge of West Nile Virus Without Poisons," J. of Pesticide Reform, Winter 2002: 22 (4) 2.
106 Rea, William, M.D., Chemical Sensitivity, Vol.3. Chapter 27, "Pollutant Injury to the Eye," pg. 1885. CRC Lewis Publishers, Boca Raton.
107 Berkowitz, Gertrude S., "Exposure to Indoor Pesticides During Pregnancy in a Multiethnic, Urban Cohort," Envir. Health Persp., January 2003:111 (1)79-84.
108 http://lists.essential.org/dioxin-l/msg00990.html.
109 Extoxnet, Extension Toxicology Network, Pesticide Information Profiles, June 1996, Oregon State University.
110 Caton, Helen and Harold E. Buttram, M.D., The Fertility Plan: A Holistic Program for Conceiving a Healthy Baby. 2000, Fireside. This book is out of print – limited availability through www.amazon.com.
111 Mahoney, Joe, "Skeeter Spray Firm Is Swatted," April 6, 2001, Daily News, Albany Bureau Chief. http://www.safe2use.com/ca-ipm/01-04-11h.htm
112 Eradication Program, Central Florida, Environmental Assessment, April 1998. Agency Contact: Terry McGovern, 4951-B, East Adama Drive, Suite 220, Tampa, FL 33605. 813.986.4356
113 Epstein, Samuel, M.D., The Politics of Cancer Revisited. 1998, East Ridge Press, USA, Freemont, NY. Cost: $17.00 (plus S&H).
114 Municipal Amendment Act (Prohibiting Use of Pesticides), 2002. http://www.ontla.on.ca/hansard/house_debates/37_parl/Session3/L068A.htm#P196_57445
115a Reichenberger, Larry, "The Billion-Dollar Blunder," Chemical Application Journal, Fall 1994.
115b Journal of the American Optometric Association, 1994.
116 Buffaloe, Adrienne, M.D., 31 E. 31st Street, #4D, New York, NY 10016. 212.685.2286. FAX: 212.725.5744.
117 Colborn, Theo, Dianne Dumanski and John Peterson Myers, Our Stolen Future: Are We Threatening Our Fertility, Intelligence, and Survival? 1996, Penguin Books, Inc. New York, NY. Cost: $15.95. www.ourstolenfuture.org, pg. 170.
118 http://www.ADHD-biofeedback.com/alternate.html
119a Silver, Nina, The Complete Guide To Sauna Therapy. 2002, 845.687.0963, www.healingheart-harmonics.com.

119b Wilson, Lawrence, M.D., Manual of Sauna Therapy, 2003, L.D. Wilson Consultants, Inc., P. O. Box 54, Prescott, AZ. 86302-0054; 928.445.7690. Larry@drlwilson.com

120 Mangan, Robert, USDA-ARS Subtropical Agricultural Research Center, Weslaco, TX. FAX: 956.565.6652. mangan@pop.tamu.edu.

121a National Resources Defense Council, "Toxic Chemicals and Health; Kids Health. In Depth Report: Growing up with Pesticides in Agricultural Communities," Chapter 6 "Confirming Exposure: Pesticides in Blood and Urine."

121b www.nrdc.org/health/kids/farm/chap6.asp.

122a ELF International, State Route 1, Box 21, St. Francisville, IL 62460.

122b The Stressbuster Circulation/Lymphatic Stimulator, CAC Inc., 3801 Pineoakyo Court, Rescue, CA 95672. 877.867.2477.

123 Pristine Products, 4626 N 57th Ave., Phoenix, AZ 85031. 800.266.4968. www.pristineorganicproducts.com

124 Wax, Paul M., M.D. and Robert S. Hoffman, M.D., "Fatality Associated With Inhalation of a Pyrethrin Shampoo," Clinical Toxicology, 1994:32 (4) 457-460.

125 CDC, "Mosquito Spraying Doesn't Harm Humans," April 4, 2003. http://www.cnn.com/2003/HEALTH/conditions/04/04/west.nile.spraying.ap/index.html

126a Cohen, Mitchell, Z Magazine, January 2003.

126b Cohen, Mitchell, Green Politix, Winter 2002.

127 First Response Kit, The Center for Occupational and Environmental Medicine, 7510 Northforest Dr., N. Charleston, SC 29410. 843.572.1600. www.coem.com.

128 McKinney, Deanna, "Meeting the Challenge of West Nile Virus without Poisons," Journal of Pesticide Reform, Winter 2002:22 (4).

129 Gilka, Libuse, M.D., of Physicians and Scientists for a Healthy World, Ottawa, Ontario, Canada: "An Open Letter by Concerned Physicians and Scientists."

130 Abu-Qare, A.W., et al. "Combined exposure to DEET (N,N-diethyl-m-toluamide) and permethrin: pharmacokinetics and toxicological effects," J. Toxicol Environ Health. B Crit Rev., Jan-Feb 2003:6(1):41-53.

131 Abdel-Rahman, A., et al. "Disruption of the Blood-brain Barrier and Neuronal Cell Death in Cingulate Cortex, Dentate Byrus, Thalamus, and Hypothalamus in a Rat Model of Gulf-War Syndrome," Neurobiol. Dis., 2002 Aug:10(3) 306-26.

132 Ben-Nathan, D., "CNS Penetration by Noninvasive Viruses Following Inhalational Anesthetics," Ann NY Acad Sci, 2000: 917, 944-50.

133 Contact Joel Kupferman, 917.414.1983. Email: envjoel@ix.netcom.com

134 Regush, Nicholas, "Virus or Environment?" ABC News.com, August 29, 2001. http://abcnews.go.com/sections/living/SecondOpinion/secondopinion010829.html

CHAPTER 9

Serious Monumental Challenges: GE, rBGH and Irradiated Foods

Our government has some current major challenges. These include:

1. Genetically Engineered (GE) or Modified Foods
2. Bovine Growth Hormone Used in the Dairy Industry
3. Irradiated or "Cold Pasteurized" Foods

1.
Our First Challenge Is Genetically Engineered (GE) Foods [1-7, 9a,b]

Of all the pressing issues discussed in this book, this is certainly one of the most frightening. In time, this may greatly overshadow the many other serious current chemical challenges that need to be addressed. Let's discuss what the concerns are and what you can do to protect yourself.

Genetically modified or bio-engineered products (GE) were introduced in 1995. Three nations produce 99% of all GE crops: The United States, 74%; Argentina, 15%; and Canada, 10%. The GE export markets from these countries are growing smaller, not larger, month by month.[8] Why would this happen?

The answer is that most of the world and public do not want to gamble with these products until more is known. At this time there appears to be ever increasing human health, environmental and socioeconomic reasons to be frightened and concerned. The methods used to create GE foods are admittedly crude and imprecise. The media is pro-genetic engineering and every positive claim is widely publicized, but the United States regulatory agencies have not given equal attention to the steady procession of red flags related to the burgeoning bioengineering industry. One of the latest flags was raised in October 2002 calling GE crops in Canada and the United States an economic disaster in relation to both the food and farming industries.[50]

What Is Genetic Engineering?

Genetic engineering means the basic DNA molecules are redesigned to create new forms of life. Genes are the DNA blueprint building blocks found in all living things. This new technology enables the manufacturers to break down genetic barriers between species and among humans, animals and plants. The genes from viruses, bacteria and antibiotics can be inserted into foods altering their genetic codes or their patterns of DNA and these changes can be passed onto future generations. The extensive potential health and economic ramifications of this type of engineering can be endless.

The seeds of many chemically engineered or modified food products, such as corn, soy, cotton etc., have already been altered, modified or spliced with foreign materials of various sorts. Think of a gene as a "string of pearls". The scientists can pick a particular pearl area and alter it in many ways. They can fuse or combine certain pearls with other genes from other plants, viruses or bacteria, or tear them apart, for example with enzymes so the connections are altered or rearranged. Individual genes of some plants can be mixed with a wide variety of other genes to create new packages of genes, which can be reinserted into the original "string of pearls". The whole process is hardly an exact science, especially when it happens outside a laboratory setting.

How Exactly Is GE Done?[23]

Let's look at an example of exactly what happens when something is genetically engineered:

Some of you may have heard of "Roundup® Ready" soy seeds. The object is to make the soybean plant tolerant to the effects of the herbicide Roundup® which is used to kill weeds. If this is not done, the soy crop can be killed along with the weeds when Roundup® is applied. Some who are unfamiliar with the gene concept might think the soy genes are combined in some way with Roundup® but this is not possible because a pesticide lacks genes. To make Roundup® Ready resistant soy, a new gene package or pearl area needs to be created and inserted into the original genetic soybean "string of pearls". The following is a most simplified version of what is basically done when soy is genetically engineered or modified to make Roundup® Ready resistant soy seeds.

1. Incorporation of the item to make the soy resistant to pesticide damage.

The first step to protect the soy crop from an herbicide or Roundup® is to create a new gene from a soil bacterium such as Agrobacterium tumefaciens or Bacillus thuringiensis or Bt. This gene is isolated and then inserted into a soy plant's normal "string of genetic pearls". The bacterium gene makes the seed tolerant of the active ingredient of Roundup® called glyphosate. Hence, once this gene is incorporated into the soy plant, it will tolerate being sprayed repeatedly with increasing amounts of Roundup® without being killed.

2. Adding a "promoter" so the soy accepts the above protective bacterium.

Now the soy plant is not anxious to have a foreign part added to its string of pearls, so a "promoter" gene is needed. This is sort of a genetic switch to turn on genes. In Roundup® Ready soy, this genetic promoter piece is the cauliflower mosaic virus. It encourages the soy plant to accept the new bacterium.

3. Next there is added a "marker" gene so you can tell which plants accepted the 1) protective bacterium and 2) promoter.

Because only one in 10,000-soy plants will accept the above combination, another gene needs to be added to the newly created pearl package. This part is called a "marker" or "antibiotic resistant" gene. This will make it possible to identify which plants have or have not accepted the gene package of the bacterium and promoter gene. Very simply this means when an antibiotic is applied to the treated soy plants, only those who have accepted the new gene with the antibiotic resistant gene package will survive.

4. Lastly the above three pieces (protective bacterium, promoter and marker package) must be forced into the original soy gene line up.

The final challenge is to get the newly created gene or DNA package (the combo of the "pesticide-tolerant" gene, "promoter" gene and "marker" gene) into the "string of pearls" in the soy plant seeds. Either a "gene gun" can be used to force the new pearl package of DNA into the plant cells or something is used to "infect" the soy plant so the new part can be inserted. Then these seeds can be sold and reproduced as GE soy seeds.

We must ask:

- How does a protective bacterium in the soy plant respond to the increased use of Roundup® or other herbicides that now appear to be needed in greater quantities than ever because of the appearance of new super strong weeds? The soy plant may withstand the use of more pesticides but will this in some way alter the soy plant so it can become contaminated with more of some pesticide that can hurt humans? What proof is there that these chemical sprays do not go below the surface of the plant or accumulate within the plant? Pesticided foods can be contaminated below the surface level. Are the chemical spray residues on the plants really all degraded by sunlight? If humans ingest the Bt bacterium and additional amounts of pesticides on the outside of the plants, can it hurt susceptible humans? No one really knows.[9a-b]

- Will stronger and different herbicides be required to control the newer more powerful weeds that inevitably seem to develop? This appears to be what routinely happens in relation to the use of the current pesticides. The newer stronger weeds seem to adapt so they are no longer affected by previously used herbicides.

This is similar to what happens when you take an antibiotic for only a couple days to kill certain germs causing an infection. The weaker germs are quickly killed off by the antibiotic leaving the stronger germs to multiply. If the antibiotic is not taken long enough to totally eliminate an infection, a few of the stronger, more resistant germs remain. You think you are well but a week after you stop the antibiotic, the infection recurs and this time that infection will no longer respond to the original antibiotic and a different one will have to be tried. The stronger "harder to treat germs" will have taken over making it progressively harder to treat the infection.

Which Specific Foods Are Presently Altered?

- The major genetically-altered foods include: milk and dairy products, soybeans, soy oil , corn, tomatoes, potatoes, squash, carrots, certain fish, sugar beets, wheat, rice, papaya, cotton and the oils of canola and cottonseed. As each day passes, there are more.

- The possible combinations for genetic alterations are immense and only limited by the imagination.

- GE products such as tomatoes, squash and papaya were modified by adding the genes of bacteria to enhance their freshness. Genes of viruses are used to control viral diseases that typically can damage these foods as they grow. They have put insect genes into potatoes, bacterial genes in corn and human genes in animals. The mix and match potential is endless.

Here are some examples of specific combinations:

The silkworm gene can be found in apples and apple juice.
The petunia gene can be in some soybeans and carrots.
The barley gene can be in walnuts.
Potatoes can have a chicken gene.
Tomatoes can have a flounder gene.
A cancer chicken virus is used as a carrier so that a growth hormone gene can be introduced or implanted into farmed fish so they grow faster.
The leukemia virus is used in chicken to carry genes into developing poultry.
Scorpion poison genes are used in cabbage to control caterpillars.
Antibiotic resistant genes are being used in foods as markers to indicate successful gene-to-gene engineering has occurred.

Can These Above Changed Products Affect Us Adversely?

The companies who produce or want GE foods say one thing, but increasing numbers of scientists are saying the opposite.[61] Who can we believe? Does this fish virus gene stay in the fish and then get into us? When we eat these GE foods, what can these combinations do to us? What proof is there that this is entirely safe for us? When foods containing antibiotic genes are eaten, can these make us resistant to certain antibiotics? If we become resistant, will we lose the ability to be protected with these specific antibiotics when we need them at some future time to treat specific types of infections?[1, 10, 11] No one knows. You would think we should have known these basics about genetically altered foods long before our government allowed our food supply to be altered.

How Much of Our Food Is Now Presently Altered?

There are presently at least 50 GE foods grown on over 70 million acres of land and sold in the United States. It is calculated that 90% of the money that Americans spend on foods is for processed products and 70% of these processed foods are now genetically modified.[1, 12, 48] The ultimate aim of the food industry is to alter up to 100% of the United States foods within five to 10 years. Dozens of new ones, such as strawberries and corn syrup, are already on the market or are about to be released.[13]

Should We Label GE Products or Not?

Mandatory labeling unfortunately is not required by our government in spite of a recent survey showing 93% of the United States public favors labeling. This means there presently is no way you can tell exactly what you are eating. Similarly, a poll in Canada found 90% want GE labeling and so do 70% to 80% of the population in Europe and Asia.[8, 19f]

In the United States, however, the government does say a food must be labeled if it contains a known allergen, such as a peanut combined with tomato. Fortunately before anaphylaxis (a most severe allergic reaction) occurred, one genetic combination of the highly allergenic Brazil nut combined with soy was recognized and that GE product was removed from the market before any possible chance of a death. We were lucky that time, but can a new one slip by? Genetic engineering can easily transfer new and unidentified proteins that can trigger allergic reactions from one food to another.

Food allergies are hardly a rarity. Who is to decide which foods are so allergenic that they should not be genetically engineered into some unrelated food product? Allergists know there is no doubt that different foods affect different individuals in different ways. There are many acknowledged highly allergic foods such as fish, milk, wheat, corn, egg, oranges and nuts, to name only a few. The challenge is that each person is so different that food items that rarely cause symptoms in many could be seriously dangerous for a few individuals. Although most allergic reactions cause only discomfort, some cause anaphylactic or potentially deadly reactions.[40] How can the many food allergic individuals be protected if no one knows what is in what? Because of biologic individuality, no one can predict which GE food mix will put some specific individual's health in jeopardy. Millions who have allergies will have no way to identify or protect themselves against GE "hidden" offending foods.

If you are sensitive, for example, to tobacco, ponder if some lettuce and cucumber, now combined with the tobacco gene, could cause you to become ill. One whiff of tobacco smoke can cause some asthmatics to be hospitalized. If they ate lettuce, however, who would be able to figure out if it was a tobacco gene in the lettuce causing their medical emergency?

Is Anyone Concerned?

Yes, more and more people are questioning what is being done. Even some food producers in the United States are beginning to show some concern.

- In May 2001, the federal United States regulators cleared the use of genetically modified beet sugar but some candy manufacturers refused to buy it.[34]

- The United States Food and Drug Administration (FDA) released modified rice for use in famine relief, but in Brazoria County where it was produced, they buried 4.75 million pounds in a landfill. They feared it was potentially unsafe for humans. Why would we want to give it to starving people? Why not give them safe food products?[32]

- Starving Africans are refusing GE corn because they fear after it is planted, it is possible for it to contaminate their regular food supply.[44]

Should Customers Be Informed?

There is a movement to keep the consumers uninformed. Some have decided to protect their businesses first. Recently, several chain stores decided *not* to accept food products that are labeled GMO-free or not genetically engineered (GE). This may be the result of a reported "no labeling intimidation" campaign said to be started by Monsanto in about 1994. Their action suggested certain store chains try *not* to tell people which foods are not GE because they might be purchased in preference to those that are genetically altered?[2, 33e] Kraft Foods, for example, are said to have GE components in many of their products, as do many other large companies.[49]

Others unquestionably want their customers to be informed. Regular health food stores such as Wild Oats, Whole Foods and Trader Joes are anxious to have their products labeled because their customers are concerned about the possible dangers of chemicals in foods. These stores prefer to carry labeled non-GE foods. Certain food companies are also taking sides. Purdue chicken producers are reported to have decided not to use GE feed and McDonald's similarly told farmers to stop growing GE potatoes.

Why Should Everyone Be Concerned?

We lack adequate studies to determine what happens in humans who eat genetically altered foods because the FDA has assumed the GE products are "equivalent" or basically the same as regular or ordinary food. The United States will only label foods if they are "significantly altered" in composition. *(How can they tell if the studies have not been conducted?)*

In 2002, one study at Newcastle University in the U.K. did show that ingested GE foods caused the bacteria in the human intestinal tract to adopt the genes of the genetically modified foods. No one knows what the long-term effects this will have in the human body. What will this do to the function of the intestines? Will the EPA consider this type of change significant enough to constitute a significant alteration so GE products will be labeled? [51a,b] At this time we do not know.

- It must be understood that the genetic engineering food industry determines if a product is safe, not our government.[4b] The industry conducts their own chemical analysis, does their own investigation and then submits a "summary" report to the FDA. The reports usually include no stringent pre-market-safety-testing, no long-term animal studies, no voluntary human feeding and no special considerations of fetal, infant, child, pregnancy or elderly issues. This final information is not shared, so the public cannot be aware or informed. More than 60% of all field test data in the past two years contains secret genes classified as "Confidential Business Information".[42] This is similar to the "trade secrets" in the cosmetic industry, which keeps you legally uninformed, even when the contents of some body products include known toxins, cancer-causing agents or other potentially dangerous chemicals.[6a,b] The public cannot even find out what is being done in nearby farms, let alone what's in our daily foods or body products.[42]

- The EPA is sometimes aware of major problem chemicals but this does not mean they will take immediate or obvious sensible action. For example, despite objections from environmentalists, the EPA approved the use of the chemical bromoxynil to be sprayed on genetically engineered bromoxynil-tolerant cotton. This chemical failed to meet the safety standards of the Food Quality Protection Act and is known to cause cancer and birth defects in laboratory mammals. In addition, it is toxic to fish and plants. This alone should have meant no approval.[15] We must ask, why was it approved? An unexpected splatter effect of the above decision became evident by mid-2001. Some Bt cotton sprayed with bromoxynil was found to be more susceptible to a widespread and serious insect nematode problem. Once again, this points out how it is possible for genetically engineered product changes to cause unanticipated consequences. In this case, it weakened a product. This points out the need for more extensive research concerning safety and the total environmental effects before decisions are made about the use of this new technology.[16] Twenty years from now who will suspect that the fabrics they wore and slept on might be a factor related to some newly detected medical problem such as cancer?

- No one knows what will happen to virus genes that are combined with foods, once they get into our bodies. Can they mutate or change into more or less virulent forms, alter our basic metabolism, interfere with cellular nutrition or act as toxins? We simply do not know.[40]

- Some plants produce substances that are naturally toxic to humans. They are generally present in levels that do not cause significant symptoms. By combining plant and animal species during genetic engineering, however, new and much higher levels of toxins can be created.[40] Will this make them more harmful to humans?

- Antibiotic-resistance markers are incorporated into nearly every genetically engineered product. No one knows if these, at some future time, will decrease the effectiveness of antibiotic therapy for the treatment of certain human diseases.[40]

- Without labels, those who have known food or other allergies, those whose religion includes food restrictions, those in favor of animal rights and those who are vegetarian have a right to complain. Does the vegetarian want to eat tomato that has been combined with fish? Does the peanut-sensitive individual want to eat hidden peanuts in some food product? Does the orthodox kosher Jew want to ingest milk in some altered meat product? Does a Hindu want to eat beef or milk in some hidden form? Does the Christian Scientist want an antibiotic marker in his intestines? There is no way of determining what is acceptable for them to ingest. They have lost a basic right of freedom of choice.

What Has Genetic Engineering Done to Farmers?[13]

- Monsanto, for example, has developed treated seeds that are sterile after one season, so each year farmers must buy and use only their new types of treated seeds. The GE industry, with a cartel of transnational corporations, in time, could potentially dominate and monopolize the global market for seeds and foods, and the farmers will be totally at their mercy. The days of saving and sharing seeds are over. They now also have to worry about medical liability, markets and cross-pollination.

- Organic crops can be contaminated by pollen from genetically modified crops grown near by. For example, Canada is fearful of the effects of genetically modified wheat grown on United States soil. Pollen from our GE wheat can easily blow across the border or the Great Lakes and contaminate Canadian regular non-modified wheat. As mentioned before, air and water do not have borders so if organic products intermingle with genetically engineered produce, Canada might not be able to sell their wheat to Europe. This could cause a potential economic crisis among the wheat farmers in Canada.

- The organic farmers in the United States are similarly at risk from cross contamination. As of May 2001, all seed corn in the United States was thought to be contaminated with at least a trace of genetically engineered material. Organic groups believe that GE pollution of American commodities is so pervasive that it is not possible for farmers to keep their sources of seeds pure.[43]

- It appears that some farmers whose land was contaminated with GE seeds are being sued because they did not buy GE seeds from Monsanto. This in turn has lead to counter suits because they claim they never planted or wanted the modified seeds.[17]

- President Bush in July 2002 signed a bill requiring taxpayers to give $4 billion dollars a year for 10 years to farmers to grow more corn. Why? Will the seeds they use be genetically engineered? Could this be related in some way to the United States loss of $400 million dollars a year in corn exports to Europe because they do not want our biotech crops? We already have a surplus of corn and farmers are selling it for a dollar less per bushel than it costs to grow. The farmers and the public will not benefit from additional production, but what about big business? Is there more here than meets the eye?[12b]

- At the present time it is reported that GE crops of soy and corn are less profitable than the naturally grown products.

- It is reported that since biotech crops came on the market in 1996, United States farm exports have declined 15%. United States genetically engineered soy is essentially boycotted in Europe, Korea and other nations. Major European corporations and food chains have begun to remove all GE corn and soy from their animal feed. In addition, the demand for non-GE soybean products is said to have grown from almost 0% to 25% in only 12 months; with further increases for GE-free grains anticipated in this next year.[18]

Of course the companies that promote GE products continue to claim that it is profitable for the farmers and safe for the public.

What Does GE Do to the Ecosystem?[39,41,44,50]

We simply do not know. The balance of nature is delicate.[52] There is some evidence that altered corn pollen can harm the monarch butterfly. There is evidence that this is also occurring with ladybugs, lacewings, etc. What about other beneficial insects? If natural predators are altered, new challenges in nature will arise. What will happen to normal wild fish if engineered carp and salmon are twice normal size and eat twice as much food? Will plants that are genetically altered to resist viruses cause certain other viruses to mutate or change into more virulent forms? Will these hurt us? One genetically altered soil microorganism was found to completely kill essential soil nutrients. Can some foods that are GE alter our soil so it becomes sterile? Several researchers in Germany have shown that genetically altered bacteria and viruses can persist in water, soil and even clothing.[29a,b]

The bottom line is that we simply do not know enough about the plant, animal or human effects of what is being done.

What Does GE Soy and an Associated Increased Use of Roundup® Do to Humans?

- No studies to date have been done on humans or animals with GE soy that has been sprayed with 72% more glyphosate (Roundup®) than usual.[39] Even if it does not enter the soy plant, this chemical will enter the air and the water. This chemical, glyphosate, is the one you need to be concerned about.[53]

- There has been an alarming increase in non-Hodgkin's lymphoma (NHL) since the early 1970s. Two Swedish scientists have recently published data showing a clear-cut relation between glyphosate exposure and NHL.[30]

- Severe digestive problems from gastrointestinal irritation had been attributed to overexposure to Roundup®. [31, 36]

- A 1983 study showed that glyphosate caused a decrease in liver enzymes. These are essential for cleansing, detoxification or elimination of chemicals from the body.[31]

- Others complain of breathing problems and difficulty thinking possibly due to the effect of Roundup® on the oxygen transport system of the blood.[25, 35]

Pros and Cons of GE

There appear to be some pros but the cons related to GE farming seem to include some immense unknowns. We have no idea what the potentially devastating dietary, environmental, health and economic ill effects can be. Decisions can be challenging because so much in this field is new, confusing, unknown and hidden. There are presently eight different agencies in the United States supposedly regulating the biotechnology of genetic engineering under 12 different sets of mostly outdated laws.[12a]

How Was the Idea of GE Sold to Our Government and Farmers?

The farmers, as well as government officials, were told that these modified crops would have less susceptibility to weeds, pests and certain plant or animal viruses or bacteria. The potential for larger crop yields was the major selling point used to sway politicians to allow GE foods on the market and to entice farmers to plant them. American farmers and the public were assured it would increase the crop yields at home and in developing countries, while decreasing the need for pesticide use.

Biotechnology chemical companies claim fewer pesticides are necessary on GE foods, but there is published research that has noted that although weeds diminish at first, this effect does not last. New types of more vigorous weeds tend to grow near crops that are genetically modified.[39] These new weeds are more resistant than ever and can require more powerful and different pesticides to keep them in check. It is estimated that GE possibly can significantly increase the use of pesticides.[39] This means chemical manufacturers will make more money because initially they will use more of the old herbicides and when these are not adequate, newer stronger ones will be designed and sold.[48]

- For example, farmers have presently altered about 80% of our soy crop genetically and the seeds are sold as "Roundup® Ready". The genetic change allows the soy plant to resist the herbicide Roundup® so these soy plants are not hurt when they are repeatedly doused with Roundup®, a toxic glyphosate herbicide. The EPA now allows three times the usual amount of glyphosate residues on crops using "Roundup® Ready" seeds.[37] But what about the humans who eat the soy? Although we are told this chemical dissipates in UV sunlight or is easily washed off, we must ask—is this really true?

- This Roundup® spray was assumed not to cause symptoms in those who ingest these food products. Even if this were true, there are many other unanswered questions.[29a,b, 38, 41, 50] Can this modified soy cause an illness, allergy or chemical sensitivity in humans? When you eat GE soy, are you also eating Roundup® or other weed killers that might have permeated into the crop? Are there any long-term studies in children, pregnant women or adults? What will it do to us, our soil, water and air?[9a,b]

- We must ask if any studies were done specifically to prove the safety of infant soy formulas prepared from a "Roundup® Ready" soy seed crop when a soy formula is needed to feed milk-allergic babies? The very young are admittedly more vulnerable to chemicals than most adults. How will this combination affect them? No one really knows. The infant food industry is well aware of GE products. Both Heinz and Gerber in July 1999 stated they wanted no GE components in their baby food.[48]

- What about genetically altered corn used to make dextrose that is used to sweeten infant formulas? Do we know how safe it is? There are no studies to my knowledge that address these important infant issues.

Controlling the Spread of GE Foods Is a Challenge

- Let's look at one example. Federal regulations have specified that GE Starlink corn can only be used in animal feed and for industrial use. It was not supposed to be allowed in human food, but because of problems controlling the GE corn, it has already admittedly contaminated some Kraft taco shells and beer.[45] This discovery led to the recall of almost 300 food products. The company that makes Starlink corn now wants the EPA to expand their regulations so a "tiny" amount of GE Starlink corn will be allowed in human food. Will this prove to be a foot in the door opening the way for more lenient restrictions? Japan has a zero tolerance for unapproved gene-altered products and will not even allow Starlink corn in animal feed. Do they know something we do not know or do their scientists more fully appreciate what is already known?[12a,b,61]

What Do Genetic Engineering Scientists Say?[61]

Many scientists agree that genetic manipulations cannot be precisely or completely controlled, particularly, outside of a laboratory setting. They admit it is not an exact science. Unwanted, unanticipated and irreversible mutations and side effects can and do appear because GE products splice or combine toxins, bacteria, viruses, antibiotics, enzymes and allergenic substances into their seeds. The potential for short and long term possible health problems from such exposures are not hypothetical, but very real. The possible long term hazards of gene splicing, in particular, can be monumental.[2, 4a,b] Because of this, increasing numbers of scientists are now stating that the presently used methods are crude and inexact making the results unpredictable.[61] They fear that genetic manipulation can increase the levels of natural plant toxins or allergens in foods or create entirely new toxins that might be harmful. A total of 599 scientists from 72 different countries have signed an open letter to all governments saying essentially what is written in this paragraph.[61]

- For example, in 1998 to 1999, researcher Dr. Arpad Pusztai from Scotland studied rats fed lectin incorporated into genetically modified potatoes. There was evidence of organ damage, especially of the stomach linings, thickening of the small intestines, poor brain development and a weakening of the rat's immune system. Once again there is evidence that the intestines can be affected.[51a,b] It was reported that he was fired for releasing this data.[19a, 31, 33, 36] *(See Chapter 7.)*

- It was reported that John Fagan, Ph.D., a molecular biologist at Maharishi University of Management in Iowa, returned a government grant of $614,000, plus other grants for over $1 million to do genetic engineering research because he feared that this pursuit could become more dangerous than nuclear power and he no longer wanted to be part of it.[9a,b]

- The CDC (Center for Disease Control) is investigating claims from 44 people who believe they became ill from eating corn products. How will most people know if what they ate was genetically engineered or modified if it was not labeled? How can they have a diagnosis of GE-induced illness when the effects or symptoms caused by these types of products have not been studied in humans?[12a,b] How will anyone know what to look for?

- Dr. Harash Naragn, microbiologist and senior research associate at the University of Leeds said as follows, "If you look at the simple principle of genetic modification it spells ecologic disaster...The solution is simply to ban the use of genetic modification in food."[41]

- Modified soybeans can have higher than normal levels of estrogen. How will these affect soy formula fed infants 20 years from now? Is this good for growing and sexually maturing youngsters? *(See Chapters 4, 5.)* In time, will we find that this modified soy in some way can alter the onset of puberty or increase the propensity for breast cancer in females or prostate disease in males? Some have theorized that this is possible but the companies producing these genetically altered foods insist there should be no concern. How can they predict what might happen when no long-term studies of the effects in children have been studied?

- A Dutch student, Hinze Hogendoorn, did a simple study.[20] He put two piles of corn (maize) in a barn full of mice. The GE corn was untouched while the regular corn was all eaten. Do the mice know something we do not know?

- He then studied 30 caged mice. One half the mice were partially fed GE food while the other ate their regular food. The GE fed mice weighed less in 10 weeks, and although they were in general less active, they had periods of time when they acted abnormally distressed, nervous and manifested strange unusual activity patterns. One of the GE fed mice died.[20]

Have humans become involuntary guinea pigs in a gigantic genetic chemical industry experiment? Gene pollution, unlike chemical sludge, cannot be buried.[12a, 19a] Once it is done, there can be no going back. The potential of genetically altered products to eventually cause irreversible harm can eventually prove to be immense. Short of a global moratorium, there is simply no way to control the hazards of the rapidly expanding genetic pollution that has presently permeated our food, water, air, soil, insects and animals. There is also no way to predict what can happen, but the effects will surely begin to become evident in the next few years.

We cannot extrapolate that what happens to mice could happen to children but we surely need some research in this area. It is highly doubtful that those who so loudly proclaim GE products are totally safe would be willing to use their own children for definitive studies.

2.
The Second Monumental Government Challenge Is the Use of the Natural Growth Hormone in the Dairy Industry

First We Must Know what rBGH Is [26]

This substance, rBGH, is recombinant bovine growth hormone. It is a genetically engineered potent variant of the natural growth hormone produced by cows. Since the FDA approved the sale of Monsanto's genetically altered rBGH in 1994, about 500,000 cows are now injected regularly with this hormone to increase milk production.[2] By 2001, less than 10% of the dairy products were labeled as "rBGH" free and about 15% of the 10 million dairy cows in the United States were being injected with rBGH.[8, 60]

The biotech industry predicts that almost 100% of U.S. food and fiber products will be genetically engineered by 2007 to 2012.[2] At this time, rBGH is said to be banned in every industrialized country except for the United States because of the potential cancer hazard and because of the antibiotic residues in the dairy products.[8]

What Does rBGH Do to Cows? [4a,b, 6, 40]

You might want to know what happens to cows when they are injected with rBGH. Reports indicate that it appears to increase milk production by 10% to 25% at first, but then the production is said to decline rapidly. Reports also indicate:

- They develop extremely swollen udders, which can become ulcerated with painful bloody lesions. They have to wear supports to hold their immense udders off the ground. Some can barely stand because the udders become so large.

- The cows tend to develop mastitis or infections in the udders so their milk contains pus and blood. They need antibiotics to control the infection. These, in turn, also can be found in the cow's milk or dairy products.

- The cows are so stressed they are given tranquilizers. These can be present in the cow's milk.

- Some cows develop cystic ovaries, uterine problems, digestion difficulties, enlarged hocks and knee lesions (50% become lame).

- They produce defective calves and become infertile.

- The cow's life span is shortened. A 1998 survey of Family Farm Defenders found the mortality rates in herds given rBGH increased to 40% per year. After two and a half years of injections, most of the drugged and supercharged cows were dead. Cows typically live for 15 to 20 years.[60]

- The milk that they produce is chemically and nutritionally different from natural milk. In particular, the milk is supercharged with IGF-1, an Insulin Growth Factor, which is thought to be a major cause of breast, colon and prostate cancer in humans.[4a,b, 6]

Why induce cows to make more milk that may not be safe for humans? In addition, it is reported that the farmers will lose money by producing more milk because there is already a surplus.[48] Pasteurization unfortunately does not make rBGH milk safer. It appears that rBGH is not good for the farmers, certainly not good for the cows and probably not good for us.

What Does rBGH Do to Rats? [21, 22]

- A Canadian government report says that 20% to 30% of rats fed rBGH in high doses develop thyroid cysts and infiltration of abnormal cells into the prostate gland. This can occur in 90 days. What happens to schoolchildren who are given this milk? Will this affect them when they become adults? Are the boys' prostates in special danger? Once again, we simply do not know.[21]

What Does rBGH Do to Pigs?

- It has been reported that human growth hormone was spliced into pig's DNA and the animals became crippled, blind and had compromised immune systems.[2, 40]

- If pigs are fed genetically altered corn, they have difficulty reproducing and when they switched back to regular corn, they are able to breed again.[24]

What Does rBGH Do to Us?[6]

- Studies indicate that producing rBGH milk can significantly increase the Insulin Growth Factor (IGF-1) in milk and dairy products. Studies from the University of Illinois Public Health Department and Harvard report that higher levels of IGF-1 in dairy products from hormone-treated cows can cause cells to divide, and this in turn has been reported to increase the risk of breast, prostate and colon cancer.[22, 26]

- Another study by Dr. Michael Pollack at McGill University with the Harvard School of Public Health found that high IGF-1 is a strong predictor of prostate cancer.[21]

- If the level of IGF-1 is high, studies indicate that men can have a four-fold increased risk of prostate cancer and adult and postmenopausal women can have a seven-fold increase of breast cancer.[21, 22]

- Another study found rBGH also could cause premature growth in infants, early breast enlargement, glucose intolerance and juvenile diabetes in children.[13]

- Many school districts have chosen to serve genetically engineered milk (rBGH). It is readily available but difficult to avoid because of the lack of mandatory labeling. It is reported that some schools in the northeast, for example, continue to contract milk from companies, which, for the most part, refuse to sign affidavits that they are selling only rBGH-free milk. If you do not know what is served in your child's school, maybe you should ask. Also ask which is less expensive.[21]

- In addition, it is reported that about 40% of the beef used for hamburgers is from old dairy cows that have been treated with rBGH. This beef probably also has more hormones, drugs such as antibiotics and tranquilizers, and possibly other harmful chemicals.[13] Should you or your children be ingesting these hormones and drugs?

Why Have Our Federal Agencies Allowed What Other Countries Have Banned?

The United States has many excellent scientists and protective administrations. If GE or rBGH products are bad, it does not seem reasonable or possible that they would not protect us.

- In the United States, the Department of Agriculture and the EPA have, in general, approved the genetic engineering of most foods and agreed to no labeling. It has been reported that the entire decision-making policy was "fast tracked" by an EPA official who had previously worked as a lawyer for Monsanto. This man also is said to have appointed others from Monsanto to the FDA.[1, 54]

- It was reported in 1993, that the FDA, without conducting

rigorous long-term health studies or pre-market safety testing, decided that treated GE and rBGH products were safe. The FDA does not even require the industry to reveal the source of their implanted genes.[38] In addition, the FDA did not require the usual 24 months of testing on large numbers of rats before rBGH was allowed to be released. Why not? Why was the raw data of the Monsanto study using only a few rats for three months never been made available for an impartial critique by American scientists outside the FDA?[1, 2, 10]

- Surprisingly Canadian scientists, who were able to eventually see and evaluate the rat studies in 1998, reported indications that rBGH was linked to both prostate and thyroid cancer and thyroid cysts in laboratory rats.[2] Maybe American politicians, farmers and scientists need to review and reevaluate what the critical and careful Canadian's scientists saw.

- In contrast, the GAO, (General Accounting Office) which is the research arm of Congress, had advised the FDA not to approve rBGH until the effects on humans were studied more extensively. In spite of this, the synthetic hormone was approved in 1993.[38]

- Other countries, including most of Europe banned GE products in 1994, Canada banned them in 1999 and later on, both Japan and India did likewise. Monsanto continues to claim there is no reason for concern. We must keep asking, if GE products are so safe, why have so many other countries banned them?[8, 21]

This entire situation is win-win for the pesticide/herbicide industry because it enables them to sell, use and develop more products. The farmer must continually buy their "one-time-use-only" seeds. The chemical companies can produce and sell more and more chemicals to combat the development of ever increasing super pests and weeds that their products are said to create. Once again, corporate interests have won over the sensible precautionary safety-first principle that Europe has adopted. Maybe there is a political big business mega-money/superhighway that needs some mega investigation.[48]

3.
The Third Potentially Serious Food Challenge: Irradiated or "Cold Pasteurized" Foods [27a,b, 55]

Radiation is recommended because it kills germs and this means it increases the shelf life of foods. Irradiated food is not radioactive but those who eat the foods are receiving an indirect exposure to the radiation used to process the foods. In this country beef, pork, lamb, chicken, eggs, mangoes and papayas, all can be irradiated. Legalized irradiation of shellfish, oysters and other meat products is pending or already here.

In 1991, the irradiation industry was poised to begin a new wave of food irradiation promotion.[27a] They believe that "consumer training" is the key to citizen acceptance. Surveys, however, by in 1990 and 1994 found 80% of the population were concerned about irradiation of foods.[27b] By 1997, about 77% of Americans still said they would not eat irradiated foods. The public appears to be more wary and wise than the food industry realizes.

What About Labeling?[47]

Your "right to know" and "freedom of choice" appears not be adequately protected.[47] Several forms of misleading deception are clearly evident in relation to irradiation.

- There is an attempt to decrease the print size on labels that warns an item is irradiated. It has been reported that there is an attempt to intentionally remove their warning logo "radura" from irradiated products. The symbol that a food is irradiated is sort of a flower in a circle.

- The expiration date requirements for irradiated foods have been extended.

- Misleading language is used such as "electronic" or "cold" pasteurization, rather than irradiation. It is possible these more acceptable sounding terms will fool many who are unaware.

- The food industry is required to label only whole items but not ingredients in items. For example, the chicken in the soup served to your child at school can be irradiated and unlabeled.

- In addition, you should be aware that stores must label meat as irradiated but restaurants, schools, hospitals and residential centers have no labeling requirement.[27b]

Again, we must ask why not? Who initiated these exceptions and why?

Let's look at the pros and cons of this entire issue[55]:

Pro

- The shelf life of a food is increased significantly.

- The food looks edible, even though it is very old. Normal ripening or decay is stopped.[55]

- The food looks the same but the living cells have been totally annihilated.[55]

- Many, but not all, germs in irradiated foods are killed.

Con

- Irradiation does not ensure safe meat. Yes, it kills most bacteria but it does not destroy the toxins created during early stages of spoilage. Some resistant strains of salmonella apparently can survive radiation. In addition, beneficial microorganisms that can produce odors to warn of spoilage are killed so you have no warning when the irradiated food is eventually spoiled.[27a,b]

- It is known that irradiation will not prevent hepatitis or kill viruses, such as the prion of mad cow disease.[27a]
- Irradiation does not reduce the feces or debris from dirty slaughter house contamination.[27a]
- Radiation causes aflotoxins to form from mold spores which are thought to contribute to liver cancer.[27b]
- It causes radiolytic products to form such as formaldehyde and benzene. These are known to cause mutation (cellular damage) and are suspected of causing cancer.[55]
- The flavor, odor and texture of the foods can be altered.[27a]
- From the nutritional perspective, exposing foods to what is equivalent to over a billion chest x-rays depletes them of vitamins, especially A, B complex, C, E, K and beta carotene. Radiation can cause a 20% to 80% loss of any of these nutrients, amino acids and the essential fatty acids.[27b, 55] Milk loses 70% of it's A, B_1, and B_2 when it is irradiated.
- Irradiation can increase or double the price of altered food produce. Irradiated meat can cost 20 to 75 cents more per pound.[27a]
- Workers in irradiation plants and those exposed to radiation leaks from factories near their homes, have shown evidence of illness from such exposures.[27b] The number of irradiation facilities will be markedly increased if irradiated foods are accepted by the American public and these could be potentially dangerous to all those who are exposed in nearby areas.

Do the FDA and Scientists Know If Irradiated Foods Hurt Animals or Humans?

- The answer is yes. They have some knowledge but certainly need more. The FDA is reported to have done no toxicology research in irradiation in the past 20 years.[27b]

- Early research conducted or funded mainly by the United States government initially reported that animals who ate irradiated foods had premature deaths, internal bleeding, cancer, reproductive and genetic problems and nutritional deficiencies.[47] Some of these claims have been confirmed by later studies.[55]

- The FDA did review 441 toxicity studies related to irradiated food safety and found that all were flawed. With shaky assurance from just five of 441 of these studies, the FDA approved irradiation of the public food system in 1986.[27b, 47]

Someone needs to ask some questions about this decision. Most of the following studies were available when they conducted their review.

Animal and Insect Studies

The Agriculture Department has been reported to claim that studies on laboratory animals for the past 30 to 40 years, not only in the United Stated but also in the entire world, have shown there is no health effect that is detrimental to humans[62]—but let's look at some of the studies in animals.

- In one study in 1960 at the University of Illinois, mice were fed irradiated foods and their breathing became so impaired they could not move in their cage. A total of 17% died. The autopsy showed heart enlargement, blood clots and heart muscle damage.[55, 56]

- In another animal study at the University of Illinois at the same time, all the mice used for the research were given nutrients. One group of these mice was fed irradiated *uncooked* milk. A total of 83% or 25 of these animals developed heart lesions within 85 days. Four animals that were fed irradiated *cooked* milk developed heart lesions. The heart muscle tore apart and the animals bled to death. None of the controls, who were not given irradiated milk, had cardiac or bleeding problems.[55, 56]

- In another study in 1960 at the Medical College of Virginia, laboratory rats were fed irradiated beef. All the male rats died of hemorrhages within 34 days.[57] If they castrated the male mice, all the males and females fed irradiated beef died by 63 days.

- In 1983, the research division of Ralston Purina reported a compilation of 12 studies. They examined the effects of feeding irradiated chicken to mice and other animal species.[55, 58] One group of rats in the study developed testicular tumors and a decreased life span.[27b] Another group of mice developed kidney disease. *(Earlier studies and some published by Russians also found evidence of kidney disease from irradiated food.[55])* They also reported more cancer than normal in the controls.[55] The studies indicated damage to the chromosomes, immune system and kidneys, as well as blood clots in the heart.[27, 55]

- Irradiation of foods were reported to cause the formation of a new class of chemicals called cyclobutanones.[27] These are reported to cause genetic damage in rats, and genetic and cellular damage in human and rat cells. The scientists emphasized the possible danger of irradiation was related to the potential to cause genetic structural changes.[27a,b]

- A study at San Diego State College found that when irradiated chicken meat was fed to fruit flies, they had fewer offspring, more stillborns and genetic mutations caused visible malformations.[55] In subsequent studies, fruit flies fed gamma-irradiated chicken had seven times fewer offspring than those fed regular chicken.[59]

- Dr. Au, an internationally recognized toxicologist from the University of Texas at Galveston, urged the FDA to "seriously and explicitly" consider repeated observations of genetic damage and reproductive toxicity in feed experiments. Reports indicate some reproductive cell damage to ova and sperm and this could potentially endanger future generations. [27a,b, 55]

In Humans

Now let us look at some of the research in humans.

- In one 15-week study in China, irradiated foods comprised 35% of the subjects' diet and there was no increase in cancer-like changes (polyploidy) in those who ingested these foods. They recognized that cancer typically requires longer than 15 weeks to become evident.[15]

- In the mid-1970s, five malnourished children in India were studied. Within one month, exposure to freshly irradiated wheat caused 80% of children to develop chromosomal abnormalities of the type that is reported to be associated with radiation.[55] (Similar changes were previously noted in monkeys and rats.) The type of abnormal white blood cells that were produced have been linked to the development of senility and cancer (polyploidy), such as leukemia.[55]

- Radiation can alter the bonds holding food molecules together causing new radiolytic compounds to form. One such substance is benzene. There is seven times more benzene, a known cause of cancer, in irradiated beef than in non-irradiated beef.

- The possible effects of other newly formed breakdown products, such as cyclobutanones, are not known at this time.[27a]

Even though irradiation is considered by our government to be only a food additive, more studies are imperative. We need studies to determine if birth defects, cancer, heart damage or other health problems in humans might be related, for example, to cyclobutanones. Until more is known about the effects of irradiated foods on humans, the government should definitely delay their approval. At the present time it is anticipated that eventually up to 37% of the American diet will be altered by this method.[27b]

It was reported in May 2003 that 28 million children will eat irradiated beef in their school lunch program in 2004.[62] The good news is that school districts can choose if they want irradiated beef or not. The bad news is that most parents will be unaware that this form of beef is being fed to their children. Budget problems of most schools, the increased costs of irradiated meat and possible decreases in food poisoning surely need consideration, but the major concern should be related to the lack of studies that unquestionably show this food product is safe for children. If you are concerned you should consider voicing your interest in your school's decision about this topic as soon as possible.

The bottom line is that our government should be doing its own evaluation of food products and know the answers regarding short and especially long term health effects on infants, children and adults before they release genetically modified or irradiated products to the public.[38] Products should not be released until such studies are completed.

Summary

From the rigid "scientific" perspective, the jury is still out in relation to genetically engineered or irradiated foods. However, no matter how you reflect on this topic, it appears to be just one more example of a potentially harmful and inadequately studied form of possible danger to humans. Again, we should err on the side of precaution until we have enough facts to make sensible and safe conclusions.

The potential ramifications of permitting genetically engineered and irradiating products on the market without adequate proof of safety is incredible.[38] By allowing this to happen, the unsuspecting public is truly being subjected to forced human experimentation. This lack of logic and discretion can potentially lead to many new types of illnesses in plants, animals and humans. When the full scope of possible repercussions finally becomes evident, it may be too late. Every knowledgeable person should become individually and globally proactive, in every possible way, to clean up our air, food, water, soil, homes, schools and workplaces.[46a,b] The bottom line is we should all try to stringently avoid or at least be immensely cautious about the use of GE or irradiated foods until we have more assurance that they are safe for the unborn, infants, children and adults. And lastly, we should be a bit suspicious of any group or person who tries to convince us that these products are entirely safe when the studies to verify this are simply not there. We must ask who has what to gain?

You can take measures to protect yourself and your loved ones by growing your own food or buying safer quality organic (*and hopefully labeled*) foods as much as possible. We must unite in urging the government to clearly label all genetically altered and irradiated food products, regardless of where they are being consumed. At the very minimum, foods that are genetically engineered or irradiated (*cold pasteurized*) should be labeled so those who are informed, aware or unsure, can avoid them if they desire to do so.[28]

CHAPTER 9 REFERENCES:

1 Rogers, Sherry, M.D., Total Wellness. May 2001, Organic Consumers Organization.
2 Cummins, Ronnie. "Hazards of Genetically Modified or Engineered Foods and Crops: Why We Need a Global Moratorium," Organic Consumers Organization. 218.726.1443; 218.226.4164.
3 www.inthesetimes.com.
4a Organic Consumer's Association, March 2002.
4b www.organicconsumers.org/rBGH/gotrBGHmilk.dfm.
5 Mothers for Natural Law. 515.472.2809. www.lisco.com/mothers.
6a Epstein, Samuel S., M.D., Got (Genetically Engineered) Milk? Seven Stories Press - it is an e-book, www.sevenstories.com. Cost: $7.00 to download to your computer.
6b Epstein, Samuel S., M.D., et al., The Politics of Cancer Revisited, 1998, East Ridge Press, USA. Cost: $21.95 (plus S&H).
7 www.inmotionmagazine.com/geff4.html.
8 "Genetically Modified Foods Update." www.mercola.com/2001/jul/25/gm_foods.htm.
9a Fagan, John, Ph.D. "Assessing the Safety and Nutritional Quality of Genetically Engineered Foods. A Science Based Precautionary Approach," Molecular Biology Dept., Maharishi University of Management, 1000 N Fourth Street, Fairfield, Iowa 52557. 515.472.8341.
9b Fagan, John, Ph.D., Genetic Engineering: The Hazards; Vedic Engineering: The Solutions, 1995, Maharishi International University, 1000 N. Fourth St., Fairfield, Iowa 52557. Cost: $12.00 (*Amazon.com*).
10 Spyker, Joan, "Assessing the Impact of Low-Level Chemicals on Development: Behavioral and Latent Effects," Current Status of Behavioral Pharmacology, Federation Proceedings August 1975: 34 (9) 1835.
11 Cummins, R. Lilliston, Genetically Engineered Foods, A Self-Defense Guide for Consumers, Natural Lifestyles, 1999. 800.752.2775; and Michael Fox, Beyond Evolution, The Lyons Press, 123 W 18th St, New York, NY 10011. 212.620.9580.
12a "GMO Food Contamination Is Forever" www.mercola.com/2002/aug/10/gmo_crops.htm
12b "All Hail the Corn! Or Should We?" http://www.mercola.com/2002/aug/10/corn.htm.
13a Memo, "In Support of Requiring Milk From Cows Treated With BGH (Bovine Growth Hormone) To Be Labeled." http://nys.greens.org/ge/memos.htm
13b Sympatico, Joseph, et al., "Genetically Manipulated Food News." http://www.Home.intekom.com/tm_info/rw10101.htm - 68k., Jan. 2001.

13c Keeler, Barbara and Shirley Watson, D.C., "Genetically-Engineered Foods: How It Is Done, What Are The Risks." Rense.com. Published: September 24, 2000.
13d Donovan, S.M. and J. Odle, "Growth Factors in Milk as Mediators of Infant Development." Annual Review of Infant Development. Annual Review of Nutrition, 1994: 14, 147-67.
13e Epstein, Samuel, "Polluted Data," The Sciences, July, August 1978: 18, 16-21.
13f Epstein, Samuel, "Potential Public Health Hazards of Biosynthetic Milk Hormones," Int. J. Health Services, 1990:20, 73-84.
13g Hanson, M.K., "Biotechnology and Milk: Benefit or Threat?" 1990, Consumer Policy Institute, New York.
14 www.green.ca/english/news/nr20020403.html.
15 EPA, "Bromoxynil Pesticide Tolerance," Federal Register, May 13, 1998: 63, 26473.
16 J. Mercola, "More Genetically Modified Food Concerns," www.mercola.com/2001/jul/7/gm_concerns.htm.
17 Weise, Elizabeth, "EPA Threatens Action Against Biotech Crops," USA Today, August 13, 2002.
18 Ag. Journal, UK, May 30, 2001.
19a J. Mercola, "Dangers of Genetically Altered Foods," www.mercola.com/2001/jul/14/gm_foods.htm .
19b www.iatp.org.
19c www.essential.org.
19d www.sustain.org.
19e www.biotech-info.org.
19f www.greenpeaceusa.org/ge/.
20 www.i-sis.org, Dr. Mae Wan-Ho, December 2001.
21 www.worldwidehealthcenter.net/article7.htm.
22 Gilbert, Susan, January 19, 1999, New York Times.
23 www.ems.org/biotech/how_to.html.
24 www.unknowncountry.com/news/?id=1689.
25 Kyvik K.R. and B.E. Morn, "Environmental Poisons and the Nervous System," Tidsskr Nor Laegeforen, June 10, 1995: 115(15) 1834-8.
26 "Canada discredits Monsanto study of Milk Hormone," The Civil Abolitionist, Spring 1999. http://www.linkny.com/~civitas/page94.html.
27a "FDA Ignoring Evidence That New Chemicals Created in Irradiated Food Could Be Harmful." www.mercola.com/2001/dec/15/irradiated_food.htm.
27b "Irradiated Food." www.mercola.com/article/diet/irradiated/irradiated_food.htm Wenonah Hauter www.mercola,com/article/diet/irradiated/nuclear_lunch.htm.
28 "Cancer, Heart Health: Making Sense of Soy," www.mercola.com/2001/may/23/soy.htm.

29a Manuela, J.J. and Beatrix Tappeser, "Risk Assessment and Scientific Knowledge," 1995, Freiburg, Germany: Institute of Applied Ecology.
29b Hill, H.R., "OSU Study Finds Genetic Altering of Bacterium Upsets Natural Order," The Oregonian, August 8, 1994.
30 Hardell, Lennart and Michael Eriksson, "A Case Controlled Study of Non- Hodgkin Lymphoma and Exposure to Pesticides," J of American Cancer Society, March 15, 1999.
31 Heitanen, et al., Acta Pharmacol Toxicol (*Copenh*), August 1983: 53(2):103-12.
32 "Biotech Rice is Headed for Landfill Burial," Houston Chronicle, May 21, 2001, www.thecampaign.org/newsupdates/may01o.htm.
33 Cummins, Ronnie, "Agbiotech Aggression," BioDemocracy News, July 2001 (34).
34 "Refiners Shun Bioengineered Sugar Beets Frustrating Plans for Monsanto, Aventis," Wall Street Journal, April 27, 2001. www.wsj.com
35 Meggs, William, M.D., Ph.D., N.V. Vigfusson, and E.R. Vyse, "The Effect of the Pesticides, Dexon, Captan, and Roundup, on Sister-Chromatid Exchanges in Human Lymphocytes in vitro." Mutation Research, 1980):79, 53-57. School of Medicine, East Carolina University.
36 Tominack, R.L., et al., "Taiwan National Poison Center Survey of Glyphosate-Surfactant Herbicide Ingestions," J. Clin. Toxicol., 1991: 29 (1) 91-109.
37 O'Neill, Sadhbh, at 01-4760360 or 087-2258599 or (*home*) 01-6774052.
38 "Got Milk? GAO Advised the Food and Drug Administration Not to Approve the Use of rBGH Until the Effects on Humans Were Studied More Extensively," www.babcn.lorg/images/news/archive/gmilk.htm.
39 Goldberg, "Environmental Concerns with Herbicide-Tolerant Plants, Weed Technology," 1994: 6.
40 The Gene Exchanges, December 1991, Food and Drug Administration 57 Federal Register 22988.
41 "Raising Risk: Field Testing of Genetically Engineered Crops in the US," Canadian J of Health and Nutrition, June 2001. www.pirg.org/ge/.
43 Cropchoice News, www.mercola/2001/may/23/gm_crops.htm.
44 www.mercola.com/2002/sep/4/gmo_corn.htm.
45 Statement by Stephen Johnson, EPA Deputy Assistant Administrator for Pesticides regarding Starlink corn. Note to correspondents October 12, 2000.
46a www.thecampaign.org.
46b www.keepnatural.org/.
47 "Labeling Requirements for Irradiated Foods," American Association for Health Freedom (Formerly The American Preventive Medical Association), Position Papers. www.apma.net/resources-pos-irradiation.htm.
48 "As You Sow - Genetically Engineered Food and Financial Risk," May 2001, www.asyousow.org/ge.pdf.
49 GE Food Alert Coalition; 202.783.7400, ext. 190; email action@foe.org; http://www.krafty.org, www.krafty.org/flash/

50 "Seeds of Doubt," Soil Association. Mail order 01179290661 or www.soilassociation.org/gm.
51a http://www.organicconsumers.org/ge/010103_biotech_problems.cfm
51b www.organicconsumers.org/gelink.html
52 Pimental, David, "Silent Spring Revisited – Have Things Changed Since 1962?" Pesticide Outlook, October 2002, pp. 205-206
53 Consumer Factsheet on: Glyphosate, U.S. Environmental Protection Agency, http://www.epa.gov/OGWDW/dwh/c-soc/glyphosa.html
54 "The Revolving Door, U.S. Government Workers & University Researchers Go Biotech…and Back Again, A Question of Ethics." http://www.mindfully.org/GE/Revo
55 Gibbs, Gary, Deadly Dining: The Food That Would Last Forever, 1993, Avery Penguin Putnam. http://www.mindfully.org/Food/Food-Last-Forever-2.htm
56 Monsen, H., "Heart Lesions in Mice Induced by Feeding Irradiated Foods," Federation Proceedings, December 1960: 1031-1034.
57 Mellette, S. and L.A. Leone, "Influences of Age, Sex Strain of Rat and Fat Soluble Vitamins on Hemorrhagic Syndromes in Rats Fed Irradiated Beef," Federation Proceedings, 1960: 19, 1045-1054.
58 "Ralston Purina Company: Final Report: A Chronic Toxicity, Oncogenieity and Multigeneration Reproduction Study Using CA-I Mice to Evaluate Frozen Thermally Sterilized, Cobalt-60 Irradiated and I -MeV Electron Irradiated Chicken Meat," The Ralston Purina Company, June 1983.
59 Lusskin, R. M., "Evaluation of the Mutagenicity of Irradiated Chicken by the Sex-linked Recessive Lethal Test in Drosophilia melanogaster." Final Report Submitted to the U.S. Army Medical Research and Development Command, June 1979.
60 Ronnie Cummins, "Market Pressure Busting BGH and Biotech, BGH: Monsanto and the Dairy Industry's Dirty Little Secret," Organic Consumers Association, BioDemocracy News, Feb/Mar02. www.mindfully.org
61 Mercola Newsletter, "Prominent Scientists Form Group to Counter GM Food." http://www.i-sis.org.uk
62 Gersema, Emily, "School Lunches Will Include Irradiated Burgers," The Arizona Republic, May 30, 2003.

CHAPTER 10

It Could Happen to Your Family!

You Could Buy a Home Poisoned with Dursban®[1-5, 12, 13a, 49]

For many years, hundreds of gallons of the termiticide Dursban® have been used in the foundations of homes. This chemical can gradually seep into the inside of your home. The EPA has reported that 82% of Americans have Dursban® in their bodies and this chemical can injure and disrupt the nervous system.[13a] This damage can lead to many illnesses including recurrent infections, allergies and possibly cancer.

Dursban® replaced chlordane after this chemical was found to be too toxic for termite treatment in homes.[36, 37] If your house was built before March 1988, when chlordane was finally banned, there is a 75% chance you still can be breathing this pesticide. There is a 7% chance that the level of chlordane in your home is still unsafe.

In addition, many homeowners routinely use a variety of similar pesticides or herbicides to control indoor and outdoor insects or weeds. It is possible for any of these to endanger the health of the inhabitants. Infants, children and pregnant women, particularly, are at a greater risk.

The Crozier family, discussed in detail in this chapter, illustrates how simply moving into a different home can drastically affect your life, health, future and pocketbook. The home they selected happened to be contaminated with toxic Dursban®. After you read their story, we must ask how long these parents will have to face the many intellectual, emotional, physical and financial challenges caused by this and other chemicals in their newly purchased home. Will they or their young son ever feel well again? How many others might be sick for the same reason and have no idea why?

As you read, consider if this could be why you or some family member is chronically ill. If you moved into a different home, how can you be sure a pesticide applicator did not make you and your family ill by not knowing how to mix it properly or how it should be applied.[24,44,45,48] Did some family member become seriously ill after a move to a trailer? Was there a major water leak, a malfunctioning furnace, a new synthetic carpet or mattress? These types of exposures can cause an amazing array of perplexing symptoms until the cause is recognized.

We must wonder if laws can be changed so new homeowners are protected *before* they purchase potentially toxic housing? One answer is to have an evaluation for environmental toxins before you buy a different home. *(Check your phone book.)*

A Dursban® Treated House

In November 1994, the Crozier family, Joe, Yvette and their four year old son, James, moved to Scottsdale, Arizona from Canada. They moved into an apartment and lived there for the first two years and remained healthy. This means the outside air in Phoenix was not a problem during that period of time. Then they decided to purchase a home in 1996. When they looked at the house they intended to buy, they noticed the smell of air fresheners, but gave it little thought. Within days after moving into their new home, each of them became very sick with a variety of respiratory and nervous system problems. In a short while they became ill indoors and, in time, the outdoor air pollution also became a factor.

The Son, James' Symptoms

Prior to the move in November 1996, James was well and as normal as any typical four-year-old boy. Nightly teeth grinding began within a week after moving into the new house and continues to be a problem. Within one month, by December 1996, he developed leg and foot pain. By January 1997, he developed nightly bed-wetting. Within three months, by February, he had bronchitis. By March, he had diarrhea, morning sneezing and coughing. Five months later, by April, he had headaches and frequent vomiting. His skin became itchy and flaky. Each of these symptoms came on gradually and his doctors did not know why. During a period of about six months, each of his complaints became worse.

The Mother, Yvette's Symptoms

Prior to the move into their home in November 1996, Yvette had some arthritis-like symptoms when it was damp and cold in Canada. They had moved to Phoenix because her joints were better in the warmer climate. By December, however, her hands had become numb in the morning and her scalp tingled. Her skin broke out on her face and body. She had frequent indigestion. By February 1997, she was tired all the time and had daily headaches. She never felt rested. Her concentration and memory deteriorated and she frequently experienced sudden inexplicable feelings of apprehension. By the spring of 1997, she began to have menstrual irregularities.

The Father, Joe's Symptoms

By January 1997, two months after the move to the new Phoenix home (and the exposure to what they later discovered as Dursban®), Joe developed extreme physical and mental fatigue. He awoke more tired in the morning than when he went to bed. At first, he would gradually regain his energy by mid-morning but, as the months passed, his extreme fatigue persisted all day.

In the past, Joe typically had a few weeks of mild ragweed hay fever when he lived in Toronto and, at times, he used one antihistamine a day for his seasonal symptoms. However, by the spring of 1997, Joe developed unusually severe hay fever with a constant runny nose, sneezing and itchy ears. By then he could not begin his day without a couple of antihistamines. He also developed ringing in the ears or tinnitus. (*This continues to be a daily problem and concern.*) For the first time in his life he also developed trouble catching his breath. He was also concerned because his wife and co-workers complained because, at times, he seemed excessively irritable. He could not understand his extreme fatigue and, at times, he was frightened because he realized he was unable to think clearly.

At first, he thought his family's symptoms were caused by pollen, molds or dust, so all the carpets and air ducts were cleaned.[27, 35] They replaced the old heating and air conditioning equipment with a new heat pump, installed an air filtration system and even used a germicidal ultraviolet light at the intake of the heat pump to kill germs and mold spores. They thoroughly cleaned all the bedrooms and bathrooms, including the walls and ceilings, with chlorine bleach.

Unfortunately, the odor in his house that was originally masked by an air freshener persisted. All the family's medical complaints not only persisted, but also became worse as time passed. In spite of their many attempts to feel better, the family's health did not improve. Each of them became sicker as each week and month passed until they finally found a physician who recognized they were all suffering from a chemical sensitivity, an illness caused by environmental exposures. Both parents had symptoms that their immune, nervous, respiratory, endocrine and reproductive systems had been affected in ways noted after toxic pesticide exposures.

What They Did Not Know

The Arizona Pest Control records showed that the previous owner treated their newly purchased home with pesticides on nine occasions from March 1993 to November 1995. Over 785 gallons of five types of pesticides, including 370 gallons of Dursban® had been applied. The records showed that 200 gallons of Dursban® alone were applied in the first month. *(See Dursban® details at the end of this chapter.)*

An Environmental Physician Finds the Cause

In May 1997, they fortunately found a physician who specialized in environmental medicine. Dr. Stuart Lanson in Scottsdale, Arizona *(480.994.9512)* quickly recognized and diagnosed the family's pesticide poisoning. He correctly predicted they would find many small open holes in the concrete slab under the house where pesticides had been placed through the foundation into the soil under the house. He believed the chemicals were continuing to leak through the holes in the cement into the house and that this was poisoning the family. He was absolutely right. They found unsealed holes in the cement below the living room and bedrooms. *(In some homes it is possible for the foundation slab to be cracked and this allows even more of the toxic chemicals to easily and quickly enter a home from the basement and through the walls.)*

What Did an Environmental Home Evaluation Reveal?

When an experienced environmental engineering firm in Phoenix evaluated their house, they found Dursban® in the soil. The levels in the hallway area were found to be 8.5 times higher than the levels allowed in residential homes. In the master bedroom, the levels were 2.5 times higher than the limit set by the Arizona Administrative Code.

Attempts to Clean It Up

The odor, which smelled similar to lard, was much worse as soon as the carpet was removed. The concrete was scrubbed and the holes were sealed with pre-mixed concrete. While doing these things themselves, the family became so much sicker that by June 1997 they were forced to evacuate the house. On one occasion, about eight months after they had initially moved in, Joe and Yvette had to return to their problem home for about 90 minutes. Later that day, Yvette had an earache and a recurrence of her original symptoms. Joe became extremely fatigued. Again, he found he suddenly could not concentrate, think clearly or use good judgment.

Since then, they have not been able to move back. The damage to their health had already occurred and as the years passed, they have all continued to remain ill. There is very little hope that they will ever be as healthy as they were prior to the move into the contaminated house in Scottsdale.

The Proper Environmental Medical Care

Dr. Stuart Lanson was able to help both parents, but James was so severely ill that in February 1998 he had to be seen in Dallas, Texas at Dr. William Rea's Environmental Medical Center *(214.368.4132)* and evaluated by Dr. Gerald Ross.[50] Both in Phoenix and Dallas, the specialists made recommendations, similar to ones detailed in many "how to" books to help those with environmental illness. [6a-f, 7a,b, 8a-e, 9] *(ERF 800.787.8780; Appendix E and in Chapter 3 of this book.)* The family did as much of the following as they could afford.[6a]

- They placed air purifiers throughout their home and in their car. *(800.787.8780; See Appendix C.3.)*

- They purchased safer bottled water for drinking and cooking, and put a water-purifying unit onto the kitchen faucet and bathroom shower. *(See Appendix C.3.)*

- They all had environmental allergy testing. Each member had developed sensitivities, particularly to chemicals and foods, as well as allergies to dust, molds and pollen.

- In addition, multiple, typical and less-frequently-recognized forms of allergies suddenly appeared or became worse after inadvertent exposures to chemicals.[6-9] *(See Chapters 2, 3.)*

- The family began to eat mainly organic non-pesticided foods.

- They followed a four-day Rotation Diet so most foods were eaten only at four-day intervals to diminish their food allergies. *(Sally J. Rockwell, CCN, Ph.D. 206.547.1814; See Appendices C.3, E.1.)*

- Mr. Crozier's tests for chemicals showed he was sensitive to chlorine, formaldehyde and auto exhaust.

- Mr. Crozier and his son began allergy injection therapy.

- The family started on an aggressive detoxification program with nutritional supplementation.[7b, 8e] *(See Chapter 3; Appendices D.2d, E.1)*

- They cleaned often and well with safer cleaning products in an effort to further minimize their chemical exposure. *(See Appendix C.3; Soapworks: 800.699.9917.)*

- They tried to wear and sleep in and on only natural fabrics. *(See Appendix C.3.)*

- Because of cost, they could not afford expensive SPECT brain image tests on the father and son. The SPECT test on James' mother, however, was surprisingly negative. *(See Appendix D.2b; Chapter 3.)* She had undergone detoxification for two weeks before this was done.

- The blood and urine laboratory tests showed abnormalities in the immune systems of each family member. *(See Appendix D.1a.)*

- Blood evaluations for chemicals showed they all had abnormally high levels of xylene. This is a very toxic solvent and nerve poison found in gasoline, paint and glues. It is frequently used as a solvent in pesticides but this type of toxic ingredient is not routinely specified on Material Safety Data Sheets. *(See Chapters 1, 6-8.)* MSD sheets do not have to list this chemical. Xylene is typically deceptively considered to be an "inert" ingredient even though it is admittedly an extremely toxic registered poison and known to cause cancer. In addition, they found seven other toxic, possible cancer causing, endocrine disrupting, immune system and/or nerve damaging chemicals in the blood of each family member.

Spreading Phenomenon [8a-e, 38-40]

Despite their many attempts to totally improve their health, they all continue to have some intermittent medical complaints and each of them developed the common dreaded "spreading chemical sensitivity phenomenon". This means that they all gradually began to notice they became sick in some way from chemical odors that never bothered them before. For the first time, after being exposed to their new house odors, they found they would suddenly become ill from the smell of perfume, conventional cleaning products, deodorants, swimming-pool chlorine, lawn pesticides, malls and restroom disinfectants. Their breathing and nervous system symptoms quickly recur whenever they stray too far from their more environmentally-safe apartment, or if they do not adhere strictly to drinking only their safer water and eating organic foods. They all had developed multiple chemical sensitivities.

Better in Canada

Because their six-year-old son James was so severely ill, his parents believed that his immune system had been so badly damaged they thought they would have to move from Scottsdale. After their exposures in the contaminated house, James was no longer able to adjust to the toxic outdoor environment as he did during his first two years in Phoenix. The major pollution was heavy traffic exhaust, chemically treated golf courses and pesticides used on local agriculture. These were well-tolerated until after the home pesticide exposure. His parents noticed when they returned to Toronto for visits that James improved greatly. He could not play outside in Scottsdale for an hour but in Toronto, he could act like other children playing outside for hours without difficulty.

How Has This Family Been Since the Chemical Exposure?

Six years later, they all feel better but *only* when they are in less contaminated environments. If they smell chemical odors, each of them will quickly becomes ill. If they are cautious at all times, they can stay well for a few days, at times even weeks, and then some unexpected unavoidable exposure will cause short periods of sudden incapacitating illness or minor lingering symptoms for days or weeks. They wonder how long they will have a "walk on egg shells" life, never knowing when another unsuspected toxic chemical will accidentally cross their paths and make them ill.

James

Six years after the initial exposure, he finds the odors in the aisles of regular drugstores cause him to develop a headache and he must run for the door. In natural health stores this does not happen. When the smell of a petroleum-based solvent used in his school to clean office equipment escaped into the air ducts in his school he became ill with a severe headache and remained unwell for four days. When his mother entered the school to bring him home, she too became ill, suddenly developing a nosebleed.

On another occasion a school friend came to visit wearing a scented hair gel. Again James developed a headache in less than a minute.

At the present time, if James is exposed to certain toxic chemicals, such as ordinary cleaning agents, he has a definite sequence of symptoms. First he develops bright red ear lobes, then dark eye circles, and this is then followed by sudden irritability. That night he will grind his teeth, wet his bed and the next morning he will begin his day with sneezing and nasal congestion.

This is his own personal pattern and it quickly alerts his parents that he has been exposed to some chemical. His parents find he does best if he can remain totally inside their apartment on Saturdays and adheres strictly to his special allergy-free diet. Regular outside play in polluted Scottsdale air is simply not possible. He continues to feel much better in the Toronto area, unless he is accidentally exposed to chemicals. (*This is possible even though the city air in Toronto is probably as polluted as the air in most large cities. Each city has pockets or areas of more intense, different or relatively less chemical pollution and, in part, this might account for this child's ability to tolerate being outside in one city and not another.*)

Yvette

Yvette continues to develop fatigue from smelling perfume and cleaning products. Her most upsetting symptom is related to her thinking. If she is exposed to cleaning agents, like her husband, she now manifests poor judgment and finds she is unable to concentrate or remember. She is an engineer who never had problems of this sort in the past. Can you imagine how difficult and embarrassing it can be to find that you cannot recall what someone said to you a few minutes ago? Sometimes when they go for a walk, she will suddenly become nauseous and light-headed. They must quickly return to their safe home. They know from experience that she has smelled some toxic chemical in the air. This sort of thing never happened until they were poisoned six years ago. This is what happens to many who have this type of illness. (*In this regard, we must ask, "How would children handle this type of problem in a school setting?"*

To what degree does the routine use of known toxic pesticides or cleaning agents in schools lead to inexplicable, erratic learning problems and behavioral upsets in today's classrooms? A quick check of the health office records for each 24 hour period after pesticide use in a school might be most informative.)

Joe

Joe continues to develop asthma-like respiratory symptoms and tingling of his scalp if he is exposed to chemicals. He cannot remain in his office when it is being cleaned. On one occasion, six years after his initial chemical exposure, he was inside a hospital when they began to mop the halls. In seconds he developed a splitting headache and then asthma. He had to leave immediately. As long as he is not exposed to chemicals, which at times can present a monumental daily challenge, he typically appears and feels well, although the ringing in his ears persists every day since they were originally exposed to the chemicals in their Scottsdale home six years ago. Nothing has relieved this complaint.

The improvement seen in this family is directly due to the fact that they eventually found out why they were ill and then adjusted their lifestyle so they could live in a more protected environment. The price they paid because of their prolonged exposure inside a contaminated house is much more than money and more than many people could possibly imagine. It is not uncommon for friends, co-workers and employers to forget, not to believe or to even purposely expose them to chemicals. If just one person does not remember and wears a scented substance or freshly dry cleaned clothing, Joe's work performance is impaired and he is unable to function at his usual capacity. The aromas of perfume or scented body preparations in libraries, restaurants, movies and stores have spoiled many pleasures of ordinary life. This family is justifiably angry and disappointed at what has happened to them. They wonder how many more lives must be ruined before people wake up to the devastation pesticides and other toxic chemicals can cause on the health and well being of families. How long will it be before politicians and legislators realize the children and adults they represent need much more meaningful protection so their health is not permanently damaged?

Did Local, State or Federal Officials Help This Family?

I am sorry to say, the answer was a resounding no. No American local, state or federal government agency helped this family. They all said they have no authority or jurisdiction. This situation has cost the Crozier family tens of thousands of dollars. A real estate appraiser told them their contaminated home must be demolished. They must continue to pay taxes on a house they cannot sell. The lawsuits against the previous owner and the pest control company are on hold until they can pay their legal fees. The family presently has barely enough money for essentials.

In contrast, the Canadian government's attitude appears to be much more helpful for those hurt from chemicals. In the long run, this government recognizes it will improve the health of its constituents and save money if it attempts to prevent and eliminate the cause of a medical illness. Their approach is totally different from that in the United States where personally vested economic interests seem to be the rule. In mid-2001, the Supreme Court of Canada ruled that the municipalities throughout Canada can regulate their own use of pesticides. Quebec has already implemented many exemplary changes to protect its community from toxic pesticides.[41, 42, 43]

It also has been reported that if an area in Canada is contaminated by some factory chemical, that factory has to clean it up and the government does not pay them for their losses. The person who sells a contaminated house must pay to correct the problem and pay the medical expenses of those who are hurt by the contamination. Why is this attitude not adopted in the United States? Instead, our politicians tend to give all types of advantages to big business and the chemical industries. They continue to knowingly allow progressively increasing toxic pollution of our water, air, soil and food—along with the American people.[10, 11]

Has This Happened to Your Family?

Do the tragic effects of this family's chemical exposure not sound a bit like the movies Erin Brockovich and Civil Action? Unfortunately, it is probable we shall all hear much more about this type of problem as time passes. An ever-increasing number of people are beginning to realize that pesticides, other toxic chemicals or molds have ruined their health and lives. Please consider the following:

- Should a family lose everything they own, including their precious health because they bought a contaminated house?
- Should there not be some laws, not only to protect them, but also to make those who were responsible pay for what they have done?
- Should laws not totally and immediately stop the use of toxic chemicals in the foundations of homes when safer, less expensive and better methods of termite control is known? [17]

In this regard, consider the following:[4, 5, 12a-d]

- Why were retail sales and home use of Dursban® allowed for almost two additional years after it was banned by the EPA?[49]
- Why can Dursban® continue to be used until 2005 in the foundations of homes? It was "banned" in mid 2001.
- Why can this toxic chemical continue to be used on certain fruits and vegetables, but not on others?

- It was taken off retail shelves in 2001 but stockpiles can be used indefinitely. Who will know if and when it is used?

- Why have provisions been made so it can continue to be used to control mosquitos on golf courses indefinitely?

- Why is it not allowed, in any amount, inside a barn where animals will eventually be used as food but allowed inside homes where there are pregnant women, infants and children?

- Why is 300 times more than the amount considered to be safe on the outside ground routinely used during inside home construction?

Wasn't Dursban® banned because it was a toxic poison and could cause serious illness? This entire situation simply makes no sense. Why do legislators quickly inform the public and ask for recalls on dangerous tires but allow the public to continue to be harmed for years by exposures to acknowledged toxic chemicals? Would the government allow us to stockpile dangerous tires and sell them in the future or use them indefinitely under certain circumstances? Is it not that dissimilar to a court ruling that would free a convicted murderer to walk the streets for a few more years before incarceration? What has happened to common sense? Should we all not be extremely concerned?

A Closer Look at Dursban® [4, 5, 12 a-d, 49]

- Dursban® is one of 40 some organophosphate type pesticides known to damage the brain and nervous system in children and adults, and particularly the unborn infant.[5, 12b,c, 13a,b]

- Dursban® can cause birth defects and damage to the reproductive and nervous systems, as well as the kidney and liver. It is toxic to birds, fish and bees.[12a-d]

- It can cause learning and memory problems, nausea, headaches, dizziness, anxiety, depression, joint pain, disorientation, rashes and fatigue in humans.[2, 12a-c]

- The long-term complaints, such as numbness, tingling, weakness and cramping can begin one to four weeks after exposure.[20b] How often would parents suspect this might be the cause of these types of symptoms in themselves or their loved ones?

- In 1992, the EPA had received 7000 reports of adverse reactions to Dursban®-like chemicals and over 17,000 reactions were reported to United States Poison Control Centers between 1993 to1996.[20a,b]

- Dursban® is a known harmful chemical routinely used in gardens and homes for pest and weed control.

- Hundreds of gallons are routinely used in the foundations of new houses during construction to control termites. An estimated total of 400,000,000 gallons has been poured mainly into the soil in California, Texas, Florida, New Mexico and Arizona. From there it can gradually seep into homes and down into the ground water. Why is this toxic chemical used for termite control when a more safe and economical method is to simply spray and dry borates into the construction wood? This would also save much time and money.[28-31]

- A 1997 study in California reported that about half the schools used Dursban® for pest control, in spite of the fact there are known safer methods. Why are these forms of pest control, such as Integrated Pest Management, not mandatory in all schools when these are safer, effective, less expensive and readily available?[17]

- Dursban® has a half-life of 30 days but inside buildings, it can contaminate the inside air for as long as eight years.

- Between 15 and 24 million pounds are used each year and 2.4 million pounds are used in homes and gardens.

- Dursban is marketed for over 800 uses in homes, schools, workplaces, hospitals and lawns.

- It is used on pets and in pet collars. Exposed dogs become ill with the same illnesses as humans.

- It is used to control roaches, even though it is a registered, proven poisonous substance and considered to be toxic in more than 88 countries. Maybe we need to consider which is worse, the roaches or the pesticide?

- The Federal Center for Disease Control and Prevention estimates that 82% of Americans presently have Dursban® in their bodies.[5, 12a]

- In one study, 92% of the children in Minnesota had this chemical in their urine.[12c]

Studies of Dursban® in Animals

- There are studies to document that minute exposures to Dursban® or organophosphates can cause brain abnormalities in the offspring of exposed pregnant animals. The mothers fortunately are not affected.[1-3, 13b] The literature repeatedly has indicated that exposure to minute concentrations of organophosphates at critical times during a rat's pregnancy can damage the formation of the fetal brain and adversely affect a variety of their behavioral patterns later in life.[13b, 33, 34]

- Studies on neonatal mice show that a single dose of an organophosphate 10 days after birth can cause hyperactivity at four months of age.[13a,c, 23]

- Exposure to Dursban® is reported to cause tremors, poor coordination, involuntary urination, listlessness, muscle weakness and inactivity in rabbits and rats.[2, 4, 5]

- From studies on rats, some Duke University scientists found that there were several mechanisms by which the brains could be damaged that were not related to acetylcholinesterase.[13a, 15, 35] The rat studies in 1999 reported that chlorpyrifos (Dursban® and Lorsban®) can attack the nervous system lowering the intelligence and causing behavior problems.[33-34] The activity and learning problems were more evident in male rats. In addition, females seemed to become more masculinized.[15, 35] Rat studies suggest that it might be possible for non-toxic childhood exposures to pesticides, such as putting toys contaminated with chemicals in the mouth, to cause difficulties later on even though symptoms were not evident at the time of the contact.[32]

Studies of Dursban® in Humans

- In 1995, Dr. Janette Sherman published an article reporting poor growth, major birth defects, weak muscle tone, profound mental retardation and genital abnormalities in four youngsters exposed to Dursban® while they were in the uterus. Animal studies have shown similar defects.[3, 20, 26]

- In 1996, birth defects were again found to be associated with prenatal exposure to this type of chemical in humans, as well as animals.[1, 2, 14, 21]

- One study reported that pilots who sprayed aerial organophosphate pesticides developed impaired coordination. They also had a loss of balance leading to increased accidents; leukemia and pancreatic cancer.[16] Pesticides affected their brains, muscles and immune systems. *(Should we not be more concerned about routine pesticide airline spraying especially before many intercontinental flights in relation to both the pilots and the passengers?)*[25, 47]

- In another study, Florida pesticide applicators with 20 years experience were found to have nearly three times the risk of lung cancer and twice the risk of brain cancer. The good news was that there was no increased risk seen in those who worked with pesticides for only five years.[18]

- Another study claimed that golf course superintendents had an increased risk of four types of cancer. Prostate cancer in this group was three times the national average.[19]

- Twelve volunteers in a correctional institution were fed Dursban® over a period of several weeks. Those on the highest dose had a runny nose, blurred vision and felt faint. Four weeks after the study was stopped, their cholinesterase blood levels had returned to normal suggesting the nerve pathways were open and functioning again.[20] *(The big question is were the inmates fed as much Dursban® as is found in routine diets and in the air outside an institution? Would directly ingesting this chemical cause a different effect than breathing it into the lungs? It is possible that the route of entrance into the body can cause different effects within the body. The study did not entail years of Dursban® exposures, as can happen in real life. It tells us nothing about immediate or delayed effects on infants, children or pregnant women.)*

- In addition, a number of genetic weaknesses can be present in humans that make them less able to process pesticides as well as others. For example, about 4% or the population are unable to process acetylcholinesterase properly with the result that they cannot handle organophosphate pesticide exposure, such as Dursban®, as well as other people.[13b]

Dow chemical company has presented data from many of *their own* studies and they contend that Dursban®is basically safe although some of their work did indicate minor problems.[20] This manufacturer believes the extrapolation of data from other scientists about Dursban® causing brain damage in rats and also to children is scientifically indefensible and reprehensible. If they believe the evidence of illness in exposed rats has nothing to do with what happens to children, why do any studies on rats? Are rat study results that show a chemical is safe applicable in relation to children, while those done by outside scientists that show a chemical is unsafe of no value? If they want the true facts, why does Dow chemical not offer to pay for extensive neurological long term studies on the brain function of unborn or young children who are accidentally exposed to Dursban®? Unfortunately, these children would not be difficult to find. Evaluations by neurologists and psychologists, as well as brain images would certainly provide essential information about what actually happens to the brains of exposed children. If the EPA had the adequate finances to conduct its own impartial research studies, this could and should be done.[15]

If this chemical damages the brains of animals, is it possibly also causing brain injuries in children? Could exposure to this common chemical be just one more unsuspected factor related to the inordinate increase in learning, behavioral and developmental problems in children, as well as the increased incidence of brain-damaged children? These topics are more fully discussed in Chapter 4 of this book and in the companion book entitled *Can Chemicals Cause Epidemics?** Some of the effects from chemicals have been documented on the video entitled Chemical Reactions in Children and Adults. (*800.787.8780. See Appendix E.5.*)

Observations in My Clinical Practice

It was not unusual for parents in my former practice to notice their child routinely became ill after a minute exposure to a wide variety of individual chemicals. It was also not uncom-

* *Can Chemicals Cause Epidemics?*, Doris J. Rapp, M.D. ERF, P. O. Box 60, Buffalo, NY 14223-0060, 800.787.8780, www.drrapp.com.

mon to see children and adults change, not only in how they felt, but also in their appearance and their actions after a single drop of a chemical allergy extract was placed in their arm. Most suspected they were ill from some chemical exposure related to a school or their home. Some could no longer attend school because of perfumes, deodorizers, synthetic carpets and cleaning or construction materials. After they developed their chemical sensitivity, some became ill whenever gasoline was placed in the family car or whenever they were exposed to heavy pollution in traffic jams or in the vicinity of congested tollbooths. Certain patients routinely needed to be seen in emergency rooms for asthma, narcolepsy (sudden inability to stay awake) or other perplexing medical illnesses whenever a lawn spray truck passed through their area or when certain factories routinely polluted the air in Niagara Falls, N.Y., especially on weekends.

Although we routinely documented most patient responses to allergy and chemical testing on videotapes for over 20 years while practicing environmental allergy, only the act of videotaping was unique. Environmental medical physicians throughout the United States and the world, as well as their many patients, have repeatedly seen all the clinical responses that have been described in my books and shown on our videotapes.[6, 22] The doctors who tried these newer methods of diagnosis and treatment and their patients have repeatedly noted:

- Chemical sensitivities are unquestionably one major unrecognized cause of many common, perplexing and challenging acute and chronic illnesses. It appears that any area of the body can be affected. *(See Chapter 2.)*

- Chemicals can cause most surprising changes in the actions, behavior and learning ability of both children and adults.[6f, g]

- There are ways to relieve the symptoms of chemical sensitivities using environmental medicine. *(See Chapter 3.)* These methods include, in particular, avoiding chemical exposures and routine allergenic substances, eating organic foods and improving digestion, drinking pure water, eliminating the toxins stored in the body, rebuilding the immune system with nutrients and Provocation/Neutralization allergy extract treatment. Although everyone is not helped, when this is done correctly, the majority of patients appear to quickly improve in many unanticipated and encouraging ways. Children respond more quickly than adults. *(There are some newer unproven possible treatments that appear to be both effective and inexpensive. See Appendix D.)*

Challenging Questions Remain

Should we not know how children and adults can be harmed before we knowingly expose them to toxic chemicals? To what degree do pesticide exposures in homes, schools and workplaces cause sudden or chronic health problems, hyperactivity, aggression, inexplicable outbursts, inordinate fatigue, recurrent infection, impaired learning, diminished productivity, absenteeism, tardiness, interpersonal friction, battering and marital problems? How much do chemical exposures contribute to or actually cause certain stresses associated with daily living?

Summary

The same toxic chemicals appear to be causing similar symptoms in humans and animals. There is abundant evidence they can cause a decreased ability to think and learn combined with increased infection, allergies, immune system malfunction, thyroid disease, diabetes, cancer and sexual changes. How can we not be concerned? We need much more help from our government to protect us. The good news is that once you are informed, there is much you personally can do to protect and treat yourself and your loved ones. Once you are aware, you are in a position to truly help many others. If we all work together, we can make a difference. We are all truly one, not only connected one human to another, but to all other forms of animal and plant life. Air and water have no boundaries, and neither does love and caring.

CHAPTER 10 REFERENCES:

1 Sherman, Janette D., M.D., "Dursban® Revisited: Birth Defects," U.S. Archives of Environmental Health, Editorial Environmental Protection Agency, and Centers for Disease Control, September/October 1997: 52 (5) 332-3.

2 Sherman, Janette D., M.D., Chemical Exposure and Disease Diagnostic and Investigative Techniques. 1994, Princeton Scientific Publishing Co., Inc. P.O. Box 2155, Princeton, NJ 08543. 609.683.4750. Fax: 609.683.0838. Cost: $28.00 (plus S& H).

3 Sherman, Janette D., M.D., "Chlorpyrifos (Dursban®)-Associated Birth Defects: A Proposed Syndrome, Report of Four Cases, and Discussion of the Toxicology," International Journal of Occupational Medicine and Toxicology, 1995: Vol. 4, No. 4.

4 "Ban Dursban®: Government Finds Excessive Risks in Widely Used Insecticide - Majority of U.S. Population Exposed - Children Found Especially Vulnerable," October 27, 1999. Environmental Working Group, 1718 Connecticut Avenue, N.W., Suite 600, Washington, DC 20009. www.info@ewg.org.

5 Feldman, Jay, "The Lowdown on Dursban®: MOEd* Down by EPA," Pesticides and You, Spring 2000:20(1)14-18.

6 Environmental Medical Research Foundation, ERF [Formerly: PARF], P. O. Box 60, Buffalo, NY 14223. 1.800.787.8780.

- **6a** Is This Your Child's World? 1996, Chapters 10 and 15. Cost: $15.00 (plus S&H).
- **6b** Is This Your Child? Cost $12.00 (plus S&H).
- **6c** The Impossible Child at School and at Home. Cost: $5.00 (plus S&H). Spanish version also available.
- **6d** Video: Environmentally Sick Schools, 90 minutes. Cost: $25.00 (plus S&H) Spanish version also available.
- **6e** Infant Food Allergy, 50 minute audio tape. Cost: $10.00 (plus S&H) (Book on this topic is in process.)
- **6f** Video: Chemical Reactions in Children and Adults. Cost: $25.00 (plus S&H).
- **6g** Video: Mold Reactions in Children and Adults. Cost: $25.00 (plus S&H).

7 Krohn, Jacqueline, M.D. and Francis A. Taylor. 1997, Hartley & Marks, Inc., Box 147, Point Roberts, WA 98281. 505.662.9620.

- **7a** The Whole Way to Allergy Relief and Prevention, 1991. Cost: $24.95 (plus S&H).
- **7b** Natural Detoxification: A Practical Encyclopedia: The Complete Guide to Clearing Your Body of Toxins, 2000. Cost: $24.95 (plus S&H).

8 Rogers, Sherry, M.D., Prestige Press, P. O. Box 3068, 3500 Brewerton Rd., Syracuse, NY 13220. 800.846.6687, 315.468.4417, Fax: 315.468.8119. www.prestigepublishing.com.

8a Wellness Against All Odds, 1994. Cost: $17.95 (plus S&H).

8b No More Heartburn, 2000. Cost: $15.00 (plus S&H).

8c "Total Wellness Newsletter," Annual Fee: $39.95 (plus S&H).

8d Depression Cured at Last, 1997. Cost $24.95 (plus S&H).

8e Detoxify or Die, 2002. Cost $ 22.95 (plus S&H).

9 Miller, Joseph, M.D., Relief At Last. 1987, Charles C. Thomas Publisher, Springfield, IL. 217.789.8980. Cost: $47.95 (plus S&H).

10, "Efforts To Fight EPA's Draft Decision to Require GE to Dredge Hudson River of PCB's Dumped Before 1977," The Washington Post and Los Angeles Times, July 27, 2001.

11 EPA Enforcement Chief Resignation, www.safe2use.com/ca-ipm/02-04-15h.htm.

12a "Ban Dursban®", epa.gov/pesticides, March 28, 2000.

12b "Ban Dursban®," www.safe2use.com/ca-ipm/00-03-30.htm.

12c www.panna.org.

12d www.enviroweb.org/hecweb/archive/pestfile/defects2.htm.

13a In Harm's Way, Greater Boston Physicians for Social Responsibility, January 2001. 617.497.7440. psrmabo@igc.org, www.igc.org/psr/. Cost: $10.00.

13b In Harm's Way, pg. 54.

13c In Harm's Way, pg. 8.

14 Archives of Environmental Health, 1996:51 (1) 5-8.

15 Slotkin, T., "Developmental Neurotoxicity of Chlorpyrifos: Mechanism and Consequences," 2000-2001. albert@niehs.nih.gov.

16 Cantor, K. and W. Silberman, "Mortality Among Aerial Pesticide Applicators and Flight Instructors," American Industrial Medicine August 1999 (362) 239-24.

17 Get Set. 800.221.6188.

18 Archives of Env. Health, March 1993:48(2) 89-93.

19 American J. of Industrial Med. July 1996:29(5) 501-506.

20a Morris, Jim, "Dursban®," U.S. News and World Report, Technology Section, November 8, 1999.

20b "People Harmed by Dursban® vs. Dow Agrosciences," www.callactionamerica.com/cases/case.asp?cid=764.

21 Blondell, J. and Dobozy V., "Review of Chlorpyrifos Poisoning, Data Office of Prevention, Pesticides and Toxic Substances," US EPA January 14, 1997.

22 American Academy of Environmental Medicine. (AAEM) 316.684.5500.

23 Ahibom, J., et al., "Exposure to an Organophosphate During a Defined Period in Neonatal Life Induces Changes in Brain Muscarinic Receptors and Behavior in Adult Mice," Brain Res. 1995 (677)13-19.

24 Malkin, Ray, "Ten Things Your Exterminator Won't Tell You," Consumer Action, July 16, 2002.
25 Winegar, Karen, "Danger in the Air, Pesticide Use on Domestic Airplanes May Make Flying Hazardous to Your Health," Mother Jones, July/August, 1998.
26 Int. J. Occup. Med. and Toxicology, 1995:4(4) 417-431.
27 Conyers, Congressman John, Jr., Introduces H.R. 5040: "The United States Toxic Mold Safety and Protection Act," (The Melina Bill). Michigan's 14th Congressional District, 2426 Rayburn House Office Bldg., Washington, DC 20515. 202.225.5125.
28 Feldman, Jay, "Hidden Pesticide Hazards Lurk in Newly Built Homes," Beyond Pesticides/National Coalition Against the Misuse of Pesticides, www.beyondpesticides.org.
29 Ott, Wayne R. and John W. Roberts, "Everyday Exposure to Toxic Pollutants," Scientific American, February 1998.
30 Immerman, F. and J. Schaum, "Final Report of the Non-Occupational Pesticide Exposure Study," January 23, 1990, U.S. EPA, Research Triangle Park.
31 www.poisonedinparadise.com/poison16.pdf.
32 Gurunathan, S., et al., "Accumulation of Chlorpyrifos on Residential Surfaces and Toys Accessible to Children," Environ Health Perspect 1998:106, 9-16.
33 Chanda, S.M. and C. N. Pope, "Neurochemical and Neurobehavioral Effects of Repeated Gestational Exposure to Chlorpyrifos in Maternal and Developing Rats," Pharmacol. Biochemical Behavior, 1996:53(4)771-776.
34 Campbell, C. G., et al., "Chlorpyrifos Interferes With Cell Development in Rat Brain Regions," Brain Res. Bull, 1998:43,179-189.
35 Avakian, Maureen D., "Mechanisms of Chlorpyrifos Developmental Neurotoxicity," August 2002: Research Brief 80, Dept. of Pharmacology and Cancer Biology, Duke University.
36 "Chlordane Causes Neurological Disorders and A.D.D. Symptoms," Envir. Health Persp., 1995:103, 390-394.
37 Moses, Marion, M.D., Designer Poisons, pp. 77, 276. 1995, Pesticide Education Center, P.O. Box 225279, San Francisco, CA 94122. 415.665.4722. Cost $19.95.
38 Ashford, Nicholas and Claudia Miller, Chemical Exposures: Low Levels and High Stakes, Chapter 2. 1998, Van Nostrand Reinhold, 115 Fifth Avenue, New York, NY 10003. Cost: $52.50.
39 Rea, William J., M.D., Chemical Sensitivities, Vols. 1-4. 1992-1997, CRC Press, Inc., 2000 Corporate Blvd., NW, Boca Raton, FL 33431. 214.368.4132. Cost: $75.00.
40 Matthews, Bonnye L., Chemical Sensitivity, pg 10. 1992, McFarland & Company, Inc., Box 611, Jefferson, NC 28640.
41 The Coalition for Alternatives to Pesticides (CAP). 450.653.7780 or 514.296.8222.

42 "West Nile Virus: CAP-Quebec Bill 15 Be Immediately Abandoned and Recommends Against Mass Sprayings," May 28, 2001, Press Release. Contact: Ms. Edith Smeesters, President, 450.441.3899.
43 The Toronto Public Health Association, http://www.city.toronto.on.ca/health/hcc_index.htm
44 "Six Applicators Sick After Spraying Anvil for Mosquito Control," Technical Report, March 2001:16(3). www.beyondpesticides.org
45 Sanbridge, Dean, "Do Your Technicians Know What to Say When?" Pest Control Magazine, July 2001.
46 www.ige.apc.org/pesticides
47 "Airline Passengers Are Sprayed for Bugs," Pesticide Action Network Updates Service, March 17, 2003.
48 Mahoney, Joe, "Skeeter Spray Firm Is Swatted," April 6, 2001, Daily News, Albany Bureau Chief. (http://www.safe2use.com/ca-ipm/01-04-11h.htm
49 "New York Sues Dow for Calling Dursban® Safe," Pesticide Action Network Updates Service, April 18, 2003. www.panna.org.
50 Ross, Gerald H., Bountiful, UT 84011.

Summary of the Entire Book

We have some clever creative scientists and greedy executives and lawyers working in industries who care more about their personal economics than the future of the human race or our planet. We have a government that appears to be protecting the economy and big business at the expense of the public. We have a medical profession that will be at a loss to help the public because there is no way that they can possibly know and understand the many ways our contaminated foods, water and air have altered the normal functioning and well being of the human body.

But we also have caring scientists with immense knowledge and an enviable amount of foresight and vision. If our governmental decision makers decide it is a priority, they unquestionably can safely clean up much of the air, water and soil contamination, and make positive efforts to control the acid rain, global warming and ozone layer problems. We have insightful and intuitive medical physicians and others in the healing professions who are willing to push the envelope and try newer potentially better modalities of therapy, because they appear to help and not hurt. Of course we must have solid research and valid science but the most academic scientist will readily admit the human body holds mysteries we cannot possibly adequately explain or understand at the present time. And finally, we do know we have many adults, especially parents and intelligent older youngsters, who truly care. They only need to know what is happening and they will unite and demand change. Will we make it? No one really knows but I sincerely believe we shall.

The bottom line is simple. If you personally resolve to clean up and stop polluting your nest, your food, your water, your air and your contacts, you and your loved ones will have a much better chance to become or remain well.

Most would agree that if chemical exposures are possibly unsafe, absolute scientific evidence of harm is not only desirable, but essential. This, however, is not and should not be the sole criterion for medical decisions. We must have a place for common sense and practical precautions. At the present time, the stakes are immense and the biological planetary clock is ticking so fast that time appears to be running out. Rachel Carson's 1962 book, Silent Spring, was supposed to be a wake-up call.[28] Its effect unfortunately was only transitory. Unless we immediately alter our present trajectory, we shall not only have a silent spring, but a silent summer, fall and winter. If you remain skeptical, put Theo Colborn's book, Our Stolen Future, in one hand and, as you read, keep your Kleenex® handy in the other.[2] Keep asking yourself: Can you afford to wait any longer before you personally begin to violently object to what is going on?

Epilogue

My Greatest Personal Fears as a Pediatric Allergist and Environmental Medical Physician

I am personally and extremely concerned about the potential challenge to correctly diagnose and treat health problems caused by chemicals. When all is said and done, we are faced with global contamination of our air, soil, lakes, oceans, homes, schools and workplaces. There is also much evidence that the plant, aquatic and wildlife kingdoms have been seriously affected. Toxic chemicals are everywhere. In each chapter I have cited examples and referred to studies that have demonstrated over and over again how many types of animals have suffered after certain adverse pesticide or chemical contacts.

- Some show evidence of smaller heads, problems learning or moving normally.

- Others have changes in their attitude and behavior with too little or too much activity, aggression or inordinate difficulty tolerating daily ordinary stresses.

- Some have developed cancer, smaller sexual organs or other sexual changes.

No area of the human body appears to be unscathed.

I am particularly concerned about the potential dangers of genetically engineered foods. When Monsanto inserted the Brazil nut gene into soy, their scientists did not realize that someone who was allergic to Brazil nut might possibly die if this type of altered soy was eaten. People have died from merely rubbing a Brazil nut on their skin and can become desperately ill from smelling a nut across a room. The potential danger of the Brazil nut and soy combination was fortunately recognized and potential tragedy was probably averted when this product was removed from the market, but what about the many other combinations with highly allergenic substances? Genetic manipulation can become potentially both a patient's and an allergist's worst nightmare.

- How can we possibly detect sensitivities to all the added components used to modify foods? Milk, corn and soy are extremely common allergens.

- How will we feed highly food allergic infants if milk substitutes, such as soy, are also potentially dangerous?

- Will allergy testing be valid when we test with these or other foods not knowing which allergy extracts contain other genetically-altered components?

In New Zealand, Australia and Great Britain there are already questions about soy-based infant formulas and whether these could spark thyroid or reproductive problems later in life. No one really knows and the only safe action is not to allow altered foods on the market until *we are very certain they are safe.*

It is a monumental challenge to try to fairly evaluate all the possible detrimental health effects caused by the multiple toxic chemicals to which we are exposed on a daily basis. Their potential harm can be immense, but in spite of all this, I urge you not to lose hope for a minute. There is much you, as one individual, can do. Simply follow as many of the sensible, practical, effective and often easy and inexpensive ways discussed in Chapter 3. You can do much to protect yourself and your loved ones by making your personal nest and daily exposures as free of chemicals as possible. You can and must do it. As an intelligent visionary society, creative Americans can and will devise new ingenious ways to effectively cope with the many environmental challenges we are presently facing.

The Ultimate Answer

Treatment Centers for Those with Chemical Sensitivities

For many years I have recognized the need for special medical centers on the cutting healing edge of medicine. They should combine the very best of traditional and alternative medicine. I have joined forces with like-minded health professionals and soon we hope to acquire the *initial* funding to begin to create these integrated centers that will eventually provide comprehensive diagnoses and treatment, as well as in-depth education and quality research.

The centers will be warm and caring and provide the answers to the basic crux of medicine, namely finding and eliminating the cause. By using the best of different types of medicine wisely, we should be able to provide faster, easier, more effective, less expensive and safer ways to help many. The centers will be the diametrically opposite of the current HMO type of "clock-watch" and drug-oriented medicine. We recognize the urgent need to share knowledge so as many as possible can be given practical help and hope.

How the Centers Will Approach Medical Problems

Each patient's care will be highly individualized and comprehensive. For example, suppose you had a liver problem. At this new type of center, a traditional doctor will do a detailed one to three hour history and physical examination. Preliminary screening laboratory liver function, blood and urine studies will be performed. Then the patient will be seen by:

- An osteopath or chiropractor to make sure there is nothing impeding the nerve impulses as they travel to and from the liver through the spine and into and out of the brain.

- An acupuncture specialist who will open the meridians or pathways to the liver according to Chinese medicine.

- A lymphatic drainage specialist to show you ways to help you to personally drain the lymph or toxins from your liver.

- A homeopath and a herbal specialist to provide some inexpensive natural liver healing and drainage remedies.

- A digestion specialist, nutritionist and dietician will adjust your diet to help your liver heal. You might need a liver, gall bladder or bowel cleanse.

- An allergist/environmental medical specialist will treat your food and other allergies using newer techniques that clearly demonstrate cause and effect relationships.

- A detoxification specialist will make recommendations so chemicals can be released from your liver and other body parts.

- A hypnotherapist to determine if you had more perks from being sick than being well, so nothing deters you from feeling better.

- A holistic dentist will help some because certain teeth, according to Chinese medicine, are directly connected to the liver. An abscessed tooth, mercury or metal fillings or an infected root canal in the "liver-related" teeth can cause problems specifically related to that organ, as well as any other organs that happened to be on the same "liver" tooth meridian. Repair or remove that tooth and all organs on the affected meridian should improve.

- When indicated, patients might receive anti-aging, aroma, sound, light or energy therapy.

- Some newer chiropractic techniques appear to be helpful for quickly detecting problem areas in the body and checking into emotional issues.

---

* *There is a River*, by Edgar Cayce; Dr. Norman Shealy and Carolyn Myss, *The Creation of Health: Merging Traditional Medicine with Intuitive Diagnosis.* See amazon.com.

The center will also evaluate medical intuitives who claim to diagnose illnesses by only knowing someone's name and birth date. Edgar Cayce did this for many years at Virginia Beach and helped hundreds of thousands of people from all over the world. (*See book There Is a River*)* In today's world, Caroline Myss worked with Dr. Norman Shealy for many years and similarly provided unusual insights to help perplexing patients. If such gifted individuals do indeed exist and have this capability and they can be shown to be at least 85% reliable, then their preliminary screening insight might drastically reduce the time and expense in relation to both diagnosis and possible choices of therapy. Their insights, of course, certainly should and could be verified by more traditional forms of diagnostic tests.

We Also Need Environmentally Safe Villages

In addition, we hope to eventually create environmentally safe villages where families can go for their yearly vacation and medical care. In the mornings, an entire family's medical concerns, including their pets, will be addressed, while the afternoons and evenings will offer a variety of intellectual, cultural and sports activities. All foods will be organic and beauty salons, restaurants, stores, schools, convention centers and all buildings in the entire facility will be as free of toxic chemicals as possible. Rooms, apartments, condos and homes will be available for those who need or want to live in a more totally chemically-free environment. Time-sharing at similar facilities throughout the world will hopefully eventually become a reality when more funding is available.

To make contributions to our center, contact E.R.F. (Environmental Research Foundation), 1421 Colvin Blvd., Buffalo, NY 14223; telephone 800.787.8780. For updates on our work, see our website: www.drrapp.com.

I sincerely pray the information discussed in this book will provide you with a new awareness of the immense potential dangers of the chemicals we all smell, ingest and touch on a daily basis. Even more importantly, I have tried to provide realistic hope and personal practical insight and choices so you can optimize the present and future health of yourself and those you love.

Doris J. Rapp, M.D.

Appendices

Appendix A
Two Diets That Help in 7 Days or Less*

Want two fast, easy and inexpensive diagnostic diets that have helped innumerable children and adults pinpoint the cause of many medical, emotional, activity or behavioral problems in a week or less? One is the Single Food Allergy Elimination Diet and the other is the Multiple Food Allergy Elimination Diet. They will help you discover what and how foods are making you or others ill. Most people think foods cause abdominal discomfort, nausea, diarrhea, constipation, belching, rectal gas, etc. They are right but rarely do they realize any area of the body can be affected, including your emotions, actions, behavior and memory. These diets can help you find specific answers very quickly and inexpensively.

Diagnostic Single and Multiple Food Allergy Elimination Diet

The diagnostic Single and Multiple Food Allergy Elimination Diets will enable you to determine if a food interferes with how you or your child feel, act, behave or learn at school or at work. It is not just "junk" foods that cause these changes. Many foods you consider "good" can be problematic for certain individuals. Each person is highly different.

The Rotation Diet

There is one other helpful diet called The Rotation Diet. This is also diagnostic but it is mainly used as a treatment diet for those who have multiple food allergies and cannot afford or simply do not want food allergy extract treatment. This diet enables you to eat different groups of foods (fruits, vegetables, meats, grains, etc.) every day for four days and then you repeat this cycle over and over again. It enables you to spot a food sensitivity very quickly so you know when you must stop eating a cer-

---

* *Can Chemicals Cause Epidemics?*, Doris J. Rapp, M.D. ERF, P. O. Box 60, Buffalo, NY 14223-0060, 800.787.8780, www.drrapp.com.

tain food. This is the diagnostic part. In time, many mild or moderate food reactions will stop because food allergies can unquestionably diminish or disappear if certain problem foods are not ingested more often that every four days. This is the treatment part. Initially, for some foods, it might not be possible to eat them more often than every eight or 12 days, sometimes even longer. For information on this diet, read Is This Your Child's World or Is This Your Child?* or contact Sally Rockwell, Ph.D. for her personalized expertise and guidance.[1, 2]

Can Eating a Food Ever Be Dangerous?

It certainly can be. Never test any food without your doctor's advice if it has caused serious medical problems in the past. For example: If eggs or peanuts cause immediate throat swelling, or if fish causes severe asthma, it can be unsafe to smell or eat a speck of these foods. Test only those food items that are routinely eaten, especially the ones you crave. Test the ones you never suspected might cause any difficulty because you eat them all the time. These diets will help you detect unsuspected, frequently eaten foods that commonly cause recurrent illness. There is no reason to check a food that you already know causes a serious medical problem.

Major Caution: Do not allow yourself or your child to eat ANY food that you already know causes a severe allergic reaction. If you're concerned at all, DO NOT EAT a speck without checking with your doctor.

Single Food Allergy Elimination Diet

If you suspect a single food causes you or your child's problem, try this diet. Merely stop eating that one frequently eaten

* *Is This Your Child's World?* or *Is This Your Child?,* Doris J. Rapp, M.D., 800.787.8780; www.drrapp.com.

or favorite single food in every form, for five to seven days. Don't be alarmed if your symptoms (such as a headache, fatigue or muscle aches) become worse during the first few days on the diet. This is common; and these "withdrawal" symptoms mean that your body craves a food to which you are sensitive. When you do not eat it, you feel ill. This is exactly what happens when a narcotics addict does not get his fix. This is why food sensitivities are considered by some to be food addictions. This happens quite often but if you stick with the diet, by the fifth day or so, after you have eliminated a culprit food, you should definitely feel better. After five to seven days (or sooner, if the symptoms disappear before that) eat one single food that has been avoided so you can see exactly what that food does to you. If a true food sensitivity exists, your symptoms should recur within 15 minutes to an hour after eating a normal-sized portion of a single food that has not been ingested in any form for about five days. Do this on "an empty stomach". This means nothing has been eaten for the previous four or more hours. (*On rare occasions, an offending food will have to be eaten on two or more consecutive days before symptoms recur.*)

This diet, in particular, helps those who have a major obvious sensitivity to such items as apples, oranges, grapes, peanut, coffee, chocolate, wheat (flour), corn, eggs, sugar or food coloring.

There are three other factors you must consider.

1. It is sometimes not a food that is a problem but what is put on or in it. (*See Table A1.*) Try organic forms of possible problem foods and if these seem to be fine, while the regular grocery store product is not, the culprit could be what is in or on the food in question.
2. If you or your child are routinely worse (impatient, angry, tired, irritable, have headaches and/or are hyperactive) before meals, think about hypoglycemia or low blood sugar. If this is the problem, merely eat a small protein snack every hour or

two all day.[3a] The snack will reduce the ups and downs.* Remember, however, that some children or adults have both food allergy and hypoglycemia. If they have both problems, they can be worse before and after eating, and the diagnosis can be missed for years.

Table A1
Common Contaminants Found in Foods

Most fruits and vegetables, root vegetables, carrots, beets, potatoes have less contamination if the soil is not pesticided. The fat in meat, in particular, stores pesticides unless the animals were raised on organic food.

Hormones that feminize: Chicken and turkey, beef and some dairy.

Fumigants: Nuts, raisins, figs, dates, prunes, dried fruits, grains, dried beans. In chips used on chocolate, carob, tapioca, arrowroot.

Bleaches: Grains (flour, rice). They also have pesticides from storage bin use.

Sulfur: Peaches, apricots, nectarines, raisins.

Sulfur dioxide (anti-brown agent): French fries, fresh fruits, molasses, marmalade.

Dyes: Citrus, cherries, sweet or Irish potatoes, butter, oleomargarine, meats such as wieners, bologna, hamburger, cake decorations, soft drinks.

Gas- such as Ethylene: Apples, pears, bananas with brown streaks
Flame exposure: Roasted coffee.
Bone char filtration: Beet and cane sugar, syrups.

Wax (Paraffin): Apples, cucumbers, eggplant, peppers, parsnip, turnips, rutabagas, citrus fruits.

Chemicals: Saccharine, artificial sweeteners, phenol in food cans, plastic, Styrofoam for packaging.

Source: Used by permission: Bonnye L. Matthews, Chemical Sensitivity. 1992, McFarland and Co., Jefferson, NC.

3. Another factor to consider is the possibility of a sensitivity to several foods. If you stop eating only one of several offending foods, you might not notice much improvement after five

to seven days. However, you can readily see if you or your child is much worse after any significant problem food is re-introduced into the diet in the manner just discussed. Imagine you have 10 nails in your shoe. You need to take out all 10 to feel really well. Now suppose you remove one nail, but there are nine nails left in your shoe. You will still limp. When you add a tenth nail again, you would be worse. This is what happens sometimes when you check for a single food allergy when a number of other foods are also bothering you.

For the reasons listed above, if you have multiple food allergies, you must remove as many of the major problem foods as possible, all at one time. Then you will see improvement, but only until you ingest a problem food or beverage again. Then you will quickly become ill again. This is why the following Multiple Food Allergy Elimination Diet has proven to be helpful. In over 40 years of medical practice in the field of allergy, I must admit I rarely saw a single food as the sole cause of a medical problem. You might suspect a few possible major problem foods, which I refer to as spikes, but the less apparent food problems are more like nails and thumbtacks. These will elude you unless you do the Multiple Food Allergy Elimination Diet below, which eliminates most major allergenic foods all at one time.

Multiple Food Allergy Elimination Diet

This diet enables you to easily detect multiple food problems. It is in two parts. During Part I you eliminate several major allergenic foods for about one week. During Part II you add each of these foods back into your diet providing it is normally or routinely eaten. It is that simple. (*See Table A2.*) If you have a food allergy and the major problem foods have been eliminated, you should feel better sometime between the fourth and seventh day. After about a week, you start Part II of the diet to detect which of the foods you stopped eating during Part I, are causing you to feel unwell. When you add them back, you will probably develop symptoms in 15 minutes to an hour and this effect will typically last only a few hours. Sometimes, however, the symptoms do not appear for six to 12 hours and eating a problem food just one time can cause illness that lasts for over a week. Read on to learn how to cope with such types of problems.

Exactly How to Do the Multiple Food Allergy Elimination Diet

Part I.

During Part I of The Multiple Food Allergy Elimination Diet, certain common allergenic foods are totally eliminated from your family's diet. This part can relieve one or many symptoms within four to seven days. During Part I of the diet, there are many foods that you can eat, as listed in Table A3. This diet includes most fruits, vegetables and meats, as well as some grains. Any item that is craved or eaten in excess can be an unsuspected cause of various medical or emotional problems. These also must be avoided during Part I. Also, be certain to avoid all the hidden sources of common problem foods. Read every label of everything you eat or drink. Specific details about unsuspected sources of corn, soy, wheat and dairy are available.*

A 90% improvement from Part I of the diet means the major cause of some physical illness or unacceptable behavior or memory problems is probably due to one or more foods. A 20% improvement means foods are probably a less important part of an illness. (*Try an air purifier. Your problem can be due to other common allergenic substances such as dust, pollen, molds, pets and/or chemicals. Call 800.787.8780.*) Rarely are food sensitivities the entire answer in severely allergic individuals. The diagnosis of food allergies, however, is certainly repeatedly missed or not even considered in spite of its prevalence. Of course, food sensitivities can be due to other possibilities that are totally unrelated to allergy. The surprise is that food allergies are so infrequently considered even though they are often obviously a cause of so many acute and chronic medical problems.

---

* *Is This Your Child?,* Doris J. Rapp, M.D., 800.787.8780; www.drrapp.com.

Remember, the answer to a food problem is not a label such as "heartburn," "irritable bowel," "diverticulitis," or "ulcerative colitis," or an array of drugs to control the associated symptoms.[4] The answer is to find the cause of illness and the challenge is to eliminate that cause so there is nothing left to treat. If that is not possible, there are effective ways to treat most non-life threatening food sensitivities as detailed in Chapter 3.[4]

Although the symptoms caused by a single food can vary in a specific individual, certain food sensitivities commonly occur in several family members. They can, however, affect each person in very different ways. Therefore, it is best if entire families try the Multiple Food Allergy Elimination Diet at the same time. A fringe benefit is that some emotional or "learn-to-live-with-it" type health problems in several family members might be relieved quickly with Part I of the diet. It is also easier to follow the diet correctly if the entire family does it. It is not unusual to see dramatic, unanticipated improvement in the health and behavior of several family members within four to seven days. Be prepared to find answers you never dreamed possible. During Part II of the diet you can find that the same food that causes violent behavior in one child, might cause another child to develop headaches or be fatigued; another to wet the bed; a mother to develop a stuffy nose, or a father to develop an allergic cough. Watch closely to see what happens each day to each person. Some reactions occur immediately; others in several hours. Remember, if a food is known to cause serious symptoms, it should not be eaten. Check only these food items you routinely eat.

If an individual feels better in a week, begin Part II of the diet on the eighth day. Improvement, noted on Day 2 often increases greatly by Day 7, so continue this part of the diet for seven days. The aim is to see the maximum amount of improvement that can be noted during the first seven days of the diet.

Table A2
Multiple Food Allergy Elimination Diet
Part I
What You Can and Cannot Eat During the First Week

ALLOWED	FORBIDDEN
CEREALS: rice (Rice Puffs® only); oats (oatmeal made with honey); barley (If someone has a gluten sensitivity, reactions will occur with any grain.).	***CEREALS***: *foods containing wheat flour (most cakes, cookies, bread, baked goods); corn, popcorn; cereal mixtures (granola).*
FRUITS: Any fresh fruit, except citrus; canned (if in their own juice and without artificial color, sugar, or preservatives).	***FRUITS***: *citrus (orange, lemon, lime, grapefruit) (Any fruit or juice could cause symptoms but citrus or possibly apple, are the most common.)*
VEGETABLES: Any fresh vegetables, except corn and peas; French fries (homemade); potatoes; soy.	***VEGETABLES***: *any frozen or canned vegetables, corn, peas, or mixed vegetables.*
MEATS: chicken or turkey (non-basted); Louis Rich® ground turkey; veal or beef; pork; lamb; fish, tuna.	***MEATS***: *luncheon meats, wieners, bacon; artificially dyed hamburger/meat; ham; dyed salmon, lobster; breaded or stuffed meats. Remember, the fat in meat stores chemicals.*
BEVERAGES: water; single herb or plain organic tea & honey; grape juice, bottled (Welch's®); frozen apple juice (Lincoln® or pure apple); pure pineapple juice (no corn or dextrose).	***BEVERAGES***: *milk or dairy drink with casein or whey; fruit beverages except those so specified; Kool-Aid®, Coffee Rich®J (yellow dye); 7-Up®, Squirt®, Teem®, cola, Dr. Pepper®, ginger ale.*
SNACKS: potato chips (no additives); RyKrisp® crackers and pure honey; raisins (unsulfured)	***SNACKS***: *corn chips (Fritos®); chocolate/cocoa; hard candy, ice cream, or sherbet.*
MISCELLANEOUS: pure honey; homemade vinegar/ oil dressing; sea salt; pepper; pure maple syrup; homemade soup.	***MISCELLANEOUS***: *sugar; bread, cake, cookies (except special recipes); eggs; dyed (colored) vitamins, pills, mouthwash, toothpaste, medicines, cough syrups, etc.; jelly or jam; Jell-O®; margarine or diet spreads (dyes and corn); peanut butter/peanuts; Sorbitol (corn); cheese*

(Read all labels of everything. Particularly any food items you frequently eat.)

Table A3
Multiple Food Allergy Elimination Diet,

Part II
How to Add Foods Back Into Your Diet

Add Milk	on Day 8	Add Food Coloring	on Day 13
Add Wheat	on Day 9	Add Corn	on Day 14
Add Sugar	on Day 10	Add Preservatives	on Day 15
Add Egg	on Day 11	Add Citrus	on Day 16
Add Cocoa	on Day 12	Add Peanut Butter	on Day 17

How to Make Part I of the Diet Easier

During the first week, as you can see in Table A2, most meats, fruits and vegetables are allowed. The allowed foods can be selected, combined and eaten in any quantity. There is plenty to eat! You will not go hungry. The foods that are not allowed are also clearly indicated. You won't have to ask if the diet is helping. You will know from the improvement. It will be clearly evident.

Most individuals with food sensitivities will respond favorably to this diet by about the fourth to seventh day. Some are better as early as the second day, or as late as the fourteenth day. Keep a food diary of exactly what is eaten during the first week. Once again, keep detailed records of the "Big Five" *(Chapter 2)* at the beginning and end of each day during the first week. If there are major changes in how someone feels or acts, be a bit suspicious of what was eaten in excess on that particular day.

It can take a bit of creativity to find some beverage children will drink. Too many drink only fruit drinks or sweet soda pop and avoid drinking water. For a beverage, you can use soy or rice "milk." (*Only organic and not genetically engineered, if possible, from a health food store.*) *(See Chapter 9.)* You can also mix the allowed organic fruits in the blender with spring water and use Stevia liquid (health food store), honey or pure maple syrup if you need a sweetener. You also can put bananas or nuts into a blender to make banana or nut milks if these are no problem. You can also combine a fruit juice with carbonated water to create pop. If you want color, use carrots for orange, beets for red, grape juice for purple and chlorophyll liquid (health food store) for green.

If a child refuses to cooperate with the diet, try offering a reward. Promise a party if there is no cheating and if it is obvious that the child is truly trying to cooperate in every way. The party should take place after both parts of the diet are completed. At that time, allow the foods which caused symptoms providing these were not severe and incapacitating. This will be a double check confirming the effect of these foods. If you prefer not to repeat some reaction, don't feed that specific food or try an alkali before the party. *(See Table A4.)*

Tips—If "Not Helped" or "Worse" on Part I of the Diet

1. If common foods are a problem for someone, this diet should help within a week. If someone is not better, recheck the records for the initial week of the diet. Were only the allowed foods eaten? Did anyone repeatedly forget and accidentally or purposely eat the wrong foods or drink the wrong beverages at school or at home? The item that was not really deleted or omitted from the diet may be the culprit. Try Part I again, but this time adhere more strictly to the diet. It is best to do the diet only one time, but do it right. School and work lunches must be packed and must contain only the allowed foods. Amazingly this fast, inexpensive method of food allergy detection can sometimes provide safe, most gratifying relief for innumerable

medical complaints, as well as an explanation for many activity or behavioral outbursts in both children and adults.

2. It is not uncommon for some individuals to become worse during the first two to three days of Part I of this diet. Withdrawal symptoms, however, usually subside by the fourth day. Most reactions will occur within an hour after a problem food is ingested, but occasionally the responses might not be evident for several hours. Typical complaints include a stomach ache or nausea, fatigue, headache, a stuffy nose or congestion, asthma, muscle aches, joint pains, irritability or some inappropriate form of activity or behavior.

3. If an individual is not worse until the fifth or sixth day, suspect whatever was substituted for milk or whatever was eaten in excess while on the diet, i.e. potato chips. Another common suspect is the beverage, such as the apple or grape juice used to replace milk. If any food is eaten in excess during the first week, it could be a reason for new or a worsening of certain symptoms by about the fifth day. If this happens, retry Part I of the diet, but this time also stop any new suspect food items that you believe might have caused symptoms.

4. On rare occasions, someone who was not helped during the first week will dramatically improve with a more prolonged diet. If you find the first week of the diet did not help at all, continue Part I of the diet for 14 days. If this prolonged version of Part I does not help, this particular diet is certainly not the answer. It is possible that the medical complaints or unacceptable behaviors are totally unrelated to foods or not related to the food items omitted on this particular diet. For instance, if aggression was due to some other frequently eaten or craved items, i.e. apple juice, grape juice, mushrooms, cinnamon, coffee, tea, mint, sunflower seeds, tobacco, alcohol, etc., there would be no improvement unless these specific items were removed from the diet. Each of these food items can be a major culprit in some children or adults.

Table A4
Alkali Preparations To Relieve Food Allergies

	Sodium Bicarbonate	Potassium Bicarbonate	Ratio	Citric Acid
Alka-Aid Tablet*	360 mg	180 mg	2:1	0
Alka-Seltzer® Antacid Formula Tablet	958 mg	312 mg	3:1	832 mg
Baking soda 1 teaspoon	952 mg	0	—	0

* Health Food Stores

Table A5
Specific Details of Part II of Diet.

See Tips before you start.

Day 8: **The day you add milk,** give the child lots of milk, cottage cheese and whipped cream sweetened with pure maple syrup or honey. Eat **no** butter, margarine or cheese.

Day 9: **The day you add wheat,** add Triscuits® or pure wheat cereal. If these are all right, but bread is not, it is possible that yeast is the problem. If you or your child had trouble from milk, be sure **not** to use any milk products. Use Italian bread or kosher bread, which should not contain milk (casein or whey), **but always read labels to be sure.** Bake if you like, but do not use eggs or sugar. Remember, no dairy product or milk is allowed if these foods seemed to cause medical problems. If you find that the milk day causes no problem, milk products, such as cheese, can be eaten but check each one separately.

Day 10: **The day you add sugar,** give sugar cubes and add granulated sugar to allowed foods. If milk or wheat caused trouble, they must be avoided or you can't tell whether sugar is tolerated. Many children react within one hour after eating four to eight sugar cubes when eaten by themselves on an empty stomach. Pure water in glass bottles is allowed.

Day 11: **The day you add egg,** give cooked eggs in their usual forms. Give custard but remember, no wheat, milk or sugar can be consumed if these caused problems. **Skip this food challenge if you already know that egg is a problem.**

Day 12: **The day you add cocoa,** give dark chocolate with water, cocoa (pure Hershey's® cocoa powder), with Stevia liquid, honey or pure maple syrup. No candy bars are allowed because most contain milk, sugar and corn. Remember, no milk, wheat, sugar, dyes or eggs are allowed if any of these caused symptoms.

Day 13: **The day you add food coloring,** give colored gelatin such as Jell-O®, jelly or artificially colored fruit beverages (soda pop, Kool-Aid®), popsicles or cereal. If you prefer, you can add food coloring to plain pure gelatin. Try to give lots of artificial yellow, purple and red items because only one of these colors might cause a reaction. Do the "Big Five" after each color to find out which food color is a culprit. Remember to avoid milk, wheat, cola, or sugar in all forms if any of these were a problem. If sugar caused symptoms, use Stevia liquid (health food store), honey or pure maple syrup as a sweetener. If milk, wheat or sugar were tolerated, they may be eaten.

Day 14: **The day you add corn,** give corn, corn meal and plain popcorn. It is not unusual for only one form of corn to cause symptoms. (*Do not feed corn flakes which contain sugar, malt and the preservative BHT.*) If milk, wheat, sugar, dyes, eggs or chocolate cause trouble, do not give any of these on the same day you give corn. If you do, and symptoms appear, you won't know which is at fault. Do not use butter on popcorn if there is a milk sensitivity.

Day 15: **The day you add preservatives,** give foods which contain many preservatives or food additives. Read every label. In particular, eat luncheon meat, bologna, hot dogs, bread, baked goods or soups which commonly contain many preservatives and additives.

Day 16: **The day you add citrus,** give fresh fruit or juice forms of lemon, lime, grapefruit or orange. Avoid artificial dyes if food colors were a problem. Fruit "drinks" contain much less juice.

Day 17: **The day you add peanut butter,** give a child lots of peanut butter or peanuts. Test for this only if it is a favorite food. Use RyKrisp® if no wheat is allowed. Use pure peanut butter without additives from a health food store or Smuckers®. **Don't test peanut or soy products if either caused serious health effects in the past.**

Tips for Part II of the Diet.

1. The aim is to eat the "typical" amount of each food on a specified day to see what effect it has upon how you feel and conduct yourself. If you are a bit suspicious, start with a tiny amount and increase it gradually during the day providing no symptoms become evident. Start with about a quarter of a cup or try a smaller amount, such as half a teaspoon, if there is any reason to be cautious. (*Once again, do not try any food that you know is a problem without your physician's advice.*) Double the amount taken every two to four hours providing no increase seems to cause any symptoms. The aim is to eventually increase the amount to a normal-sized portion. If you do the "Big Five" in Chapter 3 of this book, just before or after you eat each suspect food or different amounts of each item, you will quickly know which one causes a certain medical or emotional problem.

2. The "Big Five" can prove to be invaluable to help you find answers. Do it before and after each suspect food is added back into the diet during Part II of the diet. If there are no symptoms during that day, during the night or the next morning before breakfast, the food tested the day before is probably all right and can be eaten whenever desired. If a test food causes symptoms, stop eating it in all forms until you can secure the advice of your physician. Do not try another test food until the symptoms from the previous test food subsides. You will be surprised how often you can quickly determine the exact cause of perplexing, elusive, chronic medical symptoms. If a child or adult has a reading or arithmetic problem, you might want to check how well those particular tasks were performed before and after each food is reintroduced into the diet. You typically will see the effect of each specific food, often within15 minutes to an hour. However, some food-related symptoms such as eczema or itchy skin, canker sores, bed-wetting, tight joints, ear infections and common bowel problems (colitis) tend to cause delayed reactions. Because these appear several hours

after ingestion. Final decisions about any food cannot be made until the next day.

Watch very carefully if anyone has asthma, becomes violent or threatens suicide. Remember, if you challenge with the specific food that is the cause of these types of problem, it is possible to trigger an *exaggerated* exceptionally bad episode. Be prepared and be cautious!

3. If a family member has asthma, in particular, add the test food back into the diet with extreme care. Keep asthma medications on hand particularly during Part II of the diet and use the Peak Flow Meter[3] (*see Chapter 3*) to help find out exactly what is causing you or your child to wheeze. It is possible for an unsuspected food to precipitate a sudden, severe asthma attack even though you never realized it could be a problem. If you have some reason for concern or if asthma has been severe or frightening in the past, check with your doctor before the diet is tried. If an unanticipated response is frightening or severe, take an alkali such as baking soda as you rush to the nearest emergency room.

4. If a food causes some typical or unusual form of allergy, there is something that might help right away. Alkali preparations were designed to relieve acid indigestion such as heartburn but they also can stop many food reactions in a few minutes. (*See Table A4 for different forms of alkali such as baking soda, Alka-Aid or Alka-Seltzer Antacid Formula.*) These can be surprisingly helpful to prevent, treat and prove allergic responses to foods. (*See Chapter 3 for more information about what you can do to prevent or stop such reactions.*)

The preparations listed in Table A4 do not help all hyperactivity or other food reactions but they certainly appear to help reduce or eliminate roughly two thirds of such responses in less than twenty minutes. In general, the dose for a child is one half tablet or a half teaspoon for a three year old, one tablet or one teaspoon for a six year old and two tablets or two teaspoons for a twelve year old or adult. (*Check with your physician before using these preparations, especially if you have kidney or heart problems.)*

5. Other helpful products for food allergies include homeopathic remedies. See Table 3A or try Opsin I. It can be purchased directly from Mountain Standard Laboratory at 800.647.0074. This is usually available at less that $10 a bottle which can last for weeks.

6. Once you determine which foods cause specific symptoms, you must discuss the diet results with your physician. Some foods cannot be omitted for indefinite periods of time if proper nutrition is to be maintained. This is especially true for children. Ask your doctor for the help of a dietitian or nutritionist if you have specific diet questions.[1]

The Multiple Elimination Diet should be used only on a short term basis. It is not nutritionally balanced and should never be used for more than 2-3 weeks without consulting a physician or a certified nutritionist. The Rotation Diet can be nutritionally sound and continued indefinitely, but your individual version should also be evaluated by a nutritionist and monitored regularly by your doctor.

General Allergy Diet Tips

1. Unfortunately, too many children and adults in our world are presently acting angry, aggressive and uncontrollable. For this

reason it is best if the cause can be found and eliminated as soon as possible. The good news is this: If behavioral problems are due to food sensitivities or environmental illness, immediate help is available and possible, often without the need for any drugs by simply using allergy diets and possibly an air purifier. *(See Chapter 3.)*

2. Remember, if children or adults list their five most craved "can't live without" foods and beverages, they have just listed the ones that are most apt to be the cause of their emotional, medical or learning problems, but only if these complaints are food-related.

3. You must expect symptoms to get worse during the first two to three days of the diet when problem foods are stopped in all forms. Do not get discouraged but stick with it. The sun will shine again and things can quickly become dramatically better once you find and eliminate each unrecognized cause of various medical complaints or certain intermittent intolerable behavior patterns in some of your close family members.

4. Children and adults can have characteristic patterns of response to specific foods. When children react to a food during part II of the diet, they can become very negative. They only have to hear the word "no" and they are set off. Ask them to do something that they do not want to do and it is almost as if you lit the wick on a firecracker. They will suddenly become uncontrollable. It means they have been exposed to something that bothers them to such a degree that any mild stress, such as being denied something or being told they must comply, triggers a sudden outburst. This can be so severe, that you and others can barely believe such an emotional response is happening. Stay calm. Notice any change in appearance. Give the child an alkali and read Chapter 3 so you know what else you can do to prevent or stop such reactions. A cathartic or coffee enema can shorten the length of a food reaction, sometimes in minutes.[4]

Some children and adults do not become hyperactive or nasty, they become withdrawn and untouchable. They cover their face and hide in dark tight corners or under the furniture.
Another common reaction when foods are added back into the diet in children is the tendency to repeatedly say the same phrase or ask for something over and over again. This can persist even after the request is fulfilled. Just recognize that this is one common type of response that is possible in some children.

5. Most children will try with all their might to prevent reactions, except possibly when they are at home with their mother. Many mothers are extremely wonderful beings with amazingly forgiving natures. Allergic misbehaving children know they are so loved that they can do almost anything and their mothers will understand, tolerate and forgive. More mothers than you can imagine have bite marks all over their arms from their "out of control" allergic child. They rarely complain and this is truly unconditional love. This is unfortunately not as true for as many fathers because their role is often that of the disciplinarian. Even the very young children know when, where and with whom they dare "let it all out". Remember, you cannot demand an asthmatic stop wheezing. They cannot do it. Once angry, aggressive children or adults are set off from a food or some environmental exposure (dust, pollen, molds, chemicals), it will take a few minutes to stop the reaction, even if you know what to do and how to do it. (*See Chapter 3.)*

6. In the midst of a most upsetting episode, children and adults often appear unable to hear or comprehend a word that is said. Yelling at them has no effect. Save your energy and spend your efforts to figure out why it is happening. When they have a "spaced-out look", they are literally "out of it". Regardless of their age, if they have a demonic frightening look to their eyes, and some of them do, protect yourself. Their eyes will tell you when they will again respond to what you are saying. Some truly cannot recall what they did or said when they lost control during some severe food or allergenic reactions.

7. If someone routinely becomes uncontrollable after parties and holidays, you can bet that some commonly eaten favorite food or beverage is at fault. Consider sugar, food dyes, chocolate, milk, nuts, corn or some ingredient, such as a grain in alcohol.

8. As soon as a reaction to a food is over, try to recall and write down any clues that might help to predict the onset of a future loss of control or change in well-being. Did that person look or feel different in any way, in any area of the body, just before the signs of illness or extreme undesirable behavior began? If you can raise each individual's awareness, he or she will typically make every effort to prevent future explosions. Most children and adults do not want others to see how they sometimes behave and they try not to react in an unacceptable manner, particularly in front of strangers or friends. Discerning, knowledgeable mothers can tell exactly what their children ate or smelled from the way they feel, act or behave. (*See Chapter 2.*)

9. You can use your allergies to foods to your advantage at times. If a food makes you tired and sleepy, eat it at bedtime. If it makes you a bit hyperactive, use it before athletic activity. If one interferes with your ability to remember or express yourself, be sure *not* to ingest it prior to an examination or time when you must think clearly.

10. If you are uncertain whether or not a food causes symptoms, discontinue that item until the diet is completed. Then try that suspect food again at a five day intervals, i.e., Tuesday and Saturday. See if symptoms recur each time.

11. If an infection occurs during the diet, stop the diet. It is too difficult to interpret the results if it is continued. If someone always has an infection, the help of an environmental medical specialist may be needed. (*AAEM: 316-684-5500.*) With this type of medical care one infection after another often can be eliminated without the need for antibiotics.[1]

12. There are a number of excellent books that discuss the surprising major role of food sensitivities in relation to health and behavior.[3a,b, 10, 11] If you want to see examples of how some children and adults actually react to foods or chemicals, obtain the videos and books that discuss environmental illness in more depth. (*See Resources, Appendix E.*) This would help skeptical spouses, relatives, teachers, employers or doctors. Many of these illustrate the degree to which some children and adults can lose control after a drop or whiff of a number of common allergenic substances.

13. If your body is slightly alkaline, it is thought that you will have fewer allergic reactions. You can take an inexpensive alkali, such as Alka Aid (health food store) to control food-related symptoms of all types including inappropriate behavior, but again, check with your physician first. Certain foods cause the body to become more acid (grains, dairy, eggs, meat and sugar) or alkaline (fruits or vegetables). Some individuals have fewer allergies if they can keep their body slightly alkaline by eating fewer acid foods. (*See Table A6 for a list of foods that are acid versus alkaline.*) These can be ingested to help adjust the body pH so it is slightly alkaline.

Elson Haas, M.D., suggests that the diet contain 70% to 80% alkaline and neutral pH balanced foods in the spring and summer months. (*Staying Health with Nutrition, pg. 523, Berkeley, CA, Celestial Arts, 1995.*)[2] In the autumn and winter, he suggests at least 65% to 70% alkaline foods and pH balanced foods. In very cold climates, a higher percentage of richer acid-forming foods may be tolerated because they are higher in fat and provide more body fuel. Also, fewer vegetables and fruits are available at those times. By and large, whenever possible, most individuals need a more generous supply of vegetables and possibly whole grains to keep their bodies in balance.

Some drugstores sell relatively expensive pH tape strips which can be used to check the acidity or alkalinity of your saliva and urine. Inexpensive rolls of pH tape can be ordered through Health Treasures, 265 SW Port Saint Lucie Blvd., #146, Port Saint Lucie, FL 34984.[5a] Check your morning saliva and urine before you eat or drink and see if they are more alkaline than acid.[5b, 6] For more information contact an environmental medical physician or an informed health professional.[6] (*AAEM: 316.684.5500)*

14. Specific answers in relation to food allergies are possible without a diet (*see Chapter 3*), but some of the alternatives can be expensive. A number of blood tests can reveal certain types of food allergies, but these, at times, can be confusing, misleading, and inaccurate. Sometimes the blood studies miss important sensitivities and at other times, they indicate allergies that do not presently exist.[3a]

Other Ways to Possibly Find the Cause of a Food Reaction

It is most important to be able to tell if a food, chemical or additive on or in a food is causing symptoms. *(See Table A1.)* Sometimes this is easy to do using logic. If an organic and regular food, such as an apple, usually causes symptoms, it is probably a problem caused by an allergy to apple. For example, if you only have difficulty from the regular grocery store apple and not from an organic apple, it is probably due to some chemical in or on the food. Remember, 25% to 30% of the grocery store foods appear to be organic, while about 25% to 30% of the foods in organic stores are not really organic, so you can be fooled.

There are also some other unproven ways that might help. One is simple muscle testing while another is the use of a dowsing pendulum. For details of how to do these tests see Chapter 3 and Appendix D.5a,b. Both appear to possibly provide some insight in relation to foods. Remember our aim is to find fast, easy, inexpensive, safer and better ways to find answers so more people can be helped. We need more studies to evaluate these methods because most in the medical profession certainly do not consider these methods to be reliable, scientific or proven

Table A6
ACID-ALKALINE FOODS

Alkaline Foods (high pH)	Balanced Foods (low pH)	Acid Foods (neutral pH)
all vegetables	brown rice	wheat
most fruits	corn	oats
millet	soybeans	white rice
buckwheat	lima beans	pomegranates
sprouted beans	almonds	strawberries
sprouted seeds	sunflower seeds	cranberries
olive oil	Brazil nuts	breads
soaked almonds	honey	refined flour
	most dried beans	refined sugar
	and peas	cashews, pecans and peanuts
	tofu	butter*
	nonfat milk	milk*
	vegetable oils	cheeses*
		eggs
		meats
		fish
		poultry

*Some authors place milk products in the balanced area.

This Table is an abbreviated form of information from page 523 of Staying Healthy with Nutrition, gratefully used by permission by Elson M. Haas, M.D., Berkeley, CA, Celestial Arts, 1995.

at this time. In spite of this, however, many alternative health care professionals routinely use these methods to treat their patients and they find them to be helpful.[7, 8a,b] The bottom line is simply this: Are these methods better than a guess? Read a book on muscle testing or pendulums and then try it for yourself.[3] You may be pleasantly surprised.

Summary

If foods change how you or your child feel, act, behave or learn, the diets in this Appendix should help immensely. Leap for joy, for the first time you may be able to pinpoint exactly which food causes certain specific medical complaints. Thousands of parents have found the answers for their family by merely trying these diets. Typically, several family members are helped. These diets can be fast, easy and inexpensive. On a long-term basis, certain diets or food allergy injection treatments certainly can help better than a drug designed to merely mask a medical complaint. The aim must be to find and eliminate the cause of medical, activity, behavior and emotional problems. It avoidance is not possible or practical, other possible choices for treatment include homeopathic remedies, a long term supervised Rotation Diet, Provocation/ Neutralization allergy extract treatment for food sensitivities and the unproven alternative methods discussed in Chapter 3 and Appendix D.5a,b,c.

Appendix A References:

1 Sally J. Rockwell, CCN, Ph.D., A Rotation Diet, Rotation Diet Game, 206.547.1814, www.drsallyrockwell.com.
2 Elson Haas, M.D., Staying Healthy With the Seasons. Berkeley, CA, Celestial Arts, 2003. www.tenspeed.com
3 Environmental Medical Research Foundation ERF (Formerly: PARF or Practical Allergy Research Foundation), P. O. Box 60, Buffalo, NY 14223-0060, tel. 800.787.8780, www.drrapp.com.
 3a Is This Your Child's World? 1996. Cost: $15.00.
 3b Is This Your Child? 1991. Cost: $12.00.
4 Sherry Rogers, M.D., No More Heartburn. 2000, Prestige Press, P.O. Box 3068, 3500 Brewerton Rd., Syracuse, NY 13220, tel. 800.846.6687 or 315.468.4417, Fax: 315.468.8119. www.prestigepublishing.com. Cost: $15.00.
5a Health Treasures, 265 SW Port Saint Lucie Blvd., #146, Port Saint Lucie, FL 34984. www.healthtreasures.com/ph-paper.html.
 5b Make your own pH paper: www.miamisci.org/ph/phydrion.html.
6 Mark Force, DC, Choosing Health: Learn how to harness natural forces to restore, protect and enhance your health, tel. 480.563.4256, www.Threelementsofhealth.com.
7 Richard Gerber, A Practical Guide to Vibrational Medicine: Energy Healing and Spiritual Transformation. 2001, Quill Publishing. Cost: $15.00 (Amazon.com).
8a W. A. Tiller, Conscious Acts Of Creation, 2001, Pavior Publishing. Cost: $29.95.
 8b W. A. Tiller, Science and Human Transformation: Subtle Energies, Intentionality and Consciousness. 1997. Cost: $24.95.
9 Sherry Rogers, M.D., Wellness Against All Odds. 1994, Prestige Press, P.O. Box 3068, 3500 Brewerton Rd., Syracuse, NY 13220, 800.846.6687 or 315.468.4417, Fax: 315.468.8119. Cost: $17.95.
10 Jacqueline Krohn, M.D., Natural Detoxification- A Practical Encyclopedia: The Complete Guide to Clearing Your Body of Toxins. 2000, Hartley & Marks, Inc., Box 147, Point Roberts, WA 98281. Cost: $24.95.
11 Magaziner, Allan, D.O., Total Health Handbook, Your Complete Wellness Resource. February 2000, Kensington Pub. Corp., 888.345.2665, www.kensingtonbooks.com, Cost: $17.00.
12 Robert O. Young, Ph.D. and Shelley Redford Young, The pH Miracle Balance Your Diet, Reclaim Your Health. 2002, Warner Books, Inc., 1271 Avenue of the Americas, New York, NY 10020. www.twbookmark.com. Cost: $24.95.

Appendix B
Health Professionals

B.1 PHYSICIANS WITH ENVIRONMENTAL MEDICAL (EM) TRAINING

AMERICAN ACADEMY OF ENVIRONMENTAL MEDICINE [AAEM] 316.684.5500 FAX: 316.684.5709
7701 E. Kellogg, Suite 625, Wichita, KS 67207 www.aaem.com.

AMERICAN ACADEMY OF OTOLARYNGIC ALLERGY
www.aaoaf.org.

PAN AMERICAN ALLERGY SOCIETY www.paas.org.

B.1a DETOXIFICATION CENTERS

To cleanse the body of chemicals or toxins emitted into the air and water from industry and agriculture and from foods and beverages or their containers.

ALLERGY AND ENVIRONMENTAL HEALTH CENTER
716.833.2213, Kalpana Patel, M.D., 65 Wehrle Drive, Buffalo, NY 14225. www.medicallibrary.net/doctors/patel *Board certified in pediatrics and environmental medicine, a medical educator and author.*

CENTER FOR ENVIRONMENTAL MEDICINE
803.572.160, Allan D. Lieberman, M.D., 7510 Northforest Drive, North Charleston, SC 29420, www.coem.com. *Board certified in pediatrics and environmental medicine with specialized expertise in infectious disease and vaccine problems.*

ENVIRONMENTAL HEALTH CENTER 214.368.4132 FAX: 214.691.8432, William Rea, M.D., 8345 Walnut Lane, Suite 220, Dallas, TX 75231-4262, www.ehcd.com. *He is the "super" specialist in environmental, internal and vascular medicine and electromagnetic illness. He has vast experience with the sickest and most extremely chemically ill patients in the world.*

DETOX MEDICAL CLINIC 916.387.8252
FAX: 916.387.6977, David Root, M.D., 5501 Power Inn Road, Suite 130, Sacramento, CA 95820, www.healthmeddetox.com (For Non-Drug Abuse Chemical Exposures) www.getoffdrugsnow.com (For Drug Abuse Cases).

DOWNTOWN MEDICAL CENTER 212.587.3961
FAX: 212.587.3960, Apryl McNeil, M.D., Medical Director 139 Fulton Street, Suite 515, New York, NY 10038, www.healthmeddetox.com (Non-Drug abuse Chemical Exposure) www.getoffdrugsnow.com (For Drug Abuse Cases).

RANDOLPH-SHAMBAUGH CLINIC
847.519.7772 FAX: 847.519.7787, Marsha L. Vetter, M.D., Ph.D., Director, 2500 W. Higgins Road, Suite 1170, Hoffman Estates, Chicago, IL 60195, www.randolphclinic.com.

B1.b DIAGNOSTIC CHEMICAL TESTING IN GLASS BOOTHS

ALLERGY AND ENVIRONMENTAL HEALTH CENTER

716.833.2213 Kalpana Patel, M.D., 65 Wehrle Drive, Buffalo, NY 14225
www.medicallibrary.net/doctors/patel

ENVIRONMENTAL HEALTH CENTER

214.368.4132 FAX: 214.691.8432
William Rea, M.D. and Christopher Rea, 8345 Walnut Lane, Suite 220, Dallas, TX 75231-4262, www.ehcd.com.

B.1c AAEM PHYSICIAN WEBSITES

Majid Ali, M.D.	www.fatigue.net
Richard N. Ash, M.D.	www.ashmd.com
James R. Biddle, M.D.	www.integrative-med.com
Mary Ann Block, D.O.	www.blockcenter.com
Kenneth A. Bock, M.D.	www.rhinebeckhealth.com
Andrew M. Brown, M.D.	www.entgadsden.com
Theodore J. Cole, D.O., N.M.D.	www.drhealth.net
Michael Compain, M.D.	www.rhinebeckhealth.com
Richard B. Dawson, M.D., F.A.C.S.	www.dawsonmedicalgroup.com
William L. Epperly, M.D.	www.drepperly.com
Kendall A. Gerdes, M.D.	www.environmed.net
Robert W. Hall, M.S.	www.necnev.org
Elson Haas, M.D.	www.elsonhaas.com
James A. Hamp, M.D.	www.drhamp.com
Ronald L. Hoffman, M.D.	www.drhoffman.com
Steven F. Hotze, M.D.	www.hotzehealth-wellness.com
John G. Ionescu, Ph.D.	www.spezialklinik-neukirchen.de
Marjorie Hurt Jones, R.N.	www.nidlink.com/~mastent
Jeffrey C. Kopelson, M.D.	www.countrymedical.net
William G. Kracht, D.O.	www.woodmed.com
George F. Kroker, M.D.	www.allergy-solutions.com
Curt G. Kurtz, M.D.	www.myhealth.com/Curtis_Kurtz
Richard E. Layton, M.D.	www.allergyconnection.com
Warren M. Levin, M.D.	www.medicallibrary.net/doctors/dr_levin
Allan D. Lieberman, M.D.	www.coem.com
Allan Magaziner, D.O.	www.drmagaziner.com
Haitham Masri, M.D., F.A.C.S.	www.enthmasri.com
Mark J. McClure, D.D.S., FAGD, ND	www.thedentalgroup.com
George C. Miller II, M.D.	www.lbggynobpc.com
David L. Morris, M.D.	www.allergy-solutions.com
Gerald D. Natzke, D.O.	www.Allergy-Environmental.com
Ronald R. Parks, M.P.H., M.D.	www.macrohealthmedicine.com
Kalpana Patel, M.D.	www.medicallibrary.net/doctors/patel
Doris J. Rapp, M.D.	www.drrapp.com
William J. Rea, M.D.	www.ehcd.com

Dennis W. Remington, M.D.	www.freedommedcenter.com
Albert F. Robbins, D.O., M.S.P.H.	www.allergycenter.com
Sally J. Rockwell, C.N., Ph.D.	www.drsallyrockwell.com
Sherry A. Rogers, M.D.	www.prestigepublishing.com
F. Fuller Royal, M.D.	www.nevadaclinic.com
Vijay K. Sabnis, M.D.	www.allergy-solutions.com
Michael B. Schachter, M.D.	www.schachtercenter.com
Stephen Smith, M.D.	www.owt.com/pmc/
Tipu Sultan, M.D.	www.ehacstl.com
Wellington S. Tichenor, M.D.	www.sinuses.com
William H. VanHoogenhuize, M.D.	www.drvanhoogenhuize.medem.com
Marsha L. Vetter, Ph.D., M.D.	www.randolphclinic.com
Aristo Vojdani, Ph.D., M.T.	www.immuno-sci-lab.com
Walter A. Ward, Jr., M.D.	www.ccmed.net
Laurence S. Webster, M.D.	www.doctorwebster.com
Alan N. Weiner, D.O., C.C.N.	www.mainewholehealth.com
Ronald R. Wempen, M.D.	www.medical-library.net/doctors/dr_wempen
Randall E. Wilkinson, M.D.	www.aspenbenefits.com
John L. Wilson, Jr., M.D.	www.gsmedcen.org
Eileen M. Wright, M.D.	www.gsmedcen.org
Gerald A. Wyker, M.D.	www.wyker-md.com
Lawrence Young, M.D.	www.LawrenceYoungMd.com

B.2a <u>DENTISTS</u>

ALMAJIAN, ARA, DDS. Vancouver, British Columbia 604.876.9228

DOUGLAS L. COOK, DDS. 920.842.2083 FAX: 920.842.4203 10971 Clinic Road, Suring, WI 54174, www.dentistryhealth.com

MICHAEL MARGOLIS, DDS. 480.833.2232 FAX: 480.833.3062

NICHOLAS MEYER, DDS. 480.948.0560 7170 McDonald Drive, Scottsdale, AZ, www.milldental.com

"MY DENTIST" 1303 S. Longmore, Suite 1, Fiesta Professional Building, Mesa, AZ 85202, mydentist4@aol.com

TERRY J. LEE, DDS. 602.956.4807 4210 N. 32ND Street, Phoenix, AZ 85018, errandsG@aol.com

WALTER J. CLIFFORD, DDS. 719.550.0008 FAX: 719.550.0009 *Performs allergy testing for dentists to help them select the correct safe dental materials.*

B.2b

INTERNATIONAL ACADEMY OF ORAL MEDICINE (IAOM)

407.298.2450 Michael Ziff, DDS – Executive Director

B.3 CHIROPRACTIC MUSCLE TESTING TECHNIQUES NEWER DIAGNOSTIC AND TREATMENT METHODS

(Also see Muscle Test D.5a and Chapter 3)

VICTOR FRANK, D.C., N.M.D., D.O. 435.652.4340 FAX: 435.652.4339 Total Body Modification (TBM), 1140 E. Fortpierce Drive, Suite #27, St George, UT 84790 www.tbmseminars.com, health@tbmseminars.com. *Seminars for doctors and public.*

SCOTT WALKER, D.C. 800.888.4638 760.944.1030 FAX: 760.753.7191 524 Second Street, Encinitas, CA 92024, www.netmindbody.com Scottwalker@Earthlink.net. *Offers seminars for doctors and professionals on NET.*

DEVI NAMBUDRIPAD, D.C. 714.523.8900 FAX: 714.523.3068
Nambudripad's Allergy Elimination Treatment (NAET), www.naet.com naet@earthlink.net. *Offers seminars for doctors on NAET.*

SHEALY, C. NORMAN, M.D., Ph.D.
www.selfhealthsystems.com.

DONALD EPSTEIN, D.C. 303.678.8101 FAX: 303.678.8089 Network Care, www.donaldepstein.com/healing/12stageintro.htm www.associationfornetworkcare.com, info@associationfornetworkcare.com.

MARK FORCE, D.C. 480.563.4256 7500 E. Pinnacle Peak Road, Scottsdale, AZ 85255, 480-563-4256 FAX: 480-563-4269 www.theelementsofhealth.com.

M. TED MORTER, D.C. 800.874.1478 FAX: 501.631.8201 Bio Energetic Synchronization Technique (B.E.S.T.) www.morter.com.

STEEL ALTERNATIVE HEALTH CARE CLINIC
519.354.3656 390 Wellington Street, West, Chatham, Ontario N7M 1K4 CANADA *Uses newer techniques and nutrition to heal.*

B.4 NATUROPATHIC PHYSICIANS

AMERICAN ASSOCIATION OF NATUROPATHIC PHYSICIANS 866.538.2267 3201 New Mexico Ave., NW, Suite 350, Washington, DC 20016 www.naturopathic.org

SOUTHWEST COLLEGE OF NATUROPATHIC MEDICINE AND HEALTH SCIENCES, 2140 E. Broadway Rd., Tempe, AZ 85282 480.858.9100 Fax: 480.858.9116, www.scnm.edu, admissions@scnm.edu.

B.5a PSYCHOLOGISTS

SHARON CRAIN, Ph.D., drcrain@crain-interactive.com.

NANCY DIDRIKSEN, Ph.D. 972.889.9933 FAX: 972.889.9935 100 N. Cottonwood Dr., Suite 106, Richardson, TX 75080.

B.5b **ENERGY PSYCHOLOGISTS AND HEALERS**

ARENSON, GLORIA, M.S., M.F.T. Fireside, Rockefeller Center, 1230 Avenue of the Americas, New York, NY 10020 **CLINTON, ASHA** ASHAC @ aol.com.

SHEILA BASTEIN, Ph.D. 510.526.7391 2126 Los Angeles Avenue, Berkeley, CA 94707.

JAFFE, CAROLYN, JMT ADVANCE TECHNIQUE 610.685.1800 928 Penn Ave., Wyomissing, PA 19610. jmtseminars@aol.com. www.jmttechnique.com.

HOVER – KRAMER, DOROTHEA www.wwnorton.com W. W. Norton & Company, 500 Fifth Avenue, New York, NY 10110.

MARTIN, ART, D.D., N.D., M.A. 916.663.9178. 800.655.3846 Personal Transformation Press, 8300 Rock Springs Road, Penryn, CA 95663 www.medicalelectronicresearch.com.

NAMKA, LYNNE, Ed. D. www.AngriesOut.com Talk, Trust & Feel Therapeutics, 5398 Golder Ranch Road, Tucson, AZ 85739.

REED, STEVE B. 972.997.9955 2003www.psychotherapy-center.com.

SISE, MARY T., CSW-R, TFTdx 518.785.8576 msise3@aol.com

YORDY, JAN www.energyconnectiontherapies.com.

B.6 **HOMEOPATHY, HERBAL AND OTHER HEALTH CENTERS**

HOMEOPATHY

NATIONAL CENTER FOR HOMEOPATHY

703.548.7790 801 North Fairfax, Suite 306, Alexandria, VA 22314, www.homeopathic.org. *Books and kits on homeopathic treatment and references for nearest homeopaths.*

DESERT INSTITUTE SCHOOL OF CLASSICAL HOME-OPATHY-HOMEOPATHIC CORRESPONDENCE COURSE 602.347.7950.

ARIZONA BOARD OF HOMEOPATHIC MEDICAL EXAMINEERS 602.263.3589

It is most prudent to obtain a homeopathic license so that you can continue to practice medicine if you are interested in using alternative methods of therapy. Do it before you begin to practice integrative medicine.

HERBAL

AMERICAN HERBALISTS GUILD (AHG) 770.751.6021 FAX: 770.751.7472 1931 Gaddis Road, Canton, GA 3011. ahgoffice@earthlink.net. *AHG professional members list and for publications and herbal education program.*

AMERICAN ACADEMY OF MEDICAL ACUPUNCTURE AND ORIENTAL MEDICINE (AAMA), 4929 Wilshire Blvd., Suite 428, Los Angeles, CA 90010 323.937.5514.

AMERICAN ASSOCIATION OF ORIENTAL MEDICINE (AAOM) 888.500.7999 , 610.266.1433 433 Front Street, Catasauqua, PA 18032.

HEALERS

HEALING TOUCH INTERNATIONAL, www.healingtouch.net.

SHEALY, C. NORMAN, M.D., Ph.D. www.selfhealthsystems.com.

Appendix C
Resources for Environmental Home Evaluations

ENVIRONMENTAL HEALTH CENTER 214.368.4132 FAX: 214.691.8432, William Rea, M.D. and Christopher Rea, 8345 Walnut Lane, Suite 220, Dallas, TX 75231-4262. *Environmental evaluation and home mold remediation.*

ENVIRO-HEALTH (H/F) 602.432.1449 602.274.6624 Russell Olinsky, MS. Environmental Engineering, 3421 N. Paiute Way #4, Scottsdale, AZ 85251 stachy@earthlink.net. *Environmental evaluation and home mold remediation.*

MATRIX ANALYTICAL LABORATORIES, INC. 972.818.8155 FAX: 972.381.0348 4501 Sunbelt Drive, Suite B, Addison, TX 75001 www.matrixlabs.cc, mail@matrixlabs.cc. *Detection and identification of chemicals in items and home environmental building and medical evaluations.*

ENVIRONMENTAL CONSULTATION 305.0354.4597 **"SAFE HOMES"**, 2935 N.E. 163rd Street, #4H, N. Miami Beach, Fl 33160 www.Safe-Homes.com, artemiss@safe-homes.com. *Home check, mold remediation.*

C.2 ARCHITECTS-ENVIRONMENTALLY SAFE HOMES

DALE BATES & ASSOCIATES 208.726.3691 FAX: 208.726.3694, Living Architecture, 671 First Ave. N. Box 2012, Ketchum, ID 83340.
You select building design and they send every needed item to your builder. Their safe homes are designed to be more mold- and pest- free. The cost is 10% to 15% higher than normal. Prefab houses hopefully will be available soon.

JOHN BOWER, OWNER 812.332.5073 Healthy House Institute, 430 N. Sewell Rd., Bloomington, IN 47408 www.hhinst.com, healthy@bloomington.in.us.

C.3 ENVIRONMENTALLY SAFER PRODUCTS AND INFORMATION

GENERAL SUPPLIES- FOR HOME

AFM ENTERPRISES 619.239.0321
350 West Ash Street, Suite 700, San Diego, CA 92101-3404
Supplies non-toxic products, paints, sealers, carpet cleaners, radon testing kits, etc.

ALLEN'S NATURALLY 800.352.8971
P.O. Box 514, Farmington, MI 48332-0514 www.allensnaturally.com
Home care products for chemically sensitive people.

ALLERX (Formerly Allergy Asthma Shopper) 800.447.1100 P.O. Box 239, Fate, TX 75132 *Nontoxic products, carpet cleaners, sealers, bacteria and mold tests, computer-screen shields, radon and formaldehyde testing kits.*

CHEMICALLY SENSITIVE LIVING 508.678.7293 FAX: 419.730.6932, 377 Wilbur Ave., Suite 213, Swansea, MA 02777 www.chemicallysensitiveliving.com. *Certified organic & natural, fragrance–free.*

COSMETICS:
(See Personal Care Products).

DEHUMIDIFIERS
See suppliers in this sector.

ECOCLEAN PRODUCTS AND SERVICES 480.947.5286 The Asthma and Allergy Store, 3511 N. 70th Street, Scottsdale, AZ 85251. *Mattress/pillow dust mite protectors and many other supplies. Do local carpet and furniture safe cleaning.*

ELECTRIC HEATERS
Small Space Heaters: "Polonis", Purchase at local hardware store.

ENVIRONMENTAL RESEARCH FOUNDATION (Formerly PARF), 800.787.8780, 716.875.5578 FAX: 716-875-5399, 1421 Colvin Blvd., Buffalo, NY14223. *Books, videos and audiotapes about environmental illness, air and water purifiers, pendulums.*

ENVIROTEL 888.851.4404, P.O. Box 2413, Summerville, SC 29484 jmsjksn@msn.com. *Air cleaners, organic cotton bedding, HEPA vacuum cleaners, juicers, water etc.*

NATURE'S KEY THE DATSUN COMPANY 800.433.8929 760.480.8929 FAX: 760.746.8865, P.O. Box 668, Escondido, CA 92033 *Drain opener, spot and odor remover, organic cotton masks and ventilation filters.*

N.E.E.D.S., P. O. Box 580, East Syracuse, NY 13057, *1.800.634.1380* www.needs.com *Nutritional information and "super market" for all types of environmental shopping.*

THE NON TOXIC HOTLINE 800.968.9355 925.472.8868 925.472.8863, Daliya Robson, 3441 Golden Rain Road, Suite 3, Walnut Creek, CA 94595, www.nontoxic.com. *Organic cotton mattresses, sheets, futons, filters, air purifiers, water, paints, non-chemical wool carpets, industrial metal dehumidifiers, 99% pure rubber latex, etc.*

CLOTHING, BEDDING, MATTRESSES ETC:

ALLERGY RELIEF SHOP, INC. 800.626.2810 3371 Whittle Springs Road, Knoxville, TN 37917.

CROWN CITY MATTRESSESS: Allergy Free 626.452.8617 11134 Rush Street S., El Monte, CA 91733. *No chemicals, very good but very expensive.*

FISHER HENNEY NATURALS 800.365.6563 (Orders), P.O. Box 590336, San Francisco, CA 94159.

GREENPEACE 415.512.9025 568 Howard Street, 3rd Floor, San Francisco, CA 94105.

HARMONY 800.869.3446 360 Interlocken Blvd, Suite 300, Broomfield, CO 80021.

HEART OF VERMONT 800.639.4123, Old Schoolhouse, Route 132, P.O. Box 183, Sharon, VT 05065.

ILLINOIS STEWARDSHIP ALLIANCE 217.498.9707 John Demaree www.netins.net/showcase/megahoglaws.

JANICE'S NATURAL COMFORT COLLECTION 800.JANICES 800.526.4237 FAX: 973.691.5459 198 Route 46 – US Highway, Budd Lake, NJ 07828-3001.
www.janices.com Jswack@worldnet.att.net.
100% cotton mattresses, clothing and cleaning supplies.

K.B. COTTON PILLOWS, INC. 800.544.3752 972.223.7193 FAX: 888.829.5292, Kaye Behrens, R.N., President, P.O. Box 57, Desoto, TX 75123 www.kbcottonpillows.com.

NON-POLLUTING ENTERPRISES (NOPE) 800.323.2811 21 Winters Lane, Baltimore, MD 21228. *Cotton Shower Curtains.*

ORGANIC COTTON 818.886.7471 9760 Owensmouth Ave., Chatsworth, CA 91311.

OTIS BEDDING 800.588.6847 80 James E. Casey Drive, Buffalo, NY 14206.

PATAGONIA 800.638.6464 8550 White Fir Street, Reno, NV 89523.

ROYAL-PEDIC MATTRESS CO. 800.487.6925 341 N. Robertson Blvd., Beverly Hills, CA 90211 *Organic cotton mattresses, very good but very expensive.*

TEXAS ORGANIC PRODUCTS 806.748.8336 www.texasorganic.com.

THE NATURAL BEDROOM 800.365.6563 (orders/questions). 408.897.3018 FAX: 707.823.0106, P.O. Box 2048, Sebastopol, CA 95473

THE VERMONT COUNTRY STORE 800.362.2400. FAX 802.362.0285, P. O. Box 3000, Manchester Center, VT 05255-3000 P.O. Box 2048, Sebastopol, CA 95473-2048.
Clothing, House, Food General.

CARPETS:

NATURE'S CARPET 604.734.2758 FAX: 604.734.1512 1428 West Seventh Ave., Vancouver, BC B6H1C1, Canada, Colin Campbell & Sons. Carpet is "Best" according to Anderson Laboratory.)

CLEANING:

ECO CLEAN PRODUCTS AND SERVICES 480.947.5286 The Asthma and allergy Store, 3511 N. 70th Street, Scottsdale, AZ 85251.
Allersafe products: HEPA vacuum cleaners, carbon masks, air purifiers mattress/pillow protectors.

LIVING SOURCE 817.776.4878 7005 Woodway Drive, Suite 214, Waco, TX 76712. *They supply Nature Clean products; Purisol.*

SOAPWORKS 800.699.9917, 602-462-5320 FAX: 602.254.6916 www.soapworks.com. *Safer soap, laundry and cleaning materials.*

COMPUTERS AND COMPUTER MONITORS:

ULTRA-LOW RADIATION NON-CHEMICAL COMPUTER 800.222.3003, Monitors & Computers, www.biof.com/vibrantech. *Used by NASA and US National Institute of Health.*

ELECTRONIC PROTECTIVE DEVICES

Brian Briggs, M.D., 718 Sixth Street, SW, Minot, ND 58701 701.838.6011 *Inexpensive electromagnetic medallions.* Cost: $10.00.

Terri Newlon Holistic Consulting Co., LLC, 110 E. Cortez Dr., #203, Sedona, AZ 86351. terri@onepost.net. *Cell phone protectors.*

John Lowery, http://www.energyworks123.com/indexSwf.html.

FURNITURE:

CHARLES R. BAILEY – CABINETMAKERS 870.453.5433 FAX: 877.453.5433, Hwy. 62 East, PO Box 387, Flippin, AR 72634, www.southshore.com/~crbslf. *Formaldehyde and chemical-free.*

FURNITURE FOR THE ENVIRONMENT 617.926.0111 FAX: 617.926.3786, Division of: Brighton Upholstering, Inc. 86 Coolidge Avenue, Watertown, MA 02172 www.furniture.com.

HUMIDIFIERS: www.Sneeze.com 800.390.7867 Hepa Humidifier and Air Filter.

MOTELS/HOTELS:

PRIDE & JOY ENVIRONMENTAL RESORT 321.733.7804. Ocean Front Private Beach, 5685 South A 1 A Highway, South Melbourne Beach, FL 32951, www.pridejoyresort.com. *Owned by an MCS sufferer.*

SAFE PLACES TO LIVE + VACATIONS 561.879.4953 To Place an Ad, The Safer Travel Directory – Nancy Westrom 3828 Spatterdock Lane, Port St. Lucie, FL 34952, Mestravel.resourcez.com mcstravel@aol.com. *Travel directory for safe vacations and living.*

THE NATURAL PLACE RESIDENCE AND HOTEL 954.428.5438 1962 N.E. 5th Street, Deerfield Beach, FL 33441, www.thenaturalplace.com natural@traci.net. *Environmentally safe rooms and apartments.*

MOLD RESOURCESL (For mold consults see below and for web sites see F.3.)

ENVIROGEN TECHNOLOGIES 800.367.3634 806.559.4316 131 Pitkin Street, East Hartford, CT 06108 Email: johnfantry2@hotmail.com *Safe, effective and relatively inexpensive mold remediation.*

CENTER FOR ENVIRONMENTAL MEDICINE 315.488.2856 P.O. Box 2716, 2800 W. Genesee Street, Syracuse, NY 13220 Mold Plates: (One per room) Cost: $40.00 each. *Mold plates to measure mold contamination.*

ENVIRO-HEALTH 602.432.1449 602.274.6624 Russell Olinsky, MS. Environmental Engineering. 3421 N. Paiute Way #4, Scottsdale, AZ 85251, Stachy@earthlink.net. *Thorough home visits for environmental and mold control expertise.*

ENVIRONMENTAL HEALTH CENTER 214.368.4132 FAX: 214.691.8432 Christopher Rea, 8345 Walnut Lane, Suite 220, Dallas, TX 75231-4262 *Thorough home visits for environmental and mold control expertise.*

MOLD CONSULTATIONS:

PAULA VANCE[7b] 713.663.6888 FAX: 713.663.7722 Microbiologist, 8911 Interchange Drive, Houston, TX 77054. pv@microbiologyspecialist.com., www.microbiologyspecialist.com.

DAVID STRAUS, Ph.D.[7c] 806.743.2523, david.straus@ttuhsc.edu

CHRISTOPHER REA, 8345 Walnut Lane, Suite 220, Dallas, TX 75231-4262, 214.368.4132.

RUSSELL OLINSKY, M.S., Enviro-Health: Environmental Engineering, Mold Remediation, Environmental Investigations and Consultations, 3421 N. Paiute Way #4, Scottsdale, AZ 85251, 602.432.1449, stachy@earthlink.net.

THE MOLD SOURCE, P. O. Box 2421, Forney, TX 75126, 972.564.4245. www.themoldsource.com.

MOLD WEBSITES

1. www.aerias.org/default.asp
2. www.aerotechlabs.com
3. www.drfungus.org
4. www.epa.gov/iaq/pubs/moldresources.html
5. www.epa.gov/iaq/pubs/molds/graphics/moldremediation.pdf
6. www.themoldsource.com
7. www.mrmildew.com
8. www.moldalert.com/test.html
9. www.groups.yahoo.com/group/sickbuildings
10. www.toxlaw.com/chatboards/sickbldg/

11. www.stachybotrys.com/stachy.htm
12. www.hadd.com/toc2000.html
13. www.epa.gov/iaq/molds/index.html

PAINT: (try paint stores and general resources)

MILLER PAINT CO. 503.233.4021.

Benjamin Moore Prestige or Low-Odor Paint
Glidden Spread 2000 Low Voc Paint..

COSMETICS:
SEE PERSONAL CARE PRODUCTS.

PAPER :

HEALTH TREASURES, pH paper
265 S W Port Saint Lucie Blvd., Port Saint Lucie, FL 34984.
www.healthtreasures.com/ph-paper.html, www.sneeze.com
Inexpensive rolls of pH testing paper.

THE GREEN FIELD COMPANY 619.338.9432 *Organic non-chemically treated cotton paper* www.greenfieldpaper.com.

PERSONAL CARE PRODUCTS:
Categories include general, infants, women- (cosmetics, fragrances, tampons),

GENERAL:

COASTLINE PRODUCTS 800.554.4112 P.O. Box 6397, Santa Ana, CA 92706. *Personal care and household products.*

INFANTS:

EARTHLINGS 805.646.7770 Organic Cotton Baby and Children's Clothing - *Nordstrom's, Macy's, Neiman Marcus.*

DIAPERS, Tushies 800.344.6379, 675 Industrial Blvd., Delta, CO 81416. *Organic products, disposable diapers, shampoos and soaps for babies. Also buy in health food stores. Wipes have a chemical odor.*

WOMEN

FRAGRANCES

CHEMICALLY SENSITIVE LIVING 508.678.7293, FAX: 419.730.6932, 377 Wilbur Ave., Suite 213, Swansea, MA 02777 www.chemicallysensitiveliving.com. *Certified organic and natural fragrances.*

SANITARY PRODUCTS

TAMPONS: Try health food stores.

FEMININE OPTIONS 715.455.1652, Ridgeland, WI.

NATRACARE 303.320.1510, Denver, CO
www.indra.com/natracare.

NATURAL CHOICES 414.421.9394, Franklin, WI.

ORGANIC ESSENTIALS 806.428.3486, O'Donnell,TX www.organicessentials.com.

TERRESSENTIALS 301.371.7333, www.terressentials.com. *Disposable, organic cotton tampons and safe sanitary napkin.*

SKIN CARE

C.A.R.E.S. FOUNDATION, 866.742.3310, www.lindachae.com. *"Organic essentials" by Linda Chae: facial skin products.*

PEST MANAGEMENT:

INTEGRATED PEST MANAGEMENT (IPM) 800.221.6188 *www.getipm.com. Safer, more effective, less expensive pest control.*

SAUNA- DETOXIFICATION

HIGH TECH HEALTH (Dry) 800.794.5355 303.413.8500 FAX: 303.449.9640, Dale Peterson, Thermal Life Poplar Far Infrared Sauna , 2695 Lindon Drive, Boulder, CO 80304, www.hightechhealth.com., *2-4 person units, heats to 98 to 130 degrees. Detox chemicals, nicotine. Helps brain fog.*

*References for infrared saunas: www.hightechhealthin@qwest.net.

HEAVENLY HEAT SAUNA ROOMS 800.MY.SAUNA 800.697.2862, Bob Morgan, 1106 Second Street, Encinitas, CA 92024, www.heavenlyheatsaunas.com. *Personal to family sized units. Heats 98F–130F with far-infrared; 120F–170F with stone heat. These are used by Dr. Rea in Dallas, TX, and are built for the chemically sensitive, without adhesives.*

VACUUM CLEANERS

LESS EXPENSIVE:

Oreck Vacuum *(See telephone book).*

EXPENSIVE:

Kirby (*Look in local telephone book for Vacuum Dealers*).

OTHER:

HEPA Handvac – Dirt Tamer, Cordless.

HEPA Highpowered Vacuums.

Miele Vacuum – Solaris Turbo.

Vacuum Accessories, Replacement Filters and Bags.

(For more information see Is This Your Child's World? pg. 592, 800.787.8780.)

WATER PURIFIERS:

ENVIRONMENTAL MEDICAL RESEARCH FOUNDATION (ERF, formally PARF) 800.787.8780, 1421 Colvin Blvd., Buffalo, NY 14220. *House, kitchen and shower purifiers.*

The Pure Water Place, 3347 Longview Blvd., Longmont, CO 80504, 888.776.0056. Fax 303.772.2093. www.purewaterplace.com. Email: info@purewaterplace.com.

C.4 SOURCES OF ORGANIC FOODS

THE AUSTIN CHRONICLE: Second Helpings: Farm Stands & Farmer's Markets., www.austinchronicle.com/issues/dispatch/2001-10-12/food_second_all.html.

BOGGY CREEK FARMS: www.boggycreekfarms.com.

DIAMOND ORGANICS: 888.ORGANIC (888.674.2642) www.diamondorganics.ocm.

BOXED GREENS, www.boxedgreens.com.

Appendix D
Diagnosis and Treatment Tests, Resources

D.1a BASIC DIAGNOSTIC TESTS FOR CHEMICALS

For chemicals, immune system and hair.

ACCU-CHEM LABORATORIES 800.451.0116 972.234.5412 214.234.5412, 900 North Bowser, Suite 800, Richardson, TX 75081 *Blood, urine and water analysis for chemicals.*

AEROTECH LABORATORIES 800.651.4802; 623.780.4800 Martin Purpura, mpurpura@aerotechlabs.com. 1501 W. Knudsen Dr., Phoenix, AZ 85027. *Tests for chemicals, molds and fungi in materials and/or buildings.*

ANTIBODY ASSAY LABORATORY 800.522.2611 1715 East Wilshire, Suite 715, Santa Ana, CA 92705. *Blood, auto-antibody, antibody, immunity and chemical evaluations.*

DOCTOR'S DATA 800.323.2784 630.377.8139 FAX: 630.587.7871, 3755 Illinois Ave., St. Charles, IL 60174-2420 *Red blood cell, mineral, amino acid, hair, air and nutrients.*

IMMUNOSCIENCE LABORATORY 800.950.4686, 8730 Wilshire Blvd. Suite 305, Beverly Hills, CA 90211. *Immune function, chemicals, infection and parasite evaluations.*

METAMETRIX MEDICAL LABORATORIES 800.221.4640 404.446.5483 5000 Peachtree Industrial Boulevard, Suite 110, Norcross, GA 30071. *Immune, mineral, amino acid, hair toxic metals, nutritional and metabolic tests.*

D.1b MULTIPLE CHEMICAL SENSITIVITY
GENERAL INFORMATION REFERRALS AND RESOURCES

MAYO LABS 800.826.5561, 2326 Pickwick Road, Baltimore, MD 21207. *Contact for Protocol or Fact Sheets.*

D.2a SPECIALIZED DIAGNOSTIC TESTS FOR CHEMICALS:

BREAST MILK FOR PESTICIDE LEVELS:

ACCU-CHEM LABORATORIES 800.451.0116 972.234.5412, 214.234.5412.

AMERICAN ENVIRONMENTAL HEALTH CENTER 214.368.4132 FAX: 214.691.8432.

D.2b BRAIN IMAGE: SPECT TEST 214.528.2482 214.528.2670 Functional Imaging of Texas, Theodore Simon, M.D., 4429 Southern Avenue, Dallas, TX 75205, www.geocities.com/medicalkinetics.com/support/cv_trs.doc.

D.2c BIOASSAY LAB: ANDERSON LABORATORIES 802.295.7344 FAX: 802.295.7648, P. O. Box 323, 4967 Route 14, West Hartford, VT 05084- 0323, www.andersonlaboratories.com. *Biological studies on* *carpets, disinfectants, deodorants, mattresses, etc. and indoor air from buildings. They detect effects of chemical odors on mice instead of children. You can request videos of "before and after" responses for legal or insurance documentation.*

D.2d VITAMIN STUDIES:

PANTOX LAB 888.726.8698 858.272.3885 FAX: 858.272.1621, 4622 Santa Fe Street, San Diego, CA 92109. *CoQ10 and other nutrients.*

SPECTRACELL LABORATORIES 800.227.5227 515 Post Oak Blvd, Suite 830, Houston, TX 77027. *Complete B complex studies and nutrient testing.*

VITAMIN DIAGNOSTICS 732.583.7773, E. Vogellar, Ph.D., Route 35 and Industrial Drive, Cliffwood Beach, NJ 07735. *Nutrient, EFA and amino acid testing.*

D.2e YEAST OR PARASITES:

GREAT SMOKIES DIAGNOSTIC LABORATORY 800.522.4762 , 63 Zillicoa Street, Asheville, NC 28801-9801. *Parasites, yeast, stool and blood tests.*

D.2f HAIR ANALYSIS FOR TOXIC METALS:

DOCTOR'S DATA 800-323-2784 630.377.8139 FAX: 630.587.7871 3755 Illinois Ave., St. Charles, IL 60174-2420. *They offer analysis of red blood cell, mineral, amino acid and hair.*

ANALYTICAL RESEARCH LABS 800.528.4067 602-995-1580 FAX: 602.371.8873, 2225 W. Alice Avenue, Phoenix, AZ 85021, www.arltma.com.

LAWRENCE WILSON, M.D. 800.296.7053 FAX: 928.445.7690, The Hair Analysis Handbook, P.O. Box 54, Prescott, AZ 86302, www.drwilson.com.

D.3 NUTRIENT RESOURCES:

See detoxification remedies in Table 3 G, Chapter 3.

PAIN AND STRESS CLINIC 210.614.7246. Billie Jay Sahley, Ph.D. 5282 Medical Drive Suite 150, San Antonio, TX 78229. *Advice and nutritional booklets and products, especially for ADD, fibromyalgia.*

HEALTHCOMM INTERNATIONAL, INC. 800.843.9660 253.851.3943, Jeffrey Bland, Ph.D. & Associates, P.O. Box 1729,
Gig Harbor, WA 98335.

Ultraclear, ultrasustain and ultrakids for oral detoxification, educational audiotapes.

KLAIRE LABORATORIES 800.533.7255 FAX: 760.744.9364 1573 West Seminole Street, San Marcos, CA 92069. *Vital life nutritional supplements such as amino acids, lactobacillus and glutamine and First Response kit, www.klaire.com*

D.4 SOURCES OF USEFUL HOMEOPATHY REMEDIES:
See Homeopathic Remedies 1-11. See B6 for Homeopathic and Herbal Centers.

(As a traditionally-trained allergist, I was amazed to find how easily, effectively and inexpensively some homeopathic remedies helped certain illnesses, especially chronic ear and flu infections and sprains or joint injuries. If these remedies, however, do not quickly relieve an infection, antibiotics may need to be prescribed. Again we have to use common sense. See qualified physicians and in time more unbiased research will help us to better evaluate what helps and what does not appear to be effective.)
* Prices are subject to change

1.
Homeopathic Remedies To Detoxify Or Eliminate Chemicals

PRODUCT	COMPANY	PRICE*	DOSAGE	REMEDY
AIRLINE PESTICIDE DETOX 6X, 12X, 30X 800.952.2219	PROFESSIONAL COMPLEMEN-TARY HEALTH	$14.00 12 OZ	ADULT: 10 DROPS 3 TIMES DAILY UNDER 12 YRS 1/2 ADULT DOSE	HELPFUL FOR CHEMICAL EXPOSURES
"ALCOHOL DETOX" 800.869.9705	TYLER LABS	$30.00	ADULT: 3 CAPSULES 2 - 3 TIMES A DAY BETWEEN MEALS.	PROTECTS FROM TOXIC EFFECTS OF ALCOHOL NOT FOR USE DURING PREGNANCY /NURSING
CHEM-DEFENSE 800.815.2333	SOURCE NATURALS	90 TABS $16.98 (RETAIL) 45 TABS $ 8.98	2 TO 3 TABLETS DAILY UNDER TONGUE	NUTRIENT BLEND FOR DIETARY NEEDS OF THOSE WITH CHEMICAL SENSITIVITIES
CHEMTOX 800.288.9525	BIO ACTIVE NUTRITIONAL	$ 8.00	10 DROPS ORALLY 3 TIMES PER DAY	RELIEF OF CRAMPS BLOATING AND VOMITING
"CYTO-REDOXIN" REDOX-COUPLED ANTIOXIDANTS 800.869.9705	TYLER LABS	$32.00	1 TO 2 CAPS. ON AN EMPTY STOMACH 2 TIMES DAILY	PROTECTS CELLS AND OPTIMIZES CELLULAR FUNCTION

CONNECTIVE TISSUE LIQUESCENCE T24 800.952.2219	PROFESSIONAL COMPLEMEN-TARY HEALTH FORMULAS, INC.	$8.50	ADULT: 1 TSP 2 TIMES PER DAY UNDER TONGUE CHILD:1/2 ADULT DOSE	CONNECTIVE TISSUE REGENERATION AND DRAINAGE
"DETOXICATION FACTORS" 800.869.9705	TYLER LABS	$52.00	TAKE 1-2 CAPS. 3 TIMES DAILY BETWEEN MEALS	NUTRIENTS FOR TRANSFORMATION & TOXIN EXCRETION
ENVIRO DETOX 800.647.0074	MOUNTAIN STATES HEALTH CARE PRODUCTS	$14.00	ADULT: 10-15 DROPS 3 TIMES PER DAY	DETOXIFICATION OF HYDROCARBONS & AIR/WATER POLLUTANTS
VIROENTOX 800.288.9525	BIO ACTIVE NUTRITIONAL	$8.00	10 DROPS ORALLY, 3 TIMES PER DAY	RELIEF OF HEAD CONGESTION AND EXHAUSTION
INDUSTRITOX 800.647.0074	MOUNTAIN STATES HEALTH CARE PRODUCTS	$14.00	ADULT: 10-15 DROPS 3 TIMES PER DAY	DETOXIFICATION OF PLASTICS & MISC. INDUSTRIAL TOXINS
"NEURO-CORD" 800.990.7085	ENERGETIX	$30.00	15 DROPS, 3 TIMES PER DAY	DRAWS NEUROTOXINS FROM NERVE ENDINGS
"RECANSCOSTAT 400" with L-GLUTATHIONE 800.869.9705	TYLER LABS	$102.00	TAKE 1 CAPSULE W/ 12-16 OZS. OF WATER 1-3 TIMES DAILY, BETWEEN MEALS	MAINTAINS NORMAL CELLULAR METABOLISM AND REGULATION
TOXICLEANSE 800.334.4043	BIO ENERGETICS, INC.		ADULT: 10 DROPS 3 TIMES DAILY UNDER TONGUE CHILD: 1/2 ADULT	ASSIST ELIMINATION OF BY PRODUCTS AND TOXINS
WHOLE BODY DETOX LIQUESCENCE 800.952.2219	PROF. COMP. HEALTH FORMULAS, INC	$8.50	ADULT: 1 TSP 2 TIMES A DAY	DRAINS ALL ORGANS; ALL INCLUSIVE DETOXIFIER FOR BODY

2.
Homeopathic Remedies for Allergies

PRODUCT	COMPANY	PRICE*	DOSAGE	REMEDY
ALLERGY LIQUESCENCE T31 800.952.2219	COMPLEMEN-TARY HEALTH FORMULAS, INC.	$8.50	ADULT: 1-2 TIMES PER DAY UNDER TONGUE CHILD:1/2 ADULT DOSE	AID IN SUPPORT OF ADVERSE SYMPTOMS OF ALLERGIES
LUNG STIM LIQUESCENCE T26 503.245.2720	PROFESSIONAL COMPLEMEN-TARY HEALTH FORMULAS, INC.	$8.50	ADULT:1 TSP. 2 TIMES PER DAY UNDER TONGUE CHILD: 1/2 ADULT DOSE	LUNG REGENERATION AND DRAINAGE
MUCOSA COMP. 800.621.7644	HEEL	$4.75	1/DAY	MOLD ALLERGY

OPSIN 1 or OPSIN 2 800.647.0074	MT. STATES HEALTH PROD.	$8.00	ADULT: 10 DROPS 3X/DAY CHILD: + ADULT DOSE	OPSIN 1-FOODS OPSIN2-POLLEN/ INHALANTS
SEROTONIN DOPOMINE LIQUESCENCE T19 503.245.2720	PROFESSIONAL COMPLEMEN-TARY HEALTH FORMULAS, INC.	$8.50	ADULT: 1 TSP. 2 TIMES PER DAY UNDER TONGUE CHILD: 1/2 ADULT DOSE	REGULATION OF NEUROTRANSMITTER AND RELIEF OF DEPRESSIVE STATES
SUGAR MIX 800.952.2219	PROFESSIONAL COMPLEMENT-ARY HEALTH FORMULAS, INC.	$7.00	ADULT: 10 DROPS 3 TIMES PER DAY UNDER TONGUE CHILD: 1/2 ADULT DOSE	PROVIDES FACTORS THAT MITIGATE HYPERSENSITIVITY TO SUGARS, OR TO DECREASE CRAVINGS
ZINGERBER OFFICINALE [GINGER RHIZOME]	PROFESSIONAL COMPLEMENT -ARY HEALTH FORMULAS, INC.	$4.50	ADULT: 1 TSP. 2 TIMES PER DAY UNDER TONGUE CHILD: 1/2 ADULT DOSE	DIGESTIVE TRACT AND ANTI-INFLAMMATORY

***Other individual food extracts are also available**

3.
<u>Homeopathic Remedies for ADD and ADHD</u>

PRODUCT	COMPANY	PRICE*	DOSAGE	REMEDY
ATTENTION DEFICIT - MILD C 146 800-952-2219	PROFESSIONAL COMPLEMEN-TARY HEALTH FORMULAS, INC.	$14.00	ADULT: 10 DROPS 3 TIMES PER DAY CHILD: 1/2 ADULT DOSE	BALANCE PHYSIOLOGY OF THOSE WITH MILD FOCUSING /LEARNING /ATTENTIVENESS DIFFICULTIES
ATTENTION DEFICIT - SEVERE C 147 800-952-2219	PROFESSIONAL COMPLEMEN-TARY HEALTH FORMULAS, INC.	$14.00	ADULT:10 DROPS 3 TIMES PER DAY UNDER TONGUE CHILD: 1/2 ADULT DOSE	BALANCE PHYSIOLOGY OF THOSE WITH SEVERE ADHD

4.
<u>Homeopathic Remedies for Infections</u>

PRODUCT	COMPANY	PRICE*	DOSAGE	REMEDY
OSCILLO-COCCINUM	BOIRON	$12.00	3 DOSES 6 HOURS APART, DISSOLVE SLOWLY *UNDER TONGUE*	FOR FLU SYMPTOM (THIS ONE IS *FOR FLU* SURPRISINGLY EFFECTIVE.)
ABC 800.999.3001	MACRO PHARMA INTERNATIONAL	$6.00	5 DROPS EVERY 5 MINUTES FOR 2 HOURS	RELIEF OF MINOR EARACHE

BACTERIA DETOX 602.944.0104	BIOTICS	$18.00	1 CAPFUL 2 TIMES DAILY	RELIEF OF BACTERIAL INFECTIONS
HIGH ENERGY ECHINACEA LIQUESCENCE T33 503.245.2720	ROFESSIONAL COMPLEMENTARY HEALTH FORMULAS	$ 8.50	ADULT: 15 DROPS EVERY 2HRS UNDER THE: TONGUE. CHILD 1/2 ADULT DOSE	MINOR INFECTIONS, FEVER, CHILLS AND ACHES FOR CHILDREN
IMMPOWER-AHCC *800.824.2434* ORDER NO: 909.307.2100 909.307.2111	AMERICAN *BIOSCIENCES* TIDHEALTH	$49.95	1-2 CAPSULES *500MG PER DAY*	IMMUNE ENHANCING *SUPPLEMENT FOR:* LIVER CANCER, HEPATITIS C AND CIRRHOSIS OF LIVER
IMMUNI T 800.580.7587	LONGEVITY PLUS	$48.00 60 CAPS	1-2 CAPS PER DAY	COMPREHENSIVE IMMUNE SUPPORT
LYMPHONEST 800.999.3001	MACRO PHARMA INTERNATIONAL	$7.00 $14.00	30 DROPS IN WATER, 3 TIMES DAILY	RELIEF OF SWELLING OF THE LYMPH GLANDS
SEACURE ORDER NO: 800.735.2051 NO ADDED INGREDIENTS	PROPER NUTRITION INC.	$39.95 90	1-3 CAPSULES PER DAY 500MG	CROHN'S - LEAKY GUT PURE FISH PROTEIN -
SEA VIVE ORDER NO: 800.735.2051 OFFICE NO: 800.555.8868	PROPER NUTRITION INC.	$39.95 90 500MG	1-3 CAPSULES PER DAY	IMMUNE SUPPORT PREVENTATIVE FOR DISEASE AND INFECTIONS
VIRUS DETOX 602.944.0104	BIOTICS	$18.00	1 CAPFUL 2 TIMES DAILY	RELIEF OF VIRAL INFECTIONS

5.
Homeopathic Remedies for Immune System

PRODUCT	COMPANY	PRICE*	DOSAGE	REMEDY
"ESSIAC PLUS" CATS CLAW HERB 480.368.9355	NATURAL PARTNERS	$48.00	MIX 1-2 OZS. W/ 2-4 OZS HOT OR COLD DIS-TILLED WATER. ADULTS: 2 TIMES DAILY ON EMPTY STOMACH, 1 HOUR BEFORE EATING OR 2-3 HOURS AFTER EATING. *MAINTENANCE SCHEDULE:* 1 OZ W/ 2 OZS. WATER DAILY ON EMPTY STOMACH. CHILD: 1/2 THE RECOMMENDED ADULT MIN. DOSAGE.	STRENGTHENS THE IMMUNE SYSTEM

6.
Homeopathic Remedies for Kidneys

PRODUCT	COMPANY	PRICE*	DOSAGE	REMEDY
KIDNEY STIM LIQUESCENCE T13 503.245.2720	PROFESSIONAL COMPLEMEN-TARY HEALTH FORMULAS, INC.	$ 8.50	ADULT: 1 TSP. 2 TIMES PER DAY UNDER TONGUE CHILD: 1/2 ADULT DOSE	SUPPORT OF KIDNEY REGENERATION AND DRAINAGE

7.
Homeopathic Remedies for Lungs

PRODUCT	COMPANY	PRICE*	DOSAGE	REMEDY
"L-DETOX" HERBAL BLEND '480.632.9911	LONG LIFE BRAND PRODUCTS	$20.00	1 CAPLET TWICE DAILY	REMOVES TOXINS FROM THE BODY LIVER AND ELIMIN-ATORY SYSTEMS
LIQUID LIVER LIQUESCENCE T15 800.924.4133	PROFESSIONAL HEALTH PRODUCTS	$17.00	ADULT: 1 TSP. IN 8 OZ. OF WATER CHILD: 1/2 ADULT DOSE	AID IN SUPPORT AND DRAINAGE FOR LIVER FUNCTION

8.
Homeopathic Remedies for Skin

PRODUCT	COMPANY	PRICE*	DOSAGE	REMEDY
SKIN BALANCE LIQUESCENCE T27 800.952.2219	PROFESSIONAL COMPLEMEN-TARY HEALTH FORMULAS, INC.	$ 8.50	ADULT: 1 TSP. 2 TIMES PER DAY UNDER TONGUE CHILD: 1/2 ADULT DOSE	SKIN REGENERATION AND DRAINAGE

9.
Homeopathic Remedies for Lymph Drainage

PRODUCT	COMPANY	PRICE*	DOSAGE	REMEDY
LYMPH STIM LIQUESCENCE T16 800.952.2219	PROFESSIONAL COMPLEMEN-TARY HEALTH FORMULAS, INC.	$8.50	ADULT: 1 TSP. 2 TIMES PER DAY UNDER TONGUE CHILD: 1/2 ADULT DOSE	SUPPORT OF LYMPHATIC REGENERATION AND DRAINAGE
MUCOLYTIC DRAINAGE FORMULA T17 800.952.2219	PROFESSIONAL COMPLEMEN-TARY HEALTH FORMULAS, INC.	$8.50	ADULT: 1 TSP. 2 TIMES PER DAY UNDER TONGUE CHILD: 1/2 ADULT DOSE	DISSOLUTION AND ELIMINATION OF EXCESS MUCOUS (FOR SHORT-TERM USE)
MERCURY DETOX 800.869.9705	TYLER LABS	$26.00	2 CAPSULES 2-3 TIMES DAILY, BETWEEN MEALS	DETOXIFICATION OF MERCURY AND HEAVY METALS

These preparations can be used in conjunction with lymphatic drainage for enhanced cleansing.[73a,b,]

10.
Homeopathic Remedies for Oral Chelation

PRODUCT	COMPANY	PRICE*	DOSAGE	REMEDY
ORAL-CHELATION "MG-TAURINE FORTE" 800.323.2935	MILLER PHARMACAL GROUP, INC	$40.00	TAKE 1 CAPSULE DAILY	MAGNESIUM AND TAURINE SUPPLEMENT
ORAL-CHELATION "MG ASPARTATE" 800.323.2935	MILLER PHARMACAL GROUP, INC.	$28.00	ADULTS TAKE 1 TABLET DAILY	FOR PREVENTION OF MAGNESIUM DEFICIENCIES

11.
Homeopathic Remedies for Heavy Metal Detox or Radiation

PRODUCT	COMPANY	PRICE*	DOSAGE	REMEDY
"OPC GRAPE-GOLD" 888.666.1188	PRIMARY SOURCE	$39.00	TAKE 2 CAPSULES	DETOXIFIER: REMOVES HEAVY METALS AND RADIOACTIVE SUB-STANCES FROM BODY
RADIATION CNS "PRO ALGEN" 800.662.2544	NORDIC NATURALS	$30.00	4 TABLETS PER DAY, 1 W/ EACH MEAL; 1 BEFORE GOING TO BED	HELPS TO INHIBIT THE ABSORPTION, AND REABSORPTION OF HEAVY METALS FROM THE BODY
MERCURY DETOX "CILANTRO EXTRACT" 800.813.2118	DRAGON RIVER HERBS	$32.00	STEEP 1-15 DROPS IN HOT WATER 2 TIMES A DAY: 5 DAYS ON, 2 DAYS OFF	MOBILIZES MERCURY, TIN AND OTHER TOXIC METALS IN BRAIN FROM THESE TISSUES AND SPINAL CORD,

D.5 ALTERNATIVE DIAGNOSTIC METHODS

As is typical in the scientific literature, you can always find pro and con articles published by well-trained scientists. When there is a difference of opinion, check it out for yourself if it does not hurt and might help. In my personal experience, muscle and pendulum testing appears to be worthy of further critical unbiased evaluation.

D.5a MUSCLE TESTING[1-3]

Many of the newer approaches to healing or allergy treatment use some form of muscle testing. The following briefly shows one variation of how this can be done.*

First:
You must determine if the person to be tested responds normally.

- Have the person being tested place his/her arm *straight* out in front and you attempt to gently push it down while the person being tested tries to hold it up. The aim is not to see who is stronger but simply to sense how strong the arm is when it is pushed down against pressure. Be sure there is no shoulder problem before you select which arm to test.

- If testing a woman, you need only to use the index finger on the back of wrist to push down. For men, you might need to use your whole hand on the wrist to push the arm down. If a man is very strong, have the arm pointing down about half way between his waist and the floor. Almost always, if you test something to which someone is sensitive, the arm will *obviously* weaken. In general, the weaker the arm becomes, the more sensitive the person is to the test item. It's not a power struggle, just a rough test of strength. Try to consistently push with about the same amount of pressure when you do this type of testing. Keep your mind as blank as possible. You must remain neutral and not care if the arm stays strong or becomes weak.

- To double check if someone's body computer is working, do the following: place your fingernail down over the bridge of the nose near the forehead of the person being tested. When you try to push the arm down, if the "computer" is working correctly, the arm should be weak. When the fingernail is visible or up in that location, the arm should be strong. (*Yes, I agree, it makes absolutely no sense but try it. The bottom line at this time is not can we explain it, but does appear to provide any practical insight or help.*)

- To further evaluate the body computer, do the following. Ask the patient to say his/her real name: "I am Bill or Mary". The arm should remain strong. Then have the person being tested say someone else's

---

* Dr. Victor Frank-435.652.4340 provided this information.

name. Pick a name that is not admired, such as saying, "My name is Hitler". Most people would have their muscles weaken when they say, "I am Hitler" or some other distasteful name if the body is working correctly. The body muscles appear to quickly register a lie and become weak. (*This is also a way to check your young children. Ask if they are into drugs, alcohol, sex, hurting others, etc. See if the arm weakens. If it does, do some checking.*)

Second:
Once the patient responds normally, the following is thought by some to help in the detection of an allergy or sensitivity to some item.

- The person being tested holds a substance that is thought to possibly cause an allergy over the center of their chest with the flat of the hand. This could be a can of cola or beer, a cup of black coffee or milk, a piece of bread or fruit, a packet of aspartame, a piece of new carpet or synthetic clothing, a marking pen, your allergy extract or anything else. Check the arm again. If it becomes weak, or the arm goes down, this suggests that there is something in the test item that is not good for the person being tested.

- To double-check, then test with something that should test strong such as Vitamin C or glutathione. The arm should be stronger than normal. (*You can check out several brands of a product, such as a vitamin, in this manner and determine which one appears to make your arm the strongest. You will be surprised to see the differences a brand makes. Obviously you are looking for the one that makes your arm stronger, not weaker, than normal.*)

Third:
This is how to eliminate an allergy or sensitivity. (*Do not attempt this without personal instruction.*)*

- Once you detect an allergy or sensitivity, the following appears to be helpful according to some chiropractors. Have someone who has used this technique show you exactly how it is done. *(For someone nearby, call 435.652.4340.)* The head should be straight, not tipped to one side. The aim is to try, *ever so gently*, to pull the entire skull or head directly *straight up* towards the ceiling. The person should breathe *in* as the head is raised a millimeter. Hold the side of one hand on the forehead just below the bridge of the eyes. At the same time the back of the head is cradled with the other palm. By pulling both hands upwards, the head is moved ever so slightly straight *up* towards the ceiling. In essence, this will *very* gently separate the base of the skull from the top of the spine. When the person being tested breathes in, the head is pulled *up*, ever so gently and this is repeated three times. The item to

* Dr. Victor Frank-435.652.4340.

be tested should be held on the central chest while this is being done. Again, do not attempt this if there are *any* problems with a person's neck and you will need personal supervision to learn this technique.

Fourth:
This is how to double check to see if the treatment helped.

- With the test item on the central chest, again check the muscle strength and compare it with how it was before the treatment. If the problem has been corrected and if it was not good for that person, the arm should now be strong. When this happens, you assume the treatment for the tested item is complete. The test can be redone as often as desired to see how long the arm remains strong or the treatment helps. The above procedure can be repeated anytime for items to which you are exposed everyday. Things that cause weakness in the arm of a person can be retreated if the symptoms recur at any time, as indicated by the test.

  This effect of this procedure is said to last for an "indefinite" period of time, but if it lasts only a short while, you can retest and retreat anytime. (*My personal opinion is that it will last varying periods of times for different items in each individual.*)

For more detailed information contact Victor Frank, D.C. (*435.652.4340*). He gives a stress management course for parents that could be of benefit. He also gives a most surprising course for professionals and physicians called TBM (Total Body Modification). It will jar many of the basic medical concepts and beliefs of most doctors because much that he says does not seem possible or plausible.

Practical Examples:
A woman came in my house and my two tiny, friendly poodles jumped onto her lap. Within ten minutes it was obvious that she had developed asthma. I asked if she was allergic to dogs and she said yes. I did the above as she held the dogs on her chest. Within ten minutes the asthma was gone without medication. No, it won't help everyone or everything, but for some it appears to help quickly and effectively.
Similarly, someone smelled popcorn in my home and developed hay fever. I did the above while she held some popcorn over her chest and in ten minutes, no hay fever.

You can check out each food you are about to eat in a restaurant in this manner. This technique makes absolutely no sense but, try it for yourself and make your own decision. I hope to scientifically evaluate some of these types of techniques critically as soon as funding is available because there is so much disagreement about the validity of muscle testing. We obviously need more studies. (*See Appendix D.5a for other pro and con published research information.*)

1. International Journal of Neuroscience, 1998, December; 96 (3-4): 237-44. Schmidt W. H. Jr., Leisman G. "Correlation of Applied Kinesiology Muscle Testing Findings with Serum Immunoglobulin Levels for Food allergies." "These serum tests confirmed the 19 of the 21 food allergies (90.5%) suspected based on the applied kinesiology screening procedures."
2. Complementary Therapeutic Medicine, 2001, September: 9 (30): 141-5. Ludtke R. Kunz B, Seeber N, Ring J. "Test-Retest-Reliability and Validity of the Kinesiology Muscle Test. The results suggested that the use of kinesiology as a diagnostic tool is not more useful than random guessing." (Test of insect venom allergy.)
3. Scientific Validation of the Mind/Body Paradigm & Muscle Testing, Reprint of Research Study "Muscle Test Comparisons of Congruent and Incongruent Self-referential Statements". The Our Net Effect Research Foundation, 1991 Village Park Way, Suite 201-A, Encinitas, CA 92024, 760.633.1663.

D.5b **DOWSING AND PENDULUM TESTING**[1-4]

See Chapter 3.

"I know very well that many scientists consider dowsing, as they do astrology, as a type of ancient superstition. According to my conviction, this is unjustified. The dowsing rod (or pendulum) is a simple instrument which shows the reaction of the human nervous system to certain factors which are unknown to us at this time." Albert Einstein

Pendulums:

The basic principle of either using a pendulum or dowsing with a metal hanger to find water is energy. Like water or metals in the ground, humans radiate energy from their bodies and if we are near something that has either a good or bad effect on our energy, this can be monitored or registered with a pendulum.[1-4]

A pendulum is nothing but a crystal, stone or metal at the end of a short metal chain.[1] You can buy pendulums at stores, contact PARF1421@ aol.com on the internet, or make your own by simply dangling a paper clip on the end of a narrow chain or wire.

Using a pendulum is easy. The response of the pendulum, however, can vary from individual to individual, so you need only to know what a "yes" and "no" response is when you personally use it. It is important that you do try not to influence the movement of the pendulum so it does what you want. You must try to remain entirely neutral and see what the pendulum does on its own. You dangle it over something and merely ask a question that requires a simple "yes" or "no" answer. Then see how it moves. It is that simple. Some people seem to use a pendulum better than others but with a bit of practice, most can get consistent answers. In general, a back and forth movement means a "no" and a circular movement means a "yes". Try it and see what happens. Of course, it does not provide an unquestionably correct response but it appears possible that it can provide more insight than simply random guessing.

One interesting example is used by many bird breeders who claim that a pendulum can help determine the sex of a newborn bird. Don't laugh. This is how they can tell which newborn canaries are destined to become males or singers. *(You can even apply this to humans, Hold the end of the chain so the weight dangles over a male's wrist and it usually will go back and forth. In contrast, if you hold it over a female's wrist, it typically will go in a circle).*

Other practical examples:

- If you hold the pendulum over a vitamin or a non-pesticided organic food, it will typically go in a circle, which suggests a "yes". If there is something about the product that is not good for you, it will typically give a "no" response.
- If you have five bottles of a vitamin and want to know which is best, test each one. If, for example, a bottle causes a back and forth movement, this suggests a "no", or that the contents are not good for you. Look for the bottle which makes the pendulum go in a circle because this is the signal for a possible "yes".
- You can check pure water stored in a glass bottle. Usually it will provide a "yes" response. Then microwave this same water for a minute. It will then typically give a negative response suggesting that microwaving changed the water and made it not good for you. You can similarly check out foods you eat.
- If you hold the pendulum over a substance that contains a chemical, such as a smelly marking pen or a sugar substitute, it will usually go back and forth, suggesting a "no" response or that the item being tested is not good for you.

As impossible as the above may seem, it is anticipated that eventually scientific explanations will be found to explain the apparent successes of some novel creative methods, such as the above, for finding answers. In the meantime, if you or a loved one is never well, always on medications and sick and tired of being unwell, check out some of your daily contacts. If you can detect and eliminate the cause of an illness, there may be no symptoms left to treat.

Medical References on Energy, Dowsing and Pendulums.

RICHARD GERBER, A Practical Guide to Vibrational Medicine: Energy Healing and Spiritual Transformation. 2001. Quill Publishing. Cost: $15.00 (Amazon.com).

SIG LONEGREN, The Pendulum Kit, 1990, Fireside; Book and Access Edition. Cost: $21.95 (Amazon.com).

GREG NIELSEN, Pendulum Power, 1987, Inner Traditions Intl Ltd. Cost: $8.95 (Amazon.com).

WILLIAM TILLER, Science and Human Trans-intentionality and Consciousness. 1997. Cost: $24.95.

MIKHAIL DEKHTA AND RUTH SCOTT, Secrets of Healers, rscott11@aol.com, www.thehealingsite.com, 623.551.9073. Cost: $17.00 (plus S & H).

MASTER HONG LIU, The Healing Art of QI Gong, Warner Books, 1271 Avenue of the Americas, New York, NY 10020. 1999. Cost: $14.00 (plus S & H).

D.5c NEWER UNPROVEN ENERGY TECHNIQUES FOR DIAGNOSIS AND TREATMENT

MIKHAIL DEKHTA AND RUTH SCOTT, Secrets of Healers, rscott11@aol.com, www.thehealingsite.com, 623.551.9073. Cost: $17.00.

MASTER HONG LIU, The Healing Art of QI Gong, Warner Books, 1271 Avenue of the Americas, New York, NY 10020. 1999. Cost: $14.00.

CLINTON, ASHA, LCSW, Ph.D.
Finally! Successful OCD Treatment With Seemorg Matrix Work, 2003, Asha Nahoma Clinton©, 885 East Rd., Richmond, MA 01254.

JAFFE, CAROLYN JMT ADVANCE TECHNIQUE
610.695.1800, 928 Penn Ave., Wyomissing, PA 19610. jmtseminars@aol.com.

MARTIN, ART, D.D., N.D., M.A. 800.655.3846 916.663.9178. Your Body Is Talking; Are You Listening? 1997, Personal Transformation Press, 8300 Rock Springs Road, Penryn, CA 95663. Cost: $15.95

RADOMSKI, SANDI, N.D., L.C.S.W., M.S.S.W
215.885.7917, FAX: 215.572.1175. Allergy Antidotes™ The Energy Psychology Treatment Of Allergy-Like Reactions, 2000, 1051 Township Line Road, Jenkintown, PA 19046. SandiRadom@aol.com.

Appendix E

E.1 BOOKS FOR PUBLIC

Many books are listed in the area of the book in which the topic is discussed.

ANTONETTI, AMILYA, creator of Soapworks

Why David Hated Tuesdays (*creating a toxic free home*) Cost: $14.00
www.soapworks.com or amazon.com.

ARENSON, GLORIA, M.S., M.F.T.

Five Simple Steps To Emotional Healing. 2001, Fireside, Rockefeller Center, 1230 Avenue of the Americas, New York, NY 10020.

BATMANGHELID J. F. M.D. 703.848.2333

FAX: 703.848.2334 Global Health Solutions, Inc., P.O. Box 3189, Falls Church, VA 22043,

The Body's Many Cries For Water (1995). Cost: $14.95.

ABC Of Allergies, Asthma And Lupus:
Eradicate Asthma Now, (2000). Cost: $12.85.

CUTLER, ELLEN W., D.C.

Winning The War Against Asthma And Allergies: Cost: $17.95.
A Drug-Free Cure For Asthma And Allergy Sufferers.
Delmar Publishers 3 Columbia Circle, Box 15015, Albany, New York 12212-5015 www.delmar.com.

EPSTEIN, SAMUEL S. M.D., et al.,

The Politics Of Cancer Revisited Cost: $21.95.
East Ridge Press, USA, 1998.

FITZGERALD, PATRICIA, M.D.

The Detox Solution 2001. Illumination Press Cost: $19.95.

FORCE, MARK, D.C. 480.563.4256 FAX: 480.563.4269

Choosing Health 2003 7500 E. Pinnacle Peak Road, Scottsdale, AZ 85255. www.theelementsofhealth.com. Cost: $30.00

HAREZI, ILONKA, About electromagnetic energy, lymphatic drainage. To order books: 618.948.2393.

The Resonance In Residence: An Inner And Outer Quantum Journey
And The Science Edition, 2002. Cost: $28.00/Set.

HIGGINS, HAL A., DDS. & HIGGINS, SHARON A., RDH

It's All In Your Head: The Link Between Mercury Amalgams and Illness
Avery Penguin Putnam, Cost: $12.96.

HOROWITZ, LEONARD, G., 800.336.9266

Death In The Air-Globalism, Terorrism & Toxic Warfare,
Tetrahedron Publishing Group, 206 North 4th Ave., Suite 147, Sandpoint, Idaho 83864, Cost: $29.95.

HOVER-KRAMER, DOROTHEA

Creative Energies, Integrative Energy Psychotherapy For Self-Expression And Healing. 2002. w. w. Norton & Company, 500 Fifth Avenue, New York, NY 10110. www.wwnorton.com.

KROHN, JACQUELINE, M.D. AND FRANCES TAYLOR
800.277.5887 604.739.1771.
Natural Detoxification: An Encyclopedia Cost: $24.95.
ALLERGY RELIEF AND PREVENTION Cost: $24.95.
Hartley and Marks, Vancouver, BC, Canada.

LAWSON, LYNN
Living Well In A Toxic World, 1993
Living Well In A Toxic World – A New Millenium Update, 2003
Lynnwood Press, PO Box 1732, Evanston, IL 60202, lunword@aol.com.

MARTIN, ART, D.D., N.D., M.A. 916.663.9178. 800.655.3846
Your Body Is Talking; Are You Listening? 1997, Personal Transformation Press, 8300 Rock Springs Road, Penryn, CA 95663. Cost: $15.95

BONNYE L. MATTHEWS
Chemical Sensitivity McFarland & Company, Inc. (1992) Box 611, Jefferson, NC 28640.

NAMKA, LYNNE, ED. D.
Goodbye Ouchies And Grouchies, Hello Happy Feelings, EFT For Kids Of All Ages. 2003. Talk, Trust & Feel Therapeutics, 5398 Golder Ranch Road, Tucson, AZ 85739. www.AngriesOut.com Cost: $9.95

RADOMSKI, SANDI, N.D., L.C.S.W., M.S.S.W
215.885.7917, FAX: 215.572.1175
Allergy Antidotes™ The Energy Psychology Treatment Of Allergy-Like Reactions, 2000, 1051 Township Line Road, Jenkintown, PA 19046
SandiRadom@aol.com.

RAPP, DORIS J., M.D. 800.787.8780
Environmental Medical Research Foundation (Formerly PARF)
421 Colvin Blvd., P.O. Box 60, Buffalo, NY 14223-0060,
Is This Your Child? Cost: $12.00.
Is This Your Child's World? (hard cover) Cost: $25.00.
Is This Your Child's World? (soft cover) Cost: $15.00.
The Impossible Child At School, At Home Cost: $ 9.00.

ROGERS, SHERRY, M.D.
Prestige Press, P.O. Box 3068, 3500 Brewerton Road, Syracuse, NY 13220 800.846.6687 315.455.7862 FAX: 315.454.8119.
Detoxify Or Die, The Ultimate Healing Plan Cost: $22.95.
Depression Cured At Last! Cost: $24.95.
Wellness Against All Odds Cost: $17.95.
No More Heartburn Cost: $15.00.
Tired Or Toxic Cost: $18.75.
You Are What You Ate: Cost: $12.95.
The E. I. Syndrome Cost: $17.95.
Scientific Basis For Selected
Environmental Medicine Techniques Cost: $17.95

SAHLEY, BILLIE JAY, Ph.D. AND BIRKNER, KATHERINE, C.R.N.A., Ph.D., Pain & Stress Therapy Center Publication 282 Medical Drive, Suite 160, San Antonio, TX 78229-6043
Stop ADD Naturally Cost: $9.95.
Breaking Your Addiction Habit Cost: $9.95.
The Anxiety Epidemic Cost: $9.95.
Chronic Emotional Fatigue Cost: $9.95.
Breaking Your Prescribed Addiction Cost: $9.95.
Heal With Amino Acids And Nutrients Cost: $12.95.
Post Trauma And Chronic Emotional Fatigue Cost: $7.95.

SHEALY, C. NORMAN M.D., Ph.D.
The Methuselah Potential For Health And Longevity 2002. Brindabella® Books, 5607 S. 222nd Road, Fair Grove, MO 65648.
www.selfhealthsystems.com., Cost: 10.95.

STEINMAN, DAVID AND EPSTEIN, SAMUEL, M.D.
The Safe Shopper's Bible Cost: $15.95.
Publisher MacMillan, 1995, Simon & Schuster, MacMillan Company 1633 Broadway, New York, NY 10019.

W. A. TILLER, Pavior Publishing
Conscious Acts Of Creation 2001, Cost: $29.95.
Science And Human Transformation, Subtle Energies, Intentionality And Consciousness. 1997, Cost: $24.95.

ROBERT O. YOUNG, Ph.D., SHELLEY REDFORD YOUNG
The pH Miracle Balance Your Diet, Reclaim Your Health Warner Books, Inc., 2002, 1271 Avenue of the Americas, N.Y., NY 10020.
www.twbookmark.com., Cost: $24.95

E.2 PROFESSIONAL BOOKS FOR PHYSICIANS:

REA, WILLIAM, J., M.D.
Chemical Sensitivities VOL.1-4, 214.368.4132 FAX: 214.691.8432 CRC PRESS, INC, 2000 Corporate Blvd., NW, Boca Raton, FL 33431,
Cost: $75.00.

MILLER, JOSEPH B.
Relief At Last: Neutralization for Food Allergy, Flu and PMS. Book out of print—limited availability, Springfield, IL Cost: $47.50.

KILBURN, KAYE H., MD. & EDGINGTON, RALPH
Chemical Brain Injury Cost: $100.00.
John Wiley & Sons, Inc. (1998) Van Nostrand Reinholt New York, NY 10022.

SHEALY, C. NORMAN M.D., Ph.D.
The Methuselah Potential For Health And Longevity. 2002. Brindabella® Books, 5607 S. 222nd Road, Fair Grove, MO 65648 Cost: $ 10.95.
www.selfhealthsystems.com.

E.3a ENVIRONMENTAL MEDICAL BOOKS FOR LEGAL ISSUES:
PRICE KING, LINDA 757.546.0663 Chemical Injury And The Courts, A Litigation Guide For Clients And Their Attorneys The Environmental Health Network, P.O. BOX 16267, Chesapeake, VA 23328-6267.

E.3b ADVOCACY GROUP FOR LEGAL ISSUES:
ENVIRONMENTAL ACCESS RESEARCH NETWORK [EARN]
701.859.6363, P.O. Box 426, Williston, ND 58802-0426.
Newsletter, medical and legal briefs, plus law searches and expert witness information. Also see books for doctors by William Rea, M.D. and for the public by Bonnye L. Matthews.

E.4 VIDEOS:

MARTIN, ART, D.D., N.D., M.A. 800.655.3846
Changing Paradigms, A TV Interview With Patricia Hill On The Practice Of PsychoneuroImmunology

RAPP, DORIS J., M.D. Available from ERF (Formally PARF), 800.787.8780

Environmentally Sick Schools (90 min)* Cost: $25.00.
Video I, II, III: Allergies Do Alter Activity & Behavior (43 min)
Impossible Child or Allergic Child (20 min) Cost: $15.00.
Why A Clean Classroom? (62 min) Cost: $25.00.
Five Allergic Children (15 min) Cost: $15.00.
Violent Tendencies in Children (10 min) Cost: $15.00.
Reactions to Chemicals in Adults and Children** Cost: $25.00.
Reactions to Molds in Adults and Children** Cost: $25.00.
Sinus Drainage Video Cost: $25.00.
*Patients on this video are described in detail in book Is This Your Child's World? **Will be available late 2003, early 2004.

REED, STEVE B. 972.997.9955 Healing An Abandonment Trauma. A REMAP demonstration video, 2003. www.psychotherapy=center.com

YORDY, JAN Indigo Child, The Next Step In Human Evolution www.energyconnectiontherapies.com.

E.5 AUDIO CASSETTE TAPES AND DVD'S:

DISHINGER, RONALD C.– Audio tapes. 270.684.9233 Bad Behavior And Illness Are Caused By Biochemical Imbalances, www.medicimusic.com.

RAPP, DORIS J., M.D., Audio tapes. 800 787 8780.

Allergy Diets Cost: $10.00.
Environmental Aspects of Allergies Cost: $10.00.
Infant Food Allergies Cost: $10.00.
Typical lecture Cost: $10.00.

SISE, MARY T., CSW-R, TFTdx- DVD 518.785.8576 Transforming The Trauma Of The World Trade Center, msise3@aol.com.

APPENDIX F
Professional And Public Information Sources

F.1 NEWSLETTERS FOR THE PUBLIC & PHYSICIANS
Written by physicians:

TOTAL WELLNESS Sherry Rogers, M.D.
800.846.6687 315.468.4417 315.468.8119, Prestige Publishing, P.O. Box 3068, , 3502 Brewerton Road, Syracuse, NY 13220, Annual Cost: $39.95.

OPTIMAL WELLNESS CENTER, E-HEALTHY NEWSLETTER , Joseph Mercola, D.O. www.mercola.com.

HEALTH & HEALING: TOMORROW'S MEDICINE TODAY, Julian Whitaker, M.D., Whitaker Wellness Institute, Newport Beach, CA 800.488.1500. www.drwhitaker.com, www.whitakerwellness.com.

TOWNSEND LETTER 360.385.6021 FAX: 360.385.0699 www.tldp.com.

ALTERNATIVES, David G. Williams, D.C. 800.844.1462 Mountain Home Publishing, P.O. Box 61010, Rockville, MD 20819-1010. www.drdavidwilliams.com.

SMART PUBLICATIONS, Health & Wellness Update 800.976.2783, P.O. Box 4667, Petaluma, CA 94955, www.smart-publications.com.

OTHER KEY PUBLICATIONS

CRIME TIMES 214.373.3308 The Wacker Foundation, Dept. 132-1106, N. Gilbert Road, Suite 2, Mesa, AZ 85203.

RACHEL'S ENVIRONMENT & HEALTH NEWSLETTER
P.O. Box 5036, Annapolis, MD 21402-7036, 410.463.1584. 410.263.4894. www.rachelcarson.org.

HEALTHWORLD ONLINE - MIND / BODY HEALTH NEWSLETTER
Editors: David Sobel, MD, & Robert Ornstein, Ph.D. 4049 Lyceum Avenue Los Angeles, CA 90066, www.healthy.net.

THE NEW REACTOR: THE NEWSLETTER OF EHN
The Environmental Health Network (EHN), P.O. Box 1155, Larkspur, CA 94977-1155.

NEWS ON EARTH [MONTHLY] Public Concern Foundation. 101 W. 23RD Street, PMB 2245, New York, NY 10011.

F.2 <u>ADVOCACY GROUPS AND WEBSITES FOR PATIENTS</u>

AMERICAN CONFERENCE OF GOVERNMENTAL INDUSTRIAL HYGIENISTS [ACGIH], 6500 Glenway Ave., Building D7, Cincinnati, OH 45211. 513.742.2020., *Information about potential health workplace hazards.*

AMERICAN SOCIETY OF HEATING, REFRIGERATION AND AIR CONDITIONING ENGINEERS [ASHRACE] 800.527.4723 404.636.8400 1791 Tullie Circle, N.E., Atlanta, GA 30329., For air *limits for six indoor contaminants.*

BIO-INTEGRAL RESOURCE CENTER [BIRC] 510.524.2567 FAX: 510.524.1758, P.O. Box 7414, Berkeley, CA 94707.

BREAST CANCER ACTION (BCA) 410.922.8279 FAX: 410.922.3253, 1280 Columbus, San Francisco, CA 94133.

BREAST CANCER SURVIVAL SERVICES 480.473.4490 donna.cancer.bcss@att.net.

CITIZENS CLEARING HOUSE FOR HAZARDOUS WASTE [CCHW] 703.237.2249 FAX: 703.237.7449, P.O. Box 6806, Falls Church, VA 22040 *Assists the public in protecting the community from chemicals.*

GREEN SEAL, 1730 Rhode Island Avenue, N.W., Suite 1050, Washington, DC 20036. 202.331.7337., *Sets standards for air, water, energy and products.*

HEALTHY SCHOOLS NETWORK, INC. 518.462.0632, FAX: 518.462.0433, www.healthyschools.org.

HUMAN ECOLOGY ACTION LEAGUE [HEAL] 404.248.1898 P.O. Box 49126, Atlanta, GA 30359-1126. *Publish Human Ecologist.*

MOTHERS AND OTHERS FOR A LIVABLE PLANET 212.242.0010 X.305 FAX: 212.242.0545, 40 W. 20TH Street, NY, NY 10011.

NATIONAL AIR DUCT CLEANERS ASSOCIATION [NADCA] 202.737.2926 FAX: 202.638.4833, 1518 K Street, N.W., Suite 503, Washington, DC 20005, *Recommend air duct cleaner in your area.*

NATIONAL COALITION AGAINST THE MISUSE OF PESTICIDES [NCAMP] 202.543.5450, FAX: 202.543.4791, 701 E. Street, NW. Suite 200, Washington, DC 20003.

NATIONAL ORGANIZATION OF LEGAL ADVOCATES FOR THE ENVIRONMENTALLY INJURED 404.264.4445 FAX: 404.325.2569, P.O. Box 29507, Atlanta, GA 30329.

NATIONAL PARENT-TEACHER ASSOCIATION 330 North Wabash Avenue, Suite 2100, Chicago, IL 60611-3690.

NEW YORK COALITION FOR ALTERNATIVES TO PESTICIDES [NCAP] 518.426.8246, 353 Hamilton Street, Albany, NY 12210-1709.

OMB WATCH 202.234.8494, 1742 Connecticut Avenue, N.W., Washington, DC 20009. *Watchdog for public concerning government.*

PESTICIDE ACTION NETWORK NORTH AMERICAN REGIONAL OFFICE 415.541.9140 FAX: 415.541.1253, 116 New Montgomery Street, Suite 810, San Francisco, CA 94105.

PESTICIDE EDUCATION CENTER 415.665.4722
P.O. Box 225279, San Francisco, CA 94122
for book Designer Poisons, by Marian Moses.

PESTICIDE WATCH 415.543.2627 FAX: 415.543.1480
116 New Montgomery Street, Suite 530San Francisco, CA 94105, Pestiwatch@igc.apc.org.

SAFE SCHOOLS 318.984.2766 FAX: 318.984.3342, 205 Paddington Drive, Lafayette, LA 70508. *Irene Wilkinson offers a two-hour workshop.*

TOXIC TIMES 406.547.2255, Chemical Injury Information Network P.O. Box 301, White Sulfur Springs, MT 59645.

WASHINGTON TOXICS COALITION
206.652.1545 FAX: 206.632.8661 4516 University Way, NE, Seattle, WA 98105.

WELL MIND ASSOC. GREATER WASHINGTON, DC
301.949.8282 FAX: 301.946.1402, 3205 Wake Drive Kensington, MD 20895-0201 *Educational materials regarding mental illness especially schizophrenia.*

F.3 WEBSITES FOR PUBLIC

CALIFORNIANS AGAINST PESTICIDES- www.pesticidereform.org.
CHILDREN'S HEALTH AND PESTICIDES
www.pesticidefreesign.com/children.html.
INFERTILITY
Couples Turning To Infertility Treatments Too Early 10/8/00, www.mercola.com/2000/oct/8/fertility_treatment.htm.
LEGISLATIVE PETITIONwww.thepetitionsite.com/takeaction/165863399.
www.nospray.org. *(Mitchell Cohen)*
MOLD WEBSITES – See Mold sector Appendix C.3 .
NATIONAL COALITION AGAINST THE MISUSE OF PESTICIDES
www.ncamp.org, www.beyondpesticides.org.
NNCC PESTICIDES AND CHILDREN'S DIETS
www.nncc.org/nutrition/pestic.diet.html.
NEW YORK COALITION FOR ALTERNATIVES TO PESTICIDES
www.cehn.org/cehn/resourceguide/nycap.html.

ORGANIZATIONS FOR MISUSES OF PESTICIDES
www.dmoz.org/Society/Issues/Environmental/Health.
OVEREXPOSED
www.ewg.org/pub/home/reports/ops/oppress.htm.
PSR'S ENVIRONMENT & HEALTH PROGRAM - PESTICIDES AND KIDS, www.psr.org/pestkids.htm.
PESTICIDES AND CHILDREN
www.pesticidewatch.org/html/pestproblem/children.htm.
PESTICIDES IN SCHOOLS, www.billmurawski.com/poisonpage.html.
US EPA CONCERNED CITIZENS - PROTECTING OUR CHILDREN www.epa.gov/pesticides/citizens/children.htm.
US POSITION ON PESTICIDES AND CHILDREN ISSUES
www.consumersunion.org/food/codex200.htm.
WORRYING ABOUT MILK 7/30/00, www.mercola.com/2000/jul/30/milk.htm.

AAEM RESOURCE WEBSITES:
Allergy Research Group www.nutricology.com.
American Biologics Inc. www.americanbiologics.com.
Antigen Laboratories, Inc. www.antigenlab.com.
Aspen Benefit Group www.aspenbenefits.com.
BioTech Pharmacal www.bio_tech_pharm.com.
College Pharmacy www.collegepharmacy.com.
Chemically Sensitive Living www.chemsenlvng.com.
Doctors Data, Inc. www.doctorsdata.com.
Endometriosis Association www.endometriosisassn.org.
Environmental Health Center - Dallas www.ehcd.com.
Fibromyalgia Coalition www.fibrocoalition.org.
Great Smokies Diagnostic Lab, Inc. www.gsdl.com.
Immunosciences Lab, Inc. www.immuno-sci-lab.com.
Insta-Tape, Inc. www.instatapes.com.
K.B. Cotton Pillows, Inc. www.kbcottonpillows.com.
Klaire Laboratories www.klaire.com.
MCS Advocacy Fund www.mcsadvocacfund.org.
MCS Relief www.mcsrelief.com.
MetabolicMaintenance Products, Inc. www.metabolicmaintenance.com.
MetaMetrix Clinical Laboratory www.metametrix.com.
Nutritional Therapeutics www.propax.com.
The Pure Water Place www.purewaterplace.com.
Thorne Research, Inc. www.thorne.com.
Tyler Encapsulations www.tyler-inc.com.
Wellness Health and Pharmacy www.wellnesshealth.com.
Women's International Pharmacy www.womensinternational.com.

Comments About This Book

Dr. Doris Rapp has given us a survival manual for our civilized, which has begun to saturate itself with questionable chemicals. Her book is a MUST for world leaders, congressmen/congresswomen, legislators, family matriarchs/patriarchs, teachers, doctors and business owners to read. Her treatise helps us to (1) identify each destroyer of health and longevity, (2) learn how to deal with it, and (3) locate more information. Her exciting and frightening revelations will trigger life and habit changes for the betterment of you and your family existence.

Doris, good luck and Godspeed with your creation of many multifaceted healing centers, which will salvage and enhance lives using the guidelines of your book.

— *John F. Goodson, Esq., President of the College of Preventative Law*

I have thought for over 30 years that our greatest threat is nuclear contamination and the second is chemical pollution. To some extent, it is a question of which will destroy us first! Dr. Rapp has been at the forefront of intelligent, common-sense reaction to this menace. Everyone with an IQ of 90 or above needs to read and heed her sage wisdom.

— *C. Norman Shealy, M.D., Ph.D., President, Holos University Graduate Seminary, Founding President, American Holistic Medical Association, author of over 290 publications and 21 books, including* The Methuselah Potential

Index

Symbols

A

B

D

E

G

H

I

J

K

L

M

N

O

P

Q

R

S

T

U

V

Order Form

Our Toxic World – A Wake Up Call	_____	*x $24.95 each*
Is This Your Child's World?	_____	*x $16.00 each*
Is This Your Child?	_____	*x $14.00 each*
Environmentally Sick Schools Video (90 min.)	_____	*x $25.00 each*
Merchandise Total	______	
Shipping/Handling ($6 + $1 each add'l item)	______	
TOTAL	______	

Order Our Toxic World – A Wake Up Call by the case (18), and get 50% discount. That's only $12.50 each plus shipping and handling. Call Cindy at 1-800-787-8780 for shipping fees. Case of 10 Is This Your Child's World? (635 pages) at $10.00 each.

Name____

Address____

City/State/Zip____

Phone____

MC/Visa__________________________Exp.______________

Signature____

Send Order to:
Environmental Research Foundation
PO Box 60, Buffalo, NY 14223
Please make checks payable to: Environmental Research Foundation

Call: 1-800-787-8780 to place your order or www.drrapp.com

Order Form

Our Toxic World – A Wake Up Call	_____ *x $24.95 each*
Is This Your Child's World?	_____ *x $16.00 each*
Is This Your Child?	_____ *x $14.00 each*
Environmentally Sick Schools Video (90 min.)	_____ *x $25.00 each*
Merchandise Total	_____
Shipping/Handling	_____
($6 + $1 each add'l item)	
TOTAL	_____

Order Our Toxic World – A Wake Up Call by the case (18), and get 50% discount. That's only $12.50 each plus shipping and handling. Call Cindy at 1-800-787-8780 for shipping fees. Case of 10 Is This Your Child's World? (635 pages) at $10.00 each.

Name____

Address____

City/State/Zip_______________________________________

Phone____

MC/Visa_____________________________Exp.______________

Signature____

Send Order to:
Environmental Research Foundation
PO Box 60, Buffalo, NY 14223
Please make checks payable to: Environmental Research Foundation
Call: 1-800-787-8780 to place your order or www.drrapp.com